Papillomavirus-Induced Oncogenesis: Current Insights and Future Directions

Papillomavirus-Induced Oncogenesis: Current Insights and Future Directions

Guest Editors

G. Hossein Ashrafi
Mustafa Ozdogan

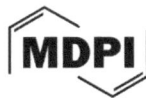

Basel • Beijing • Wuhan • Barcelona • Belgrade • Novi Sad • Cluj • Manchester

Guest Editors

G. Hossein Ashrafi
Biomolecular Sciences
Kingston University London
London
United Kingdom

Mustafa Ozdogan
Division of Medical Oncology
Memorial Hospital
Antalya
Turkey

Editorial Office
MDPI AG
Grosspeteranlage 5
4052 Basel, Switzerland

This is a reprint of the Special Issue, published open access by the journal *Viruses* (ISSN 1999-4915), freely accessible at: www.mdpi.com/journal/viruses/special_issues/papillomavirus_oncogenesis.

For citation purposes, cite each article independently as indicated on the article page online and using the guide below:

Lastname, A.A.; Lastname, B.B. Article Title. *Journal Name* **Year**, *Volume Number*, Page Range.

ISBN 978-3-7258-3796-0 (Hbk)
ISBN 978-3-7258-3795-3 (PDF)
https://doi.org/10.3390/books978-3-7258-3795-3

© 2025 by the authors. Articles in this book are Open Access and distributed under the Creative Commons Attribution (CC BY) license. The book as a whole is distributed by MDPI under the terms and conditions of the Creative Commons Attribution-NonCommercial-NoDerivs (CC BY-NC-ND) license (https://creativecommons.org/licenses/by-nc-nd/4.0/).

Contents

About the Editors vii

Preface ix

Philip E. Castle
Looking Back, Moving Forward: Challenges and Opportunities for Global Cervical Cancer Prevention and Control
Reprinted from: *Viruses* 2024, 16, 1357, https://doi.org/10.3390/v16091357 1

Georgios Konstantopoulos, Danai Leventakou, Despoina-Rozi Saltiel, Efthalia Zervoudi, Eirini Logotheti and Spyros Pettas et al.
HPV16 *E6* Oncogene Contributes to Cancer Immune Evasion by Regulating PD-L1 Expression through a miR-143/HIF-1a Pathway
Reprinted from: *Viruses* 2024, 16, 113, https://doi.org/10.3390/v16010113 41

Mary C. Bedard, Cosette M. Rivera-Cruz, Tafadzwa Chihanga, Andrew VonHandorf, Alice L. Tang and Chad Zender et al.
A Single-Cell Transcriptome Atlas of Epithelial Subpopulations in HPV-Positive and HPV-Negative Head and Neck Cancers
Reprinted from: *Viruses* 2025, 17, 461, https://doi.org/10.3390/v17040461 52

Arsenal Sezgin Alikanoğlu and İrem Atalay Karaçay
Detection of High-Risk Human Papillomavirus (HPV), p16 and EGFR in Lung Cancer: Insights from the Mediterranean Region of Turkey
Reprinted from: *Viruses* 2024, 16, 1201, https://doi.org/10.3390/v16081201 72

Ömer Vefik Özozan, Hikmet Pehlevan-Özel, Veli Vural and Tolga Dinç
Relationship Between Human Papilloma Virus and Upper Gastrointestinal Cancers
Reprinted from: *Viruses* 2025, 17, 367, https://doi.org/10.3390/v17030367 83

Beliz Bahar Karaoğlan and Yüksel Ürün
Unveiling the Role of Human Papillomavirus in Urogenital Carcinogenesis a Comprehensive Review
Reprinted from: *Viruses* 2024, 16, 667, https://doi.org/10.3390/v16050667 97

Miriam Latorre-Millán, Alexander Tristancho-Baró, Natalia Burillo, Mónica Ariza, Ana María Milagro and Pilar Abad et al.
HPV-Associated Sexually Transmitted Infections in Cervical Cancer Screening: A Prospective Cohort Study
Reprinted from: *Viruses* 2025, 17, 247, https://doi.org/10.3390/v17020247 113

José L. Castrillo-Diez, Carolina Rivera-Santiago, Silvia M. Ávila-Flores, Silvia A. Barrera-Barrera and Hugo A. Barrera-Saldaña
Findings and Challenges in Replacing Traditional Uterine Cervical Cancer Diagnosis with Molecular Tools in Private Gynecological Practice in Mexico
Reprinted from: *Viruses* 2024, 16, 887, https://doi.org/10.3390/v16060887 123

Melvin Omone Ogbolu, Olanrewaju D. Eniade, Hussaini Majiya and Miklós Kozlovszky
Factors Associated with HPV Genital Warts: A Self-Reported Cross-Sectional Study among Students and Staff of a Northern University in Nigeria
Reprinted from: *Viruses* 2024, 16, 902, https://doi.org/10.3390/v16060902 135

Jobran M. Moshi, Aarman Sohaili, Hassan N. Moafa, Ahlam Mohammed S. Hakami, Mohsen M. Mashi and Pierre P. M. Thomas
Short Communication: Understanding the Barriers to Cervical Cancer Prevention and HPV Vaccination in Saudi Arabia
Reprinted from: *Viruses* **2024**, *16*, 974, https://doi.org/10.3390/v16060974 . . . . **149**

About the Editors

G. Hossein Ashrafi

Dr. G. Hossein Ashrafi is an Associate Professor/Reader of Pathology at Kingston University London, where he leads the MSc Cancer Biology programme. He is a Fellow of the Institute of Biomedical Science (FIBMS) and a Fellow of the Higher Education Academy (FHEA), and serves on editorial boards of several peer-reviewed journals, including *Scientific Reports – Nature*.

He received his PhD in 1998 from the Beatson Institute for Cancer Research, University of Glasgow, focusing on viral causes of cancer. The same year, he was awarded a postdoctoral fellowship at Glasgow University Medical School, followed by a Royal Society Developing World Study Visit Fellowship for his research on the immune response to papillomavirus.

Dr. Ashrafi's research has contributed significantly to understanding HPV-induced carcinogenesis. His collaborative work with Professor Campo was the first to experimentally demonstrate that the papillomavirus E5 oncoprotein downregulates MHC-I, facilitating immune evasion. This finding has informed subsequent studies and secured national and international funding.

His current work focuses on virus–host interactions and therapeutic strategies for HPV-associated cancers. In collaboration with Kingston Hospital NHS Trust, he recently provided the first evidence of HPV DNA in fresh human breast, prostate, and bladder cancer tissues in the UK, published in *Scientific Reports – Nature*. These findings have led to further grants from Kingston Hospital Charity, the Laurie Todd Foundation, and the Medical Research Centre, Doha-Qatar. Dr. Ashrafi actively supervises PhD students and teaches a range of medical science modules. His research is supported by the Medical Research Council (MRC), the Royal Society, and other organizations, contributing to advancements in cancer virology and translational medicine.

Mustafa Ozdogan

Prof. Dr. Mustafa Ozdogan is a leading Medical Oncologist and Professor of Medicine with a distinguished career in cancer research, clinical oncology, and academic leadership. He currently serves as the Head of Antalya Memorial-Medstar Cancer Center and oversees the Medical Oncology Clinics. Prof. Ozdogan's expertise spans immunotherapy, genomic testing in cancer, minimally invasive treatments, and patient-centered care models in oncology.

He completed his medical education at Erciyes University and his specialization in Internal Medicine and Medical Oncology at Akdeniz University, where he began his academic career in 2003. In 2004, he conducted advanced studies in Germany on complementary cancer therapies and hyperthermia treatment. He was appointed Associate Professor in 2006 and became a Full Professor in 2011.

Prof. Ozdogan has published over 112 peer-reviewed articles and has received 17 academic awards for his innovative research and contributions to oncology education. He is a member of leading scientific organizations including the European Society for Medical Oncology (ESMO) and the American Society of Clinical Oncology (ASCO). His pioneering work includes introducing the concepts of "Oncology Nursing" and "Art House in Chemotherapy Units" in Turkey. He is the founder of several oncology-focused associations and projects, such as the Oncology Nursing Education Project and Oncotrust Health Tourism.

In addition to his clinical and academic work, Prof. Ozdogan is a science communicator, having published over 4500 articles on his public platform, aimed at enhancing cancer literacy. His research interests include the integration of personalized medicine, supportive oncology, and the development of patient-oriented cancer treatment strategies.

Preface

Papillomaviruses are among the most studied oncogenic viruses, recognized for their etiological role in a broad spectrum of human malignancies. Since the discovery of the causal link between human papillomavirus (HPV) and cervical cancer, our understanding of HPV's involvement in various cancers—including those of the anogenital tract and head and neck—has grown exponentially. This Reprint, derived from the Special Issue "Papillomavirus - Induced Oncogenesis: Current Insights and Future Directions" published in *Viruses*, brings together original research articles, reviews, and short communications that provide a comprehensive perspective on the state of HPV-related cancer research.

The subject matter of this volume spans from molecular biology to public health, offering in-depth insights into mechanisms of HPV-induced oncogenesis, novel diagnostic and screening approaches, immunological evasion strategies, epidemiological patterns, and prevention challenges. The aim of this compilation is to bridge fundamental science with clinical and societal applications, while fostering a deeper understanding of the biological complexity and global health significance of HPV.

The motivation behind curating this Special Issue was driven by the persistent global burden of HPV-associated cancers. Despite the availability of effective prophylactic vaccines and diagnostic tools, significant disparities remain in implementation, particularly in low- and middle-income countries. Through this collection, we hope to encourage interdisciplinary collaboration and innovative thinking to close these gaps and promote equitable health outcomes.

This reprint is intended for a diverse readership, such as of virologists, oncologists, molecular biologists, epidemiologists, public health professionals, and students alike. It also serves as a valuable reference for educators, healthcare policymakers, and advocacy groups committed to cancer prevention and control.

We extend our sincere gratitude to all contributing authors for their high-quality submissions and dedication to the field. We are also grateful to the editorial staff of *Viruses* for their ongoing support and professionalism. In particular, we would like to acknowledge Mr Muharrem Okan Cakir, who served as an Assistant Guest Editor. His close involvement in coordinating submissions, supporting peer review, and ensuring timely communication was instrumental to the successful delivery of this Special Issue.

We trust that readers will find this Reprint informative, timely, and thought-provoking. It is our hope that the work presented here will inspire future research and reinforce global efforts to reduce the burden of HPV-associated cancers.

G. Hossein Ashrafi and Mustafa Ozdogan
Guest Editors

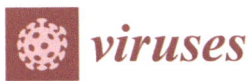

Review

Looking Back, Moving Forward: Challenges and Opportunities for Global Cervical Cancer Prevention and Control

Philip E. Castle

Divisions of Cancer Prevention and Cancer Epidemiology and Genetics, US National Cancer Institute, National Institutes of Health, 9609 Medical Center Dr., Room 5E410, Rockville, MD 20850, USA; philip.castle@nih.gov; Tel.: +1-(240)-276-7120; Fax: +1-(240)-276-7825

Abstract: Despite the introduction of Pap testing for screening to prevent cervical cancer in the mid-20th century, cervical cancer remains a common cause of cancer-related mortality and morbidity globally. This is primarily due to differences in access to screening and care between low-income and high-income resource settings, resulting in cervical cancer being one of the cancers with the greatest health disparity. The discovery of human papillomavirus (HPV) as the near-obligate viral cause of cervical cancer can revolutionize how it can be prevented: HPV vaccination against infection for prophylaxis and HPV testing-based screening for the detection and treatment of cervical pre-cancers for interception. As a result of this progress, the World Health Organization has championed the elimination of cervical cancer as a global health problem. However, unless research, investments, and actions are taken to ensure equitable global access to these highly effective preventive interventions, there is a real threat to exacerbating the current health inequities in cervical cancer. In this review, the progress to date and the challenges and opportunities for fulfilling the potential of HPV-targeted prevention for global cervical cancer control are discussed.

Keywords: Human papillomavirus (HPV); cervical cancer; HPV-related cancers; Pap testing; cytology; vaccination; gynecologic oncology

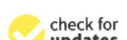

Citation: Castle, P.E. Looking Back, Moving Forward: Challenges and Opportunities for Global Cervical Cancer Prevention and Control. *Viruses* **2024**, *16*, 1357. https://doi.org/10.3390/v16091357

Academic Editors: Hossein H. Ashrafi and Mustafa Ozdogan

Received: 5 August 2024
Revised: 21 August 2024
Accepted: 22 August 2024
Published: 25 August 2024

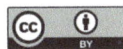

Copyright: © 2024 by the author. Licensee MDPI, Basel, Switzerland. This article is an open access article distributed under the terms and conditions of the Creative Commons Attribution (CC BY) license (https:// creativecommons.org/licenses/by/ 4.0/).

A. Part 1: Looking Back
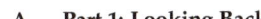

1. Introduction

Cervical cancer is highly preventable. The implementation of widespread Pap testing, starting in the mid-20th century in high-income countries (HICs), led to significant declines in cervical cancer incidence, saving millions of lives. Unfortunately, these same benefits were not fully realized in underserved populations living in those same HICs and those living in low- and middle-income countries (LMICs). This was due to social inequities, geographical barriers, complexity, lack of quality control, and/or resource limitations, the latter of which include the lack of healthcare infrastructure, resources, and trained medical personnel to provide screening, i.e., testing and follow-up care. Consequently, cervical cancer became the "poster child" for cancer health disparities, with an order-of-magnitude difference in cervical cancer burden between the wealthiest and poorest countries [1] and significant differences between well-served and underserved populations in the wealthiest countries like the USA [2,3] and others [4–10]. Cervical cancer incidence and mortality were inversely correlated with gross domestic product *per capita*, and the ratio of cervical cancer mortality to incidence increased with greater the incidence (Figure 1).

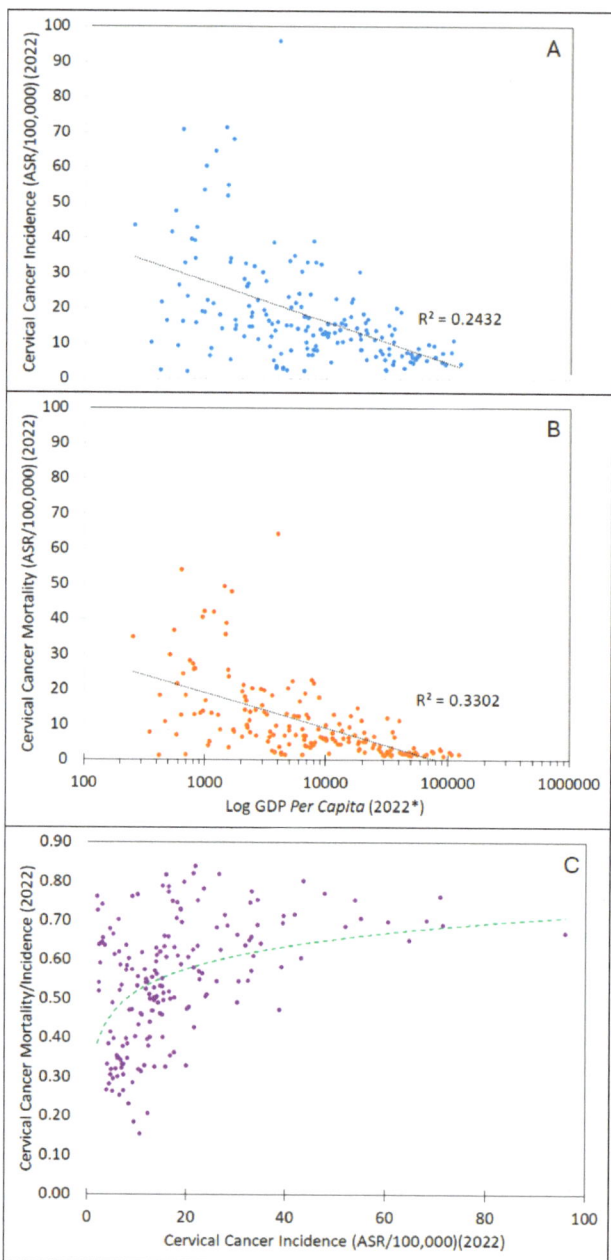

Figure 1. (**A**) country-specific relationship between 2022 cervical cancer incidence [1] and gross domestic product (GDP) *per capita* (on a log scale) in 2022 [11] (black dotted line shows the linear trend); (**B**) country-specific relationship between 2022 cervical cancer mortality [1] and GDP *per capita* in 2022 (black dotted line shows the linear trend); and (**C**) country-specific relationship between the ratio of cervical cancer mortality to incidence and 2022 cervical cancer incidence [1] in 2022 (green dashed line shows the logarithmic trend). * If GDP *per capita* was not available for 2022, the most recent data were used.

It is now accepted that high-risk human papillomavirus (HPV) is the nearly obligate viral cause of cervical cancer [12]. This discovery catalyzed the development of two complementary, highly efficacious precision prevention strategies, i.e., those that directly target HPV including prophylactic HPV vaccination for primary prevention and HPV testing-based screening for secondary prevention. Despite these advances, more than two decades after their development and validation, cervical cancer remains a major cause of morbidity and mortality in women globally, with an estimated 662,000 new cases and 349,000 deaths attributed to cervical cancer in 2022, with the vast majority occurring in LMICs [1].

In 2018, the World Health Organization (WHO) announced a global call to action for the elimination of cervical cancer as a public health problem. In 2020, the World Health Assembly launched a Cervical Cancer Elimination Initiative [13]. Its strategy includes the following WHO "90-70-90" targets to be reached by 2030: 90% of girls fully HPV vaccinated by age 15 years, 70% of women screened twice using a high-performance test by the ages of 35 and 45 years, and 90% of women diagnosed with pre-cancer and 90% of women with invasive cancer treated. The "90-70-90" targets were designed to meet the "elimination" metric of incidence rates below four cases per 100,000 women. Of course, the target of treating 90% of invasive cancer will not contribute to the goal of reduced incidence but will benefit the population by reducing cervical cancer-related mortality and morbidity.

Together, these three interventions, cancer prophylaxis through HPV vaccination, cancer interception through HPV-based screening and treatment of cervical pre-cancers, and cancer mitigation through detection and treatment of early cancer, will have profound impacts on cervical cancer control, but each works on a different time horizon [14]. Mitigation will measurably benefit the population on the earliest time horizon through reduced mortality and morbidity, screening-based interception next, and finally, prophylaxis, which may take decades to observe its impact on cancer incidence. From modeling exercises, combining primary prevention through HPV vaccination and secondary prevention through HPV testing-based screening and treatment of pre-cancer and cancer will achieve the most rapid risk reduction towards achieving the WHO goal [15,16]. In order to accelerate mortality reductions and prepare for the anticipated sharp increase in screen-detected cancers needing treatment, should screening programs go to scale, mortality reduction targets also need to be set and included in the WHO's goals.

At this juncture, as the field moves from basic and translational science to dissemination and implementation, it is a good time to review what has been achieved, why, and consider the challenges ahead to achieve global cervical cancer prevention and control. I provide my own perspective from my 25 years in the field. These lessons learned—and to be learned—can and should inform future efforts to control other cancers globally.

2. A Brief History

How did we arrive at this unique opportunity? The evolution of our understanding of cervical cancer is well described and discussed by others [17–19] and will be only recapitulated here briefly as it relates specifically to this discussion. It began with Hippocrates, at the beginning of the era of modern medicine and before the Common Era, who first documented and described HPV-related diseases of genital and skin warts, cervical precursors or lesions, and cervical cancer. He observed that cervical abnormalities, which he called "ulcers", could progress to cervical cancer, providing the earliest insight into carcinogenesis [18]. Namely, cancer does not arise spontaneously but through intermediate, pre-cancerous changes that precede invasive cancer, which is still a foundational concept of carcinogenesis today.

Almost 2000 years later, 19th-century surgeon Domenico Antonio Rigoni-Stern made his famous observation about people engaged in sex work being more likely to die from cervical cancer than celibate nuns (the opposite for nulliparity and breast cancer deaths) [18,19], implicating a sexual factor in the development of cervical cancer. More than a century later, this observation fueled research to find the sexually transmitted causal factor, now known to be HPV.

In the early 1920s, physician George Papanicolaou first observed cancer cells in a cytology smear made from vaginal samples. Refinements in this method occurred over the next two decades [20], including improved staining [21] and sampling directly from the cervix [22], leading to what is known as the "Pap smear" for cervical cytology screening. Widespread adoption of annual Pap testing followed recommendations first in the mid-1940s, resulting in significant reductions in cervical cancer incidence and mortality in those places that could implement it effectively [23].

In the 1960s and 1970s, epidemiologic research hotly pursued the causal sexually transmitted infection, with a focus on herpes simplex virus. The discovery by Nobel-Laurate Harald zur Hausen and colleagues in the late 1970s into the early 1980s [24,25] of HPV genomes in cervical cancers revolutionized our understanding of the cause and the natural history of cervical cancer. Over the next decades, international, transdisciplinary teams of researchers, including but not limited to basic and clinical laboratory scientists, clinicians, epidemiologists and statisticians, public health scientists, and other disciplines, worked collaboratively to deepen our understanding of HPV and its role in cervical cancer as well as develop and validate prophylactic HPV vaccination and HPV testing-based screening, which are now seen as the standard of care for cervical cancer prevention and control worldwide [26,27].

3. HPV and Cervical Cancer

It is now understood that the sexual transmission and persistence of high-risk HPV genotypes ("types") are the almost obligate cause of virtually all cervical cancer worldwide. Approximately 13 HPV types (HPV16, 18, 31, 33, 35, 39, 45, 51, 52, 56, 58, 59, and 68) have been designated as "high-risk". In reality, there is a continuum of risk for HPV types. HPV16 and HPV18, the two high-risk HPV types targeted by first-generation HPV vaccines, cause approximately 70% of cervical cancer; HPV16 is the most carcinogenic HPV type, causing approximately 55–60% of cervical cancer, and HPV18 is the second most carcinogenic HPV type, causing approximately 10–15%. HPV31, HPV33, HPV 45, HPV52, and HPV58 together cause another 20% of cervical cancer. On the other end of the spectrum of high-risk HPV types, HPV68 is only considered a probable carcinogen, and the risk of cancer is considerably less than HPV16 [28–30]. Some HPV types, especially those phylogenetically related to the high-risk HPV types, can rarely cause cervical cancer [28–32]. This includes HPV66, which was mistakenly classified as high-risk [33] and now, unfortunately, is included in all second-generation HPV tests, providing very little benefit but reducing specificity, as it is commonly detected in low-grade abnormalities [32].

HPV infection also causes most cancers of the anus and a high percentage of cancers of the vagina, vulvar, penis, and oropharynx [34–36]. Almost 5% of cancers globally are attributable to HPV infection [36].

Other HPV types, notably HPV6 and HPV11, cause *condyloma acuminata* (genital warts) and recurrent respiratory papillomatosis. Still, other HPV types have no known link to human disease, and some appear to have some tissue tropism for vaginal epithelium [37–40], just as some non-genital HPV types have tropism for different skin locations [41]. Genital types unrelated to cervical cancer and not targeted by or protected from current HPV vaccines make for useful intrapersonal controls since they are all sexually transmitted concomitantly and may allow for single-arm, non-randomized HPV vaccine trials [42] by serving as markers for total HPV exposure.

The same 13 high-risk HPV types generally cause the same percentages of cervical cancer everywhere in the world [43] but with some notable variations in different racial/ethnic populations, such as higher percentages of HPV35-related cervical cancers in women of African descent [44–46] and HPV52-related cervical cancers in women of Asian descent [47–49], likely because of the evolutionary selection of viral variants within those populations. While HPV35 causes only about 2% of cervical cancer in the general population [28], it causes approximately 10% in women of African descent [44–46]. Although HPV35 is not currently included in prophylactic HPV vaccine formulations, hopefully, it will be included in future vaccines [50]. The relative public health importance of individual HPV types cannot be determined by their prevalence in the general population, or even in precursors to cancer, but must be determined in cancer itself.

HPV-negative cervical cancers do occur but are exceedingly rare once the denominator of cervical cancers is corrected for the HPV-related cervical cancers that are prevented (censored) by screening and treatment of HPV-related precursors. These HPV-negative cancers are pathologically defined as cervical but have molecular features that are shared with—and mostly resemble those of—endometrial cancer [51].

High-risk HPV prevalence is similar in exfoliated specimens from the vagina and the cervix [38–40]. However, despite the vagina having a much larger surface epithelial area to infect than the cervix (≤ 360 cm^2 vs. ≤ 33 cm^2, respectively [52,53]), cervical cancer is 20-fold more common cancer than vaginal cancer. That is, the cervix is at least 200-fold more susceptible to HPV-induced carcinogenesis than the vagina, which does not account for the vagina possibly being more exposed to HPV than the cervix, as the former is the first mucosal epithelium exposed to it. The physiological nature of the susceptibility to HPV-induced carcinogenesis of the annulus of tissue known as the cervical transformation zone, where cervical cancer primarily occurs, is not completely understood. However, a specialized stem cell, the cervical reserve cell, found under the columnar epithelium has been implicated as the susceptible cell for HPV transformation [54].

Cervical cancer develops along a simple, robust causal pathway with four reliably measured, natural history stages including the following: normal epithelium, hrHPV-infected epithelium, cervical pre-cancer (defined best as histologic diagnoses of cervical intraepithelial neoplasia CIN) grade 3 (CIN3) or adenocarcinoma in situ (AIS)), and invasive cancer [55]. HPV is the most common sexually transmitted infection. Indeed, among those who have ever been sexually active, it seems likely that nearly everyone has had an HPV infection, given that there are hundreds of HPV types and epidemiologic studies of incidence only detect a subset of those, infections can be acquired and cleared/controlled in the interval between observations, there are no observations over the entire sexually active life, and the entire lower genital tract can be infected but we typically only sample a small portion of it for HPV testing. In prospective cohorts, a high percentage of women test positive for HPV within a few years of observation, but the range of cumulative HPV positivity (approximately 30–80%) is wide, likely the result of differences in populations, the HPV test used, frequency of testing, and length of follow-up [56–61]. Natural history modeling estimated the lifetime probability of at least one HPV infection to be 85% for women and 91% for men [62], but, given the aforementioned factors, it could be higher still.

HPV persistence is the key determinant in the natural history of disease and is required for progression to pre-cancer and then invasive cancer [63–65]. However, not all persistent HPV infections develop into detectable CIN3/AIS, although it is probable that long-lasting, persistent HPV infection is essentially a "molecular" pre-cancer whether there is an accompanying histopathologic diagnosis of CIN3. CIN2 grade 2 (CIN2), the standard threshold of severity for treatment, is now understood to be an equivocal high-grade abnormality that is highly regressive, especially in younger women [66–68].

The transition probabilities between stages are difficult to observe directly, except for the acquisition of HPV infection, but they have been modeled [69]. The transition from HPV infection to CIN3/AIS is typically observed following prevalent HPV infection and, therefore, "left-censored", i.e., the HPV infection has already persisted for some unknown amount of time. Likewise, the CIN3/AIS transition to invasive cancer is left-censored. The "Unfortunate Experiment" in New Zealand, in which treatment was purposely withheld from approximately 150 women with CIN3, found approximately 35% of CIN3 progressed to invasive cancer [70]. However, the median age of these women was 38 years, approximately 5–10 years after the peak of CIN3 in a screening cohort, and, therefore, their CIN3 was relatively "mature" [71]. The median time from HPV acquisition to cervical cancer detection ranges from 17.5 to 26 years, depending on the model used and its assumptions [69]. The age distribution of cervical cancer tracks with population behaviors and exposure to HPV, i.e., those populations that initiate sexual activity at a younger age tend to develop cervical cancer at younger ages, while those that start at an older age develop cervical cancer at older ages [72–74], although the effects of the latter may be muted by the effects of reduced circulating estrogen in peri- and post-menopausal women on hormonally responsive cervical tissue [72].

Condoms, when used correctly, are effective in blocking HPV transmission in women [75,76]. Male circumcision also reduces HPV carriage in men [77,78], and females with circumcised male partners are lower risk of getting HPV than those with uncircumcised male partners [77,78]. There is also some evidence that topical microbicides with carrageenan, a commonly used seaweed extract used as a thickening agent in food, provide broad-spectrum, safe protection against cervical HPV acquisition [79,80].

Despite 40 years of studying the natural history of HPV and cervical cancer and its clinical and molecular correlates, there are still important gaps in our knowledge. While we know that women who are immunosuppressed because of HIV or receiving a solid organ tissue transplant are at significantly higher risk of cervical cancer compared with immunocompetent women [81–83], the specific immunologic factors that play a role in determining the outcome of an HPV infection and clearance/control vs. persistence/progression in the general population are unknown. A better understanding of the immunological determinants of persistence would contribute to the development of effective HPV therapeutic vaccines, which, to date, have demonstrated effectiveness against CIN2/3 [84] that is much less than current standard-of-care physical (excisional or ablative) treatments [85]. A highly effective pan-HPV therapeutic vaccine or anti-viral, combined with HPV-based screening, could facilitate and accelerate global control of cervical cancer, especially in LMICs, where there is a huge gap in medical and health-system capacity to provide care and treatment to support the scale-up of screening [86].

There is also evidence of latency in HPV infections [87,88], which is a sub-clinical infection that is maintained and presumably controlled by the host immune system [87]. However, the clinical significance of latent HPV infections and how frequently they occur vs. true clearance remain unknown. A greater understanding of its role if any in cervical cancer diagnosed in older women would inform decisions about the age and other criteria for stopping screening.

4. Precision Prevention: Targeting HPV for Prophylaxis and Interception

A targeted, precision prevention approach of prophylactic HPV vaccination and HPV testing-based cervical cancer screening is now widely accepted as the new standard of care for the prevention of cervical cancer. The two strategies are complementary and combined can accelerate the control of cervical cancer [15] as follows: (1) HPV vaccination for long-term and perhaps lifetime cervical cancer risk reduction by preventing HPV acquisition and (2) HPV testing-based screening to detect and intercept pre-cancer through treatment before it becomes invasive to reduce cervical cancer risk immediately.

Prophylactic HPV vaccines produce high titers of HPV-neutralizing antibodies that block cervical HPV infection [89]. Antibody titers following HPV vaccination are an order of magnitude or greater than those that occur following natural infection, which provides partial protection against re-infection against the same type [90,91]. First-generation vaccines targeted HPV16 and HPV18; one product also targeted HPV6 and HPV11 to prevent genital warts and RRP. Different HPV vaccine formulations have been shown to provide different levels of cross-protection against untargeted but phylogenetically related high-risk HPV types [92–94]. A next-generation HPV vaccine includes additional five high-risk HPV types plus HPV16 and HPV18 [95]. A summary of HPV vaccines, the projected health benefits, and related biosimilars are shown in Table 1. Ignoring any future secular trends in HPV, it is reasonable to assume that the first- and second-generation of HPV vaccines could prevent approximately 3.5% and 4.5% of all cancers worldwide.

Table 1. Overview of HPV vaccines.

	Quadrivalent HPV Vaccines	Bivalent HPV Vaccines	Nonavalent HPV Vaccines
U.S. FDA-approved product name	Gardasil	Cervarix	Gardasil-9
Manufacturer	Merck	GSK	Merck
Virus-like particle type and dosing	40 mg HPV16; 20 mg HPV18; 20 mg HPV6; 40 mg HPV11	20 mg HPV16; 20 mg HPV18	60 mg HPV16; 40 mg HPV18; 30 mg HPV6; 40 mg HPV11; 20 mg HPV31; 20 mg HPV33; 20 mg HPV45; 20 mg HPV52; 20 mg HPV58
Adjuvant	225 mg amorphous aluminum hydroxyphosphate sulfate	500 mg aluminum hydroxide and 50 mg 3-O-desacyl-4′ monophosphoryl lipid A (MPL)	500 mg amorphous aluminum hydroxyphosphate sulfate
Projected, estimated prevention benefits	70% of cervical cancers; 90% of warts	84% of cervical cancers [†]	90% of cervical cancers; 90% of warts
Biosimilars	Cervivac ™ [96] (Serum Institute of India, Pune, India)	Cecolin ® [97,98] (Xiamen Innovax Biotech Co. Ltd.; Xiamen, China); Walrinvax (Walvax Biotechnology Co.; Yunnan, China)	Cecolin 9 ® [99] (Xiamen Innovax Biotech Co. Ltd.; Xiamen, China)

[†] Assuming cross-protection against untargeted HPV types [92–94].

Registration clinical trials of HPV vaccines demonstrated nearly 100% reduction in cervical pre-cancer [89,100]. Recent reports from Finland, Denmark, Sweden, England, and Scotland have provided real-world evidence that HPV vaccination significantly reduces the incidence of cervical cancer [101–105]. HPV vaccination has been shown to be safe [106–108].

There is now evidence that protection against HPV endures for a decade or more with no evidence of waning immunity [109,110]. Importantly, there is a growing body of evidence that a single dose of an HPV vaccine is sufficient to provide long-lasting protection against targeted HPV types [110–115] and even cross-protection against untargeted but related types [92].

HPV vaccination of women living with HIV (WLWH) is well tolerated, safe, and generates adequate titers, albeit lower than populations without HIV [116–118]. However, there is currently no evidence that HPV vaccination is effective in protecting WLWH against HPV, cervical pre-cancer, or cancer [116–118].

HPV testing-based screening has replaced Pap testing/cervical cytology as the recommended method for secondary prevention of cervical cancer through the detection and treatment of cervical pre-cancer [26,119–121]. HPV testing is more sensitive but less specific for cervical pre-cancer and early cancer than cytology [121,122]. As a result of its greater sensitivity compared with other methods of screening, HPV testing more efficiently/effectively reduces cervical cancer incidence [123] and mortality [124], and a negative HPV test provides a more effective "rule-out", i.e., reassurance against cancer [123–126], than cytology and other screening methods. The greater safety following a negative HPV test can be used to extend screening intervals, thereby reducing the harms of screening, or, in the same interval (as cytology), to reduce the risk further in screen-negative women. The U.S. Preventive Service Taskforce currently recommends routine quintennial HPV testing alone or concurrently with cervical cytology ("co-testing") [119], although co-testing offers very little in terms of clinical performance above what HPV testing alone can [126].

Importantly, HPV testing-based screening permits the use of self-collection of cervicovaginal specimens or urine for HPV testing. In controlled research settings, HPV testing of self-collected cervicovaginal specimens performs comparably to provider-collected cervical specimens when a DNA amplification method of HPV testing is used [127–129].

Self-collection increases participation and acceptability of cervical cancer screening by not requiring an initial clinical visit for cervical screening and obviates the need for a pelvic exam with a speculum. Consistently, women prefer self-collected cervicovaginal specimens over provider-collected cervical specimens [130–132]. However, one of the primary barriers to the acceptance of self-collection is a lack of self-efficacy (i.e., women are concerned as to whether they can complete it "as well as the clinicians"), and women cite this as a reason that they might prefer provider-collected cervical specimens [130–132].

Urine collection for HPV testing obviates the need to insert a device vaginally and therefore may be more acceptable to some women, as well as some transgender men and nonbinary people with a cervix [133], in need of screening. Urine-based HPV testing may overcome cultural barriers to cervical cancer screening. Although there are few data for the HPV testing of urine, a similar comparability to provider-collected cervical specimens when a DNA amplification method of HPV testing is used has been shown [134]; however, further research is needed to optimize its use. Several studies report preference by women for, and greater confidence in the use of, urine over self-collected cervicovaginal specimens [135–138].

HPV-positive women can be triaged with a second, more specific test (also known as adjunctive or reflex testing) to "rule-in" those who need immediate further management (colposcopy and biopsy or treatment). The addition of secondary testing trades off immediate sensitivity for better specificity, with the goal of allowing some benign HPV infections to clear on their own. Thus, the population is stratified into low-risk (HPV-negative), who return to routine screening, intermediate-risk (HPV+/Triage−), who are followed at shorter intervals (increased surveillance), and high-risk (HPV+/Triage+), who need immediate care. Programmatic sensitivity and effectiveness depend on the sensitivity of the second test to identify immediately those who have cervical pre-cancer and cancer and losses in the follow-up of those who are HPV+/Triage−.

Cytology testing was the first method used as a triage test for HPV+, either performed concurrently ("co-testing") or sequentially following an HPV+ result. Second-generation HPV tests have included some degree of HPV genotyping to identify those with HPV16 and HPV18 who are at the highest risk of cervical cancer [139–141] and warrant immediate clinical action or those with lower risk types that may be managed less aggressively/invasively [142–144].

New biomarkers have emerged that may replace or complement cytology and HPV genotyping as triage methods for the management of HPV-positive women. The most promising include p16/Ki-67 immunocytochemistry [145–147] and methylation of the HPV and host genomes [148–150]. p16/Ki-67 immunocytochemistry is now recommended for the management of HPV-positive women in the U.S. [145]. Molecular triage methods such as genome methylation might be particularly suited for self-collected specimens [151], which may not be collected in a way to preserve whole cells or have fewer diagnostic whole cells than found in a provider-collected specimen. New sequencing technologies that measure methylation without the need for bisulfite conversion may make methylation biomarkers more practical for clinical applications [152–154]. Another emerging approach is machine learning algorithm-based analyses of cervical images [155–157].

HPV E6 and E7 oncogene products remain an intriguing target for detection since low levels of E6 and E7 are necessary for genomic replication and amplification, but their overexpression is a biomarker for cervical pre-cancer and cancer [158,159]. Thus, a quantitative mRNA test with a low- and high-level cut point could function as both a screening and triage test, respectively. Detection of low levels, such as those achieved by commercial qualitative mRNA tests [160,161], would indicate the presence of HPV infection, and a negative result would rule out HPV infection, allowing for extended screening intervals. High levels of HPV E6/E7 mRNA are expected to have a high positive predictive value for cervical pre-cancer and cancer and should be more common among the more carcinogenic types, i.e., high levels of HPV16 E6/E7 mRNA should be much more common than HPV68 E6/E7 mRNA. An HPV16, HPV18, and HPV45 E6 oncoprotein test (now just HPV16 and HPV18) was shown to be less sensitive but highly specific for cervical pre-cancer compared with DNA detection [162], but this does not include a broad enough group of types to be clinically useful. It also needs further development so that it is scalable and reliable since it takes ~2.5 h to run a single test and is impacted by ambient testing conditions, respectively (personal observation).

However, the increasing number of tools for the prevention of cervical cancer may have the unintended consequence of increasing the complexity of providing care, leading to its suboptimal provision. To ensure appropriate care, the following strategies should be implemented: (1) risk-based decision-making to ensure equal care for equal risk [163] and (2) a risk calculator/decision support tool to guide providers [164,165].

Importantly, as discussed below, many of the barriers (access to healthcare, home and work obligations, financial toxicities, stigmatization, marginalization of/discrimination against racial, ethnic, sexual/gender minorities, etc.) to screening will impede follow-up care of HPV-positive women. These barriers must be addressed to realize the full benefits of adding self-collection, HPV testing, and other strategies to increase participation in routine cervical cancer screening.

5. Cervical Cancer: The Low-Hanging Fruit

It is worth noting that cervical cancer has some unique characteristics that make it uniquely preventable and controllable. Table 2 summarizes the following reasons why advances towards the prevention of cervical cancer have been exceptional: (1) a single etiologic agent, (2) slow development of cancer, (3) ease of tissue accessibility, (4) a small area of cancer susceptibility, and (5) a proven surrogate for cancer. While there are other cancers with one or more of these characteristics, no others have all five of these specific characteristics or are common enough that population-level interventions are warranted and potentially cost-effective.

Table 2. Characteristics that make cervical cancer uniquely preventable.

	Characteristic	Comment
A.	Single etiologic agent	Approximately 13 HPV types cause virtually all cervical cancer worldwide. There are no other cancers for which there is a single, identifiable causal agent.
B.	Slow-growing cancer	Average sojourn time from HPV exposure (initiation) to cancer is ~25 years.
C.	Tissue accessibility	The cervix can be sampled directly by a brush for cytology and molecular testing for screening and by biopsy forceps to collect tissue for diagnosis with an outpatient speculum exam. The relative acceptability of sampling from this tissue allowed the early development of Pap testing, which was key to elucidating the natural history of cervical cancer, including the identification of a good surrogate (see D). Cervicovaginal sampling collects sufficient amounts of HPV for detection that self-collection is feasible.
D.	Small area of susceptibility	The vast majority of HPV-related genital cancers occur in a very small annulus of tissue, the cervical transformation zone, with the most distal (from the vaginal opening) boundary defined by the squamocolumnar junction, which can be visualized, making sampling and diagnostic biopsies much simpler.
E.	Proven surrogate for cancer	CIN3/AIS have some characteristics of invasive cervical cancer, most notably an HPV-type distribution. A proven surrogate permitted the more rapid validation of novel, HPV-targeted intervention strategies including HPV vaccination and HPV testing-based screening.

Some of the key lessons learned from studies of cervical cancer include the following:
- Natural history informs interventions. The elucidation of the natural history of cervical cancer has guided the development and use of prevention strategies. It is now clear

that younger women—and men—should be vaccinated against HPV before exposure to it but not screened because they have very little true pre-cancerous lesions and almost no cancer. However, mid-adult women need screening for long-persisting HPV infections that have developed into cervical pre-cancer and cancer but will benefit very little from HPV vaccination as they will acquire relatively few incident HPV infections that will go on to become cancer [166,167].

- Surrogates accelerate progress. Having a good surrogate of cancer allows for rapid cycling through novel interventions to identify those that are most promising without requiring an incidence or mortality endpoint. CIN3 and AIS have HPV genotype distributions that closely resemble that of invasive cervical cancer [144,168–171]; the positivity for biomarkers associated with cervical cancer increases with increasing certainty of pre-cancer [172,173]. Conversely, CIN2, which has been included in combined endpoint (CIN2 or more severe abnormality ("CIN2+")) to help power prevention and screening trials, is highly regressive and is often caused by low-risk HPV, as a result of likely being an admixture of manifestations of HPV infection (e.g., CIN1) and CIN3 rather than a true biological entity [66,174–176]. Thus, its inclusion in a composite endpoint must be interpreted with caution. As a result of including CIN2 in endpoints, the clinical importance of certain HPV types can be overestimated. For example, HPV66, which commonly causes CIN2 and low-grade abnormalities [32], is included in all current HPV tests because of one influential study [33], despite the fact that it rarely causes cancer [28,29,32] and is not considered a high-risk HPV type [30,177]. Conversely, HPV18 is often under-represented in CIN3 compared with its prevalence in cervical cancer [32,168,170,178]. Thus, a weighted average based on histology and HPV genotype fraction based on cancer may better predict the impact of an intervention on cervical cancer risk than simple HPV type prevalence when a surrogate endpoint of CIN2+ is used [174].
- Screening works best as a two-step process. First rule out, then rule in. Typically, diagnostic tests are used to confirm a disease in a selected population enriched for the disease of interest, e.g., someone has a symptom, such as fever, and then a diagnostic test is run to determine the underlying cause. In the case of cancer screening, the intervention is performed in a population in which cancer and even precursors are relatively rare. In this scenario, a single-test screening algorithm will have poor positive predictive value (PPV) unless the test is extremely specific [179], which usually then sacrifices sensitivity. In the two-step, rule-out/rule-in algorithm, the first, more sensitive test (HPV) rules out disease in the healthy population. An important but underappreciated benefit of the rule-out algorithm is providing reassurance against disease, i.e., telling healthy people that they are healthy and at low risk of cancer. In the case of HPV testing, testing negative for the cause of cervical cancer allows screening intervals to be safely extended, reducing screening harms.

When the triage test is applied to the sub-population of screen positives to risk stratify and determine who needs further evaluation (rule-in), the PPV is much better because the endpoint of interest is enriched [179]. Using a two-step, rule-out/rule-in algorithm, populations are stratified into three distinct risk groups, i.e., higher risk (rule-out+/rule-in+), intermediate risk (rule-out+/rule-in−), and lower risk (rule-out−), that can be managed according to clinical action thresholds. For example, HPV+/Pap+ women are sent to colposcopy, HPV+/Pap− are placed under active, annual surveillance (until there is evidence of increased risk in follow-up), and HPV− return to routine, 5-year screening. The results of the screening test can be combined with the triage test results for further risk stratification. For example, if HPV genotyping for HPV16 and HPV18 is available as part of HPV testing, the three tiers of risk are (1) HPV16+, HPV18+, or Pap+ go to colposcopy (rule-out+/rule-in+), (2) HPV+ but HPV16−, HPV18−, and Pap− undergo active annual surveillance (rule-out+/rule-in−), and (3) HPV− return to routine screening. As a consequence, more high-risk women are sent for immediate colposcopy, likely increasing programmatic sensitivity.

Clinical action thresholds (CATs) can be established to guide the optimal management of women by maximizing the population benefits-to-harms ratio as well as promoting the principle of equal care for equal risk. CATs, based on risk, are used to guide clinical decision-making and are informed by sociocultural acceptance of tradeoffs in benefits and harms. Operationally, both biological (e.g., HPV16 detection) and non-biological risk factors (e.g., social determinants of health) are integrated into an individual risk estimate, and the CAT determines whether more (above the CAT) or less (below the CAT) aggressive intervention is warranted, e.g., colposcopy vs. surveillance, respectively.

- Implementing best practices is very difficult and slow. Even when the science and evidence are robust, adoption is slow, especially in "disorganized" healthcare systems, like cervical cancer screening in the U.S. It has been known that HPV testing is a better screening test than cytology for 20+ years, but, even now, very few women living in the U.S. get screened at the recommended screening intervals [180], screening tests are overused [181], and most U.S. cancer centers do not recommend HPV testing as the front-line cervical cancer screening test [182]. Vested interests almost certainly played a role in the slow change from cytology to HPV testing. Without HPV testing, self-collection will not be an option, which is key to reaching many women who cannot or will not undergo a pelvic exam or obtain care in the clinic. Implementation research on how to bring HPV testing into practice and de-implementing cytology-based screening and over-screening is greatly needed. By comparison, national, publicly funded healthcare programs, such as those in many European countries like The Netherlands, tend to be more efficient and have better adherence to guidelines, thereby reducing costs and harms of screening compared with the U.S. [183,184].

- Systematic Bias. The development of new technologies is subject to systemic biases. The HPV35 story is an example of such a bias. The formative epidemiological studies of cervical cancer did not include enough cases of cervical cancer in women of African descent to detect this important relationship and, consequently, HPV35 is not included in any current HPV vaccine formulations. Those studies that did include cases of cervical cancer from WLWH of African descent from sub-Saharan Africa and differences in type distribution were first attributed to HIV co-infection. Whether current multivalent HPV vaccines generate enough cross-protection to protect against untargeted HPV35 is unknown. However, it was recently announced that one vaccine manufacturer will develop a multivalent (> nine-valent) HPV vaccine that hopefully will include HPV35 [50].

- New technologies can exacerbate health disparities. The role of Pap in accelerating global cervical cancer prevention cannot be overstated. Millions of cervical cancers, and deaths due to cervical cancer, were averted worldwide because of Pap testing, though these benefits were concentrated in high-resource populations. Another important contribution of routine Pap testing was helping to elucidate the natural history of cervical cancer, which had profound consequences for the subsequent development of newer, more effective technologies directly targeting HPV. Having a Pap as a predicate test facilitated the development of HPV testing. In addition, Pap testing-based screening identified and validated CIN2/3 as precursors to cervical cancer, which allowed clinical trials to use them as an early, surrogate endpoint for invasive cervical cancer, which accelerated approvals of HPV testing and HPV vaccines. That said, it is time to sunset Pap/cytology for the next-generation test for screening, HPV testing, which, in addition to better sensitivity and negative predictive value, offers greater flexibility for screening through self-collection, allowing more women to get screened. Unfortunately, as discussed below, we are in danger of repeating the same mistakes as the wealthiest women are given preferential access to these new, more effective, HPV-targeted technologies for cervical cancer prevention.

6. Discussion

Despite the successes of Pap testing, the geographical variation in cervical cancer incidence and mortality in the U.S. and globally highlights important health inequities due to differential access to high-quality screening and follow-up care. In the U.S., the unequal burden of cervical cancer is related to many factors including but not limited to social, racial, sexual, and ethnic discrimination, low income/poverty, stigma, and geographic isolation such as rurality [3]. Communities with higher rates of cervical cancer mortality have poorer access to health care in general [185]. State- and county-level cervical cancer mortality is correlated with increased mortality of other preventable cancers, such as colorectal cancer, and they are inversely correlated with average *per capita* income [186]. Counties with persistent poverty (counties that have had at least 20% of their residents living below the federal poverty line continuously since 1980) experience significantly higher mortality rates in several cancers, including cervical, than those with non-persistent poverty [187].

Although HPV-based interventions have the potential to "close the gap" in the cervical cancer burden in the U.S., they also have the possibility of exacerbating it if the underlying causes of those disparities are not addressed [3]. The uptake of HPV vaccination, which was first approved by the FDA in 2006 and recommended by the Advisory Committee on Immunization Practices in 2007, has been unacceptably low. HPV vaccine coverage with at least one dose was 25.1% in 2007 and 54% in 2012 [188]. As of 2022, 78% and 65% of females aged 13–17 years received at least one and all recommended doses of HPV vaccine, respectively, which was similar to the coverage in 2021 (79% and 64%, respectively) [189]. The percentage of adolescents with at least one HPV vaccine dose declined in those insured by Medicaid and remained lowest among the uninsured [189]. By comparison, Australia achieved >70% coverage with three doses of the HPV vaccine in female children in its first year of introduction in 2007; differences across economic groups were significant [190] but less pronounced than in the U.S. By 2017, Australia achieved nearly 90% coverage for at least one dose and 80% coverage for three doses [191]. As of 2018, Australia had not yet reported a decline in the age-standardized annual rate of cervical cancer incidence [192].

There are several factors that have likely influenced the uptake of HPV vaccination in the U.S. and perhaps other places in the world. HPV vaccination is mandated only in Virginia, Hawaii, Rhode Island, and Washington D.C. By comparison, measles, mumps, and rubella vaccination and diphtheria, tetanus, and pertussis vaccination are mandated by all states and Washington D.C., and the coverage in 2021 was 91% and 80%, respectively. Hepatitis B vaccination, which requires three doses, is required by colleges and universities in about 30% of states and the coverage in 2021 was 91% [193,194]. So, while requiring vaccination undoubtedly improves coverage, its impact is somewhat variable.

Another factor that appears to influence HPV vaccine updates is the link between HPV and sex. Parents are still concerned that HPV vaccination may promote high-risk sexual behaviors in their children [195,196] despite the evidence that HPV vaccination does not promote compensatory sexual behaviors [197,198]. Messaging to parents and providers that de-emphasizes HPV vaccination as prevention for a sexually transmitted infection (STI) and emphasizing its cancer prevention benefits may help [199–201]. Delivering HPV vaccination as part of the early childhood vaccination schedule, as discussed in Part 2, would not only simplify HPV vaccine delivery but could help to distance it as an STI vaccine being delivered to preteens and early teens "before sex starts".

The role of HPV vaccination in males warrants discussion. In general, gender-neutral (males and females) will prevent more cancers than female-only HPV vaccination. Importantly, men who have sex with men (MSM) may not benefit from the herd protection of HPV vaccination of females, as was demonstrated early following the introduction of HPV vaccination in women in Australia, where genital warts declined rapidly and sharply in women and heterosexual men but not MSMs [202]. However, while gender-neutral HPV vaccination is estimated to be a good value, it is generally less cost-effective than female-only HPV vaccination because females gain the majority of the benefits [203–207].

Thus, gender-neutral HPV vaccination might be a reasonable healthcare investment in HICs but rapid, high-coverage HPV vaccination in females should be the priority in LMICs.

Expanding cervical screening in the U.S. via self-collection and HPV testing is a promising, complementary approach to reaching the sub-population of women who do not participate in current clinic-based programs. Yet, many of the underlying social determinants of health (SDoH)-related barriers to cervical screening remain [3] and will not be solved using self-collection alone. Figure 2 highlights some of those delivery barriers for self-collection-based cervical cancer screening. In the U.S. context, the optimal health service delivery model has not been established. Community health worker-based/door-to-door approaches to delivering self-collection devices consistently show greater increases in screening participation than more passive approaches (e.g., opt-out) [129,208] but they also require a greater commitment of resources. A recent trial in the U.S. among those receiving care at a U.S. integrated health care delivery system demonstrated a 17% increase in screening with mailed self-collection kits in women overdue for screening [209], but these women are not representative of those who are most underserved by the U.S. healthcare system.

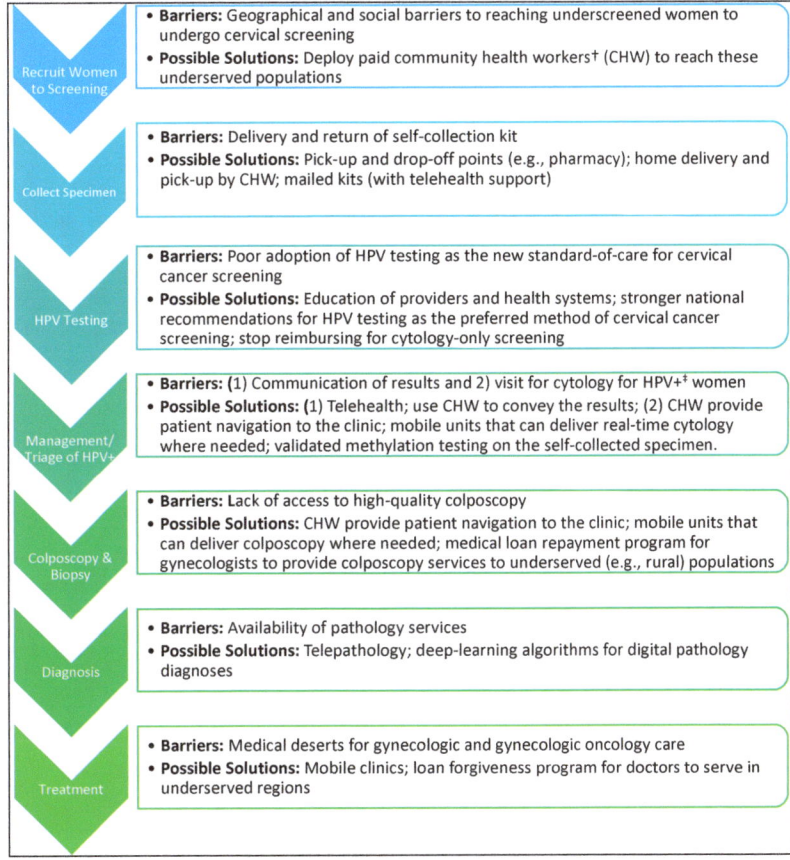

Figure 2. Some of the barriers and possible solutions for delivering self-collection and HPV testing for cervical cancer screening along the care continuum in the U.S. [†] Need to be paid members of the medical home, which will require a billable CMS code for their services. [‡] Women who test HPV positive (HPV+) but are negative for HPV16 and HPV18 will need an extra visit for cytology in the U.S. Self-collected specimens cannot be used for cytology because there are not enough diagnostic cells, and it is unlikely that the medium used for the self-collected specimen will preserve whole cells.

There are obvious financial barriers to those who do not have insurance or have insurance but cannot afford the co-pay for any screening or follow-up care. Of note, recommended cervical cancer screening in the U.S. starts (age 21 years) and ends (age 65 years) largely before Medicare eligibility begins (age 62 years); therefore, other types of medical insurance coverage are necessary to pay for care. While the CDC's National Breast and Cervical Cancer Program provides screening and diagnostic services [210], and treatment for cervical pre-cancer and cancer is made available to Medicaid-eligible women through state Medicaid programs under the Breast and Cervical Cancer Prevention and Treatment Act of 2000 [211], less than 7% of the 5.3 million eligible women accessed the program in 2017 [212]. Moreover, there are medical provider deserts, primarily in rural settings, of gynecologic and radiation oncologists to manage invasive cervical cancers [213–215] and gynecologists to biopsy and manage pre-cancerous abnormalities [216,217]. Because follow-up of screen-positives requires clinical visits and pelvic exams, these remain barriers to the completion of care.

In summary, highly effective tools to prevent cervical cancer are in hand. However, as discussed in Part 2, the hard work begins now, which is how to make these tools available to all.

B. Part 2: Moving Forward

Although HPV-targeting interventions for global prevention and control of cervical cancer have been identified and are robust, their implementation presents many challenges. Most of these challenges are related to the lack of healthcare infrastructure and financial and human resources to implement them in LMICs. Investments to address these gaps lag far behind the technological advances and will be the bottleneck to achieving WHO goals to reduce the cervical cancer burden worldwide. Some of these barriers for each of the three target goals are discussed below and summarized in Table 3.

Table 3. Some of the challenges and potential solutions to implementing WHO interventional targets to achieve cervical cancer elimination. Bold type highlights areas in need of additional research.

HPV Vaccination	Challenge	Potential Solution (s)
Financial	• Cost of vaccines.	• One-dose HPV vaccination. • Expand GAVI eligibility and include Gardasil-9. • Use lower cost biosimilars.
Technical/Logistical	• Lack of adolescent health platform.	• Develop adolescent health platform. • **Include HPV vaccination of infants WHO EPI vaccine schedule.**
Human Capacity	• Expand the providers who can provide HPV vaccination.	• Training and certification of community health workers to vaccinate.
Infrastructure	• Cold chain for vaccine delivery.	• Develop cold-chain infrastructure. • **Develop temperature-resistant VLP vaccine.**
HPV Testing-Based Screening	**Challenge**	**Potential Solution(s)**
Financial	• Test cost.	• **Development of low-cost testing technology.** • Establish a global procurement strategy for laboratory tests and testing.
	• Cost of disposables (pipet tips, PPE, etc.).	• Tests that require minimal specimen handling and processing. • Global procurement strategy for laboratory tests and testing.

Table 3. Cont.

HPV Testing-Based Screening		Challenge	Potential Solution(s)
	Technical/logistical	• Getting the specimen to the HPV test.	• Development and validation point-of-care or near point-of-care HPV tests. • Use pre-existing or develop specimen courier networks to transport specimens to central testing laboratory.
		• Management of HPV-positive women.	• **Develop and validate deep learning algorithms for image analysis to distinguish those with and without cervical pre-cancer.** • **Develop a robust methylation assay that works from a self-collected specimen.**
	Human capacity	• Number of trained technicians,	Expand training and retention of laboratory technicians; develop assays that require minimal training.
	Infrastructure	• Lack of qualified labs with "clean rooms" for PCR-based testing.	• Develop assays that do not require PCR safe testing environments.
	Other		

Management/Treatment of Precursors		Challenge	Potential Solution (s)
	Human capacity	• Limited capacity for gynecologic services including colposcopy and treatment of precursors.	• Increase gynecology training. • **Develop pan-HPV Therapeutics**
		• Limited capacity for pathology.	• Screen and treat; screen, triage (non-pathology methods), and treat. • **Develop an AI-based digital pathology platform.** • Increase human capacity in histotechnology and pathology.
	Infrastructure	• Lack of clinics to provide services.	• Mobile clinics.

Cancer Treatment, Management, and Care			
	Financial	• Cost of treatment.	• Subsidized care based on ability to pay.
	Technical/logistical	• Long distances to reach health care facilities with cancer care capacities.	• Dedicated transportation for cancer care.
	Human capacity	• Lack of gynecologic oncologists. • Lack of radiation oncologists and technologists. • Lack of pathologists.	• Training and mentoring programs for staffing of gynecologic oncology, radiation oncology, and pathology services.
	Infrastructure	• Lack of LINACs. • Lack of brachytherapy.	• Place more LINACs. • Increase availability of brachytherapy. • Validate the use of neoadjuvant therapy and surgery.
	Policy	• Access to and acceptance of morphine/opioids for pain management [218].	• Policy changes and de-regulation of morphine/opioids. • Education and training on their use and abuse.

7. Achieving 90% HPV Vaccination

Prophylactic HPV vaccination is the ultimate cervical cancer risk reduction strategy, but it is not a panacea because there are several generations of adult women who will benefit little or not all from HPV vaccination. As a result, adult women generally will not be targeted by public health programs for HPV vaccination, especially those living in LMICs, because of the relatively poor cost-effectiveness compared with vaccinating younger females [219,220]. There has been some consideration of delivering HPV vaccination to adult women undergoing screening [221,222]. Such an approach would primarily reduce the endemicity of HPV in the population rather than prevent cervical cancer, since most HPV infections that ultimately cause cervical cancer are acquired before the age of 30 years [166]. It is also unknown whether multiple doses of HPV vaccine would be needed in this older population, which would logistically complicate its delivery. The cost and the cost-effectiveness of such an approach have yet to be determined and, given the significant barriers to delivering screening, this "faster HPV" approach may be limited to certain settings and target populations.

Relatively few women living in LMICs have received HPV vaccination compared with HICs [223], further exacerbating the cervical cancer health disparities rather than narrowing the gap. One-dose HPV vaccination should greatly increase its availability, deliverability, and affordability for LMICs. Yet, even with one-dose HPV vaccination, GAVI The Vaccine Alliance ("GAVI") [224] subsidies, and Pan American Health Organization Revolving Fund discounted vaccine pricing [225], cost may still be a significant barrier, especially for those countries ineligible for support through these programs. Indeed, lower-middle-income countries, which are not eligible for GAVI support, have had much lower HPV vaccine uptake than low-income countries [223]. Strategies to increase the availability of lower-cost HPV vaccine doses, including access to biosimilars, expanding GAVI eligibility, and/or the development of a complementary global procurement mechanism, should help accelerate HPV vaccine coverage.

Perhaps a more significant challenge is the delivery of HPV vaccination to preteens and adolescents in some LMICs, especially those in sub-Saharan Africa (SSA), where health service delivery to this large segment of the population is typically limited and focused on reproductive health needs, although that is slowly changing [226–232]. Notably, as of 2020, 20% of the world's population of adolescents, an estimated 250 million people, live in SSA, and that percentage of the world's adolescent population is expected to grow to 25% by 2030 [233,234]. Thus, investment in the infrastructure, particularly in SSA, to develop more comprehensive adolescent healthcare, especially to deliver preventive services, could facilitate the delivery of HPV vaccination and have a broad impact on adolescent health. This could be school-based, although not all adolescents attend secondary education, and there is a significant decrease in school attendance with increasing age of adolescents, especially in low-income countries [235], so a secondary system may be needed to achieve high population coverage of HPV vaccination.

An alternative or complementary strategy is to deliver one-dose HPV vaccination, if proven safe and highly immunogenic, as part of routine infant/early pediatric ("early childhood") vaccination, integrating it with other scheduled vaccines as part of WHO's Expanded Programme on Immunization [236,237]. The approach is highly plausible. Many countries throughout the world have an early childhood immunization program, most of which have policies that recommend or mandate childhood vaccination, although vaccine coverage varies by country and correlates with country wealth [238–242]. Nevertheless, many countries have at least some capacity and infrastructure to deliver HPV vaccination to these young children. Moreover, existing data indicate long-term, age-specific anti-HPV titers are higher the younger a person is vaccinated [243–245], suggesting that the protective anti-HPV antibody titers could be even greater than those seen in preteens. Importantly, demonstrating that HPV vaccination delivered to infants and young children generates comparable immunity in adolescence to that generated by the current schedule in pre-adolescents would give vaccination programs more flexibility in the delivery of HPV vaccination at the age that is most convenient.

Those countries that have not introduced HPV vaccination then could choose the most convenient age group to deliver HPV vaccination for their context. For those countries in which adolescent HPV vaccination is already offered, two implementation strategies might be considered. The first is to continue vaccinating preteens and early adolescents while initiating HPV vaccination in infants and young children. When the first cohort of infants and young children reach the age of 9 years, vaccination of preteens is phased out. The second option is campaign-style outreach to vaccinate children from infant and early pediatric ages to the age at which female children are currently vaccinated, and then subsequently continue HPV vaccination only of infant/early pediatric females. Of course, other strategies might be considered and tailored to local needs and resources.

8. Achieving 70% HPV Testing-Based Screening

Globally, the varying ability to effectively implement Pap-based cervical cancer screening across the world has led to the current large disparities in cervical cancer burden. Pap testing under the best circumstances is only a moderately sensitive and reproducible screening method (compared with HPV testing) [122,246], and clinical performance can only be accomplished when robust, extensive quality assurance and control measures are taken [247]. There are now decades of experience demonstrating that Pap testing cannot be successfully and effectively implemented at a population level in LMICs [248–252], as indicated by the 10-fold disparities in cervical cancer burden worldwide [1], despite claims to the contrary [253,254]. Whether Pap testing is more affordable than HPV testing is irrelevant if it cannot be successfully implemented to scale in LMICs, and advocacy for it gives false hope and delays the implementation of technologies that can realistically reduce the burden of cervical cancer. In addition, the infrastructure, technical, and human capacities to provide Pap testing are specialized and cannot be adapted to address other healthcare needs in LMICs, thereby limiting the value of investing in it. Efforts should focus on bringing HPV testing technologies to everyone, rather than investing in Pap technology that cannot be scaled or sustained [253,255]. Or, as discussed below, resources should be devoted to other preventable/controllable diseases that burden the population even more than cervical cancer.

HPV testing is now considered the recommended method of cervical cancer screening [26,256] and, where available, should be considered the preferred, standard-of-care method. Modeling studies show that a program of HPV testing-based screening offers greater benefits and reduced harm compared with other methods in the general population of women and WLWH [257,258].

However, many countries do not have a recommended screening test and others still recommend cytology and/or visual inspection after acetic acid (VIA), not HPV testing [259]. Worldwide, most adult women have never been screened for cervical cancer with the following large differences in those who have ever been screened by any method by World Bank Economic Classification: 84% in high-income, 48% in upper-middle-income, 9% in lower-middle-income, and 11% in low-income countries [259]. As a first step towards achieving higher coverage for screening worldwide, national cancer control plans might consider including recommendations for cervical cancer screening, with HPV testing as the preferred method and a secondary method of choice as the stop-gap method until HPV testing becomes available and affordable.

Although HPV testing is more feasible than some methods and more effective than other methods for routine cervical cancer screening, there are formidable barriers to its global implementation, especially in LMICs. Importantly, screening is not a test but a multi-step process, the effectiveness of which is limited by the weakest step. Barriers in this process include the following: (1) the availability of LMIC-ready, robust, and effective HPV tests; (2) the limited number of gynecologists and clinicians who can provide colposcopic services and treatment of precursors; (3) the lack of pathology services; (4) weak health systems to identify, call, and recall women for screening and care, etc.; and (5) the lack of gynecologic oncologists to surgically remove early cancers and guide care and radiotherapy services to treat more advanced cervical cancers. A major limitation of the Cervical Cancer Elimination Initiative [13] is that it did not come with a plan to facilitate access to HPV testing and treatment.

Technical challenges for implementing HPV testing in LMICs have been discussed extensively and will be only briefly revisited here [260]. First, tests must have the necessary characteristics to perform well in many LMIC settings where there is only basic laboratory infrastructure and limited ability to run complex tests, and they must be performed under a wide range of environmental conditions. Second, these tests must be validated and easy to use, have a rapid sample-to-answer turnaround for some health service delivery models, and minimize biomedical waste, which many LMICs do not have the capacity to manage. Third, the testing cost, which includes not just the HPV test but all reagents, disposables, equipment (amortized over its lifespan), and personal protective equipment, must be low either because of the low cost of the technology itself or a global procurement strategy (e.g., a GAVI-like program or organization for in vitro diagnostics). Finally, the test must require very limited or no equipment; otherwise, all the technical issues related to equipment use and maintenance will be very problematic over time.

The ideal characteristics for an HPV test may differ by the care delivery model. Fundamentally, the three general delivery models include the following: (1) bring a test to a person; (2) bring a person to a test, i.e., a central facility that has testing capability; or (3) bring a specimen to a centralized testing laboratory.

In the first scenario, a single-use point-of-care (POC) test, such as a lateral flow test, might be well suited for a low-volume setting, whereas a small (e.g., 96-well) batch test on a clinical testing platform might be necessary for medium and higher volumes. In either case, testing will need to be performed in the most basic setting (e.g., rural health clinic), likely without any real laboratory infrastructure, and all testing (one or several tests) must be performed within an hour to minimize the time burden on the women being screened. In this setting, if it takes several hours to collect the necessary minimum number of specimens to run a batch test, or the batch test is run with fewer specimens, thereby increasing the testing costs, this approach becomes less attractive. Alternatively, campaign-style screening events (i.e., mobile screening units) could be performed with a batch test, but this would require the necessary logistics to move to different locations and provide comprehensive follow-up care.

In the second scenario, individuals come to a clinical facility to get tested and care on the same day. Like the first scenario, testing must be performed in short order to allow the completion of care in a timely manner, especially since women may travel significant distances/expend significant time coming to a facility, and there is a real risk of loss-to-follow-up if they are required to return for a second visit.

However, same-day screen-and-treat is challenging to implement at any scale, except in the context of research projects with dedicated personnel. In a real-world scenario, there are many barriers to same-day screen-and-treat, e.g., laboratory personnel have other tests to run and are not dedicated to HPV testing.

In the third scenario, specimens are collected remotely and tested centrally. Unlike the first two scenarios, rapid testing is not necessary since screening is not completed on the same day, but it would require linking the results back to the women and getting HPV-positive women back to a clinic for follow-up care. Some LMICs may have a specimen transport network, such as those used to transport blood for HIV and TB testing, which HPV testing specimens could leverage, as was the case with COVID-19 testing during the pandemic [261].

Screening algorithms usually rely on pathology to identify those at high risk, but that is not possible in many LMIC settings. In many LMICs, especially SSA, pathology services are very limited and unreliable, if available at all [262–264], and will not be able to handle any increased workload corresponding to scaled-up screening any time soon. Indeed, it is not uncommon to find stacks of unread cytology and histology slides in pathology labs throughout LMICs (personal observations). Machine-learning algorithms for the diagnosis of histopathology slides might provide a solution in the future [265–268]. However, many pathology labs do not have access to high-quality chemicals or equipment to fix and process biopsies, well-maintained equipment to section biopsies, or histotechnologists to prepare tissues. Therefore, scaled-up screening in these settings cannot rely on cytology as a triage test or biopsy for diagnosis to guide the management of HPV-positive women.

Non-pathology-based algorithms to manage HPV-positive women will trade programmatic sensitivity vs. specificity and pragmatic vs. accuracy. The most sensitive and simple algorithm is to treat all HPV-positive women immediately, but this leads to significant overtreatment by methods that may increase the risk of pre-term delivery [269]. Treating those only with the highest-risk HPV types such as HPV16, HPV18, and/or HPV45, which all next-generation HPV tests identify separately, would reduce overtreatment by roughly 70–80% while treating HPV types responsible for approximately 60–75% of cervical cancer. An alternative strategy that has been proposed is to screen with only the eight or so most carcinogenic HPV types that cause approximately 90% of cervical cancer, which is more specific than tests that include 13 or 14 HPV types. Speculatively, adding VIA to detect the highest-risk HPV types and find visually concerning abnormalities and cancer might incrementally increase the sensitivity of the triage step, but it may be subject to the same intra- and inter-provider variability that limits its effectiveness and at the "cost" of performing many more pelvic exams.

New technologies hold promise in identifying which HPV-positive women are at the highest risk of cervical cancer more effectively than VIA and could be combined with HPV genotype information to further risk stratification [155,157]. These methods also require a pelvic exam and so must be considered in the context of the aforementioned tradeoffs in performance vs. pragmatism. These include deep-learning/artificial intelligence optical image analysis of cervical images [155,157] and the use of optical fiber technology to provide an in situ, in vivo diagnosis [270,271]. Importantly, these technologies work in real time and thus, packaged with rapid sample-to-answer HPV testing, hold promise for one-visit, same-day screening algorithms, with only one pelvic exam and completion of care in under two hours. For remote specimen collection, an LMIC-ready host and/or viral methylation panel reflex test from the same HPV testing specimen could identify only the high-risk women who would need to come to the clinic to undergo a pelvic exam for treatment.

The issue of HPV test affordability is best addressed immediately through a global procurement strategy that buys HPV tests in large quantities to keep prices low as well as subsidizes costs to the end users, just as vaccines through GAVI [224] and other medications through The Global Fund. The currently available HPV vaccines would not be affordable otherwise; so, perhaps it should come as no surprise that neither are current HPV tests. In the future, lower-cost POC tests [272], near point-of-care batch tests [273], and high-throughput centralized testing will be more affordable and, therefore, sustainable, and the appropriate HPV-testing technology can be matched to the care delivery model. Still, these new HPV testing technologies will need an orchestrated procurement and subsidization to make them available, especially to those populations of women with the greatest need. Importantly, HPV testing implementation, especially using clinical testing platforms that are multi-analyte or adaptable to other diagnostic targets, will build important capacity in molecular diagnostics for other disease prevention, control, and management.

9. Achieving 90% Treatment

Regardless of the screening modality and delivery model, there must be a linkage to care to treat cervical cancer precursors and invasive cervical cancer. Otherwise, the full benefits of screening will be unrealized. Unfortunately, this component of the WHO strategic plan is the least developed, as it requires significant investment in building human and infrastructure capacities. Effective treatment of invasive cervical cancer requires human capacities in pathology, gynecology, gynecologic surgery/oncology, and radiotherapy [274,275]. To incentivize the investment and development of these capacities and infrastructure, the WHO cervical cancer elimination plan should include mortality reduction targets, e.g., reduce cervical cancer mortality by 50% by 2050, akin to President Biden's aspirational and inspirational Cancer Moonshot goal of reducing all cancer mortality by 50% in 25 years [276].

Consider that there are approximately 8.1 billion people in the world now, if 7.5% of the world population are women aged 35–45 years, and only 10% of those have had even a single high-quality cervical screening in a lifetime, there are approximately 550 million women who need cervical cancer screening today. Assuming a 20% HPV prevalence and 0.2% cervical cancer prevalence, this will translate into an *additional* 110 million women in need of gynecologic care and 1.1 million women with screen-detected cancers that will need cancer therapeutic services.

There are few surgeons, anesthesiologists, and obstetricians in LMICs [277,278], which should be taken as a proxy for a lack of gynecology services for the treatment of cervical cancer precursors. There is also a lack of sufficient expertise to deliver tissue destructive (excision or ablation) treatment of cervical cancer precursors, which will result in both over- and under-treatment and sub-optimal effectiveness [279].

Few women with cervical cancer living in SSA receive the cancer care they need [280–282]. In fact, few African countries have the adequate human capacity, equipment, and supplies to treat cervical cancer. In a survey of African countries, where 43 of 57 responded and provided data, only 20% were deemed to have adequate gynecologic and radiation oncology staffing [283]. Twelve countries (22%) reported having no gynecologic oncologists while 24 of 31 countries (77%) with gynecologic oncologists had ≤ five gynecologic oncologists per 1000 cervical cancer cases [283]. Fourteen countries (26%) reported having no radiation oncologists, while 21 of 29 countries (72%) with radiation oncologists had ≤ five radiation oncologists per 1000 cervical cancer cases [283]. In comparison, for the approximately 14,000 cervical cancer cases diagnosed in the U.S. in 2023, there were approximately 1300 gynecologic oncologists (~93 per 1000 cervical cancer cases) and 5800 radiation oncologists (~412 per 1000 cervical cancer cases) [284]. A recent study of publicly available databases from 175 countries estimated that 57% of cervical cancers would require surgery, so an estimated 630,000 of the 1.1 million screen-detected cases would need surgery if screening was to scale up globally [215].

Effective treatment of advanced cervical cancer requires radiotherapy, which is best accomplished using a linear particle accelerator (LINAC) and brachytherapy. Yet, some LMICs do not have a LINAC, and those that do have insufficient numbers, often only one or two, to manage the total number of in-country cancer cases, including but not limited to cervical cancer, needing radiotherapy [280,283,285,286]. Indeed, the International Atomic Energy Agency ideally recommends four radiotherapy units per million people, with a minimum of at least 1.5 units per million, and most LMICs fall well short of that capacity [287–289]. In addition, when a LINAC is in disrepair, it might be years before it is repaired or replaced. Even when there is LINAC availability, there are also significant geographical and financial barriers to providing radiotherapy in many of these settings [280,290–292]. Likewise, brachytherapy is in short supply in Africa [283].

The situation in Uganda a few years ago provides an illustrative example. Starting in 2016, Uganda's only LINAC, which provided the necessary radiotherapy for only 2.6% of those in need (1 LINAC vs. the minimum of 60 LINACs needed for a Uganda population of 39 million in 2016), was broken beyond repair, and Uganda had no in-country radiotherapy available [293]. Cobalt-60 radiotherapy was introduced in 2018–19 as a stopgap [294] until a single LINAC machine was available in 2021.

Several organizations [295–297] are working to address these gaps in cancer care by building human capacity and increasing access to radiotherapy. However, at the current scale of these admirable efforts, the demand is already well beyond the ability of these activities to address them, that is, before the substantial scale of screening in many countries.

Therefore, a concomitant increase in the capacity to treat pre-cancer and cancer in LMICs and low-resourced settings in HICs will need to accompany the scaling-up of HPV testing-based screening. However, while a commitment to increase treatment and diagnostic capacities is necessary, it will take years if not decades to achieve them, and alternative strategies should be considered in the interim. Neoadjuvant chemotherapy (NACT) followed by hysterectomy has been suggested as an alternative treatment regimen in the absence of standard-of-care cisplatin-based chemoradiation to treat locally advanced cervical cancer [290,298,299]. Yet, the evidence for the effectiveness of this alternative therapy is inconsistent and/or lacking [298–303]. Further research on NACT followed by hysterectomy is needed to establish its efficacy, for whom it works best, the best practices, and the training on how to implement it.

Is it ethically acceptable to scale up HPV testing and the treatment of pre-cancer without the concurrent capacity to treat invasive cancer? On one hand, it violates a well-accepted doctrine that care must be provided for all who are screened. Yet, many women would be spared from developing cervical cancer if there is sufficient capacity to treat pre-cancers even if most cancers could not be appropriately treated. The decision to introduce screening without the capacity to treat screen-detected invasive cervical cancer is an ethical dilemma, but the decision must be left to informed, in-country policy makers.

Although the WHO calls for two rounds of screening at ages 35 years and 45 years, perhaps it is worth considering only screening once in a lifetime for now and targeting women in a slightly younger and more narrow age group, e.g., 30–35 years of age, in whom there will be fewer screen-detected cancers and more but smaller pre-cancers that are more easily and effectively treated [304]. As noted, many countries have never had population screening for cervical cancer, and it will take time to build the human and infrastructure capacities to support it. Targeting a smaller population for whom it will be easier to provide care will give programs a greater chance at early success while building up the capacity to screen a larger population and treat more advanced disease.

There is a great need for effective HPV therapeutics, which could be coupled with HPV testing in a simplified screen-and-treat strategy. Unfortunately, there has been little success to date in developing a therapeutic HPV vaccine with efficacy against cervical pre-cancer that approaches that of current standards-of-care treatments (e.g., excision or ablation) (>80%) [84,305,306]. The efficacy of these experimental vaccines has been limited to approximately 20% and only against HPV16- and/or HPV18-related cervical pre-cancers, meaning that the population effectiveness for preventing invasive cancer is no more than ~15%. A study of topically applied artesunate showed approximately two-thirds of CIN2/3 regressed, but approximately half of those CIN2/3 retained the causal HPV infection, which means that it may not have cleared at all [307].

Notably, those trials included CIN2, which often regresses without treatment, especially in younger women [66]. Thus, even those additional CIN2 observed to regress during the trial period of observation in the intervention arm may be subject to time interval bias, and, had the cohort been observed sufficiently long, there would have been no difference in the regression between the intervention and control arms. In addition, CIN2 is an admixture of CIN1 and CIN3, i.e., either misclassified CIN1 or CIN3, and a CIN2 diagnosis is poorly reproducible [176,308], so the transition from CIN2 to CIN1 may not be truly regression but reclassification. Thus, the population effectiveness in reducing cervical cancer risk of these HPV therapeutics may be significantly overestimated.

A recent meeting was convened to describe a preferred product profile for an HPV therapeutic vaccine [86]. Local priming at the cervix may be necessary to recruit effector T-cells across the basement membrane of the cervical epithelium to the site of the abnormality [309]. However, as noted, an HPV therapeutic vaccine may be less effective in WLWH, in whom 6% of cervical cancer occurs [310], because they are immunocompromised. Thus, a complementary strategy to develop a non-immune-related biological against HPV, such as an antiviral, should be considered.

More fundamentally, what is the minimum acceptable effectiveness of such biological agents as a substitute for standard-of-care tissue-destructive treatments? The aforementioned meeting [86] suggested that 50% direct efficacy against targeted HPV16- and HPV18-related CIN2/3 and 50% cross-efficacy against CIN2/3-related types is the minimum. By inference, this would suggest an efficacy of 50%, but that assumes equal efficacy against CIN3 and CIN2, the latter of which is more likely to regress on its own [66], and that women get the full regimen of multiple treatments. Nor is cross-efficacy assured, at least for a therapeutic vaccine, given that they typically target E proteins that are less well conserved between types than L proteins, which do show some cross-protection as prophylactic vaccines, but not so much that it stopped the development of next-generation prophylactic vaccines are multivalent to provide broader protection. Thus, it is reasonable to assume that effectiveness might be significantly less than 50% for the base-case product. When used correctly, tissue-destructive methods, such as excision and ablation, are highly effective (~5–10% failure rate, i.e., 90–95% effective) [311], but, as discussed, they are much more difficult and more resource-intensive to deliver effectively. Is it ethical to deliver the lesser therapeutic option knowingly, given that it is likely to be less efficacious but potentially more effective? Ultimately, should such a biological therapeutic emerge with lower efficacy, local policy makers will need to weigh those tradeoffs and decide.

10. Cancer Care

Although not included in the WHO's targets for cervical cancer control, palliative care is a critical component in the cancer care continuum and cannot be overlooked. Women living in LMICs and identified clinically or by screening with incurable late-stage cervical cancer will need palliation for the highest quality of life for as long as possible. However, like with the other components of a comprehensive cervical cancer control program, there are huge health inequities between HICs and LMICs in terms of access to palliative care and opioid medications for pain control and cancer care [218,312–315]. As of 2013, no African country had all seven essential opioid formulations (immediate-release oral morphine; controlled-release oral morphine; injectable morphine; oral immediate-release oxycodone; transdermal fentanyl; oral methadone) recommended by the International Association for Hospice and Palliative Care [218]. A number of factors impact access to these medications, including eligibility restriction, physician prescriber restrictions, no emergency prescriptions by fax/phone or non-medical prescribing, limited prescription duration, no pharmacist authority to correct prescription, and increased bureaucratic burden of prescriptions, restricted dispensing sites, and negative language in laws.

11. Other Barriers

Another very underdeveloped capacity for delivering a comprehensive cervical cancer elimination plan is the maintenance and repair of equipment. As noted, LINAC machines fall into disrepair, and there must be a plan in place to maintain them [316], especially in the lowest-resourced countries in the world, where LINAC availability is already well below what is needed. Human and infrastructure capacities to provide preventive maintenance and repairs for equipment are greatly lacking in LMICs [317]. It is very common to walk through clinics and hospitals and see hallways cluttered with broken donated state-of-the-art equipment that may never be repaired (personal observation) because often the equipment needs to be shipped to another continent, usually the U.S., Europe, or Australia, for repair and that just does not happen. Thus, the cost is more than the equipment itself, and investment in the infrastructure to provide maintenance and repair services locally will be critical for the sustainability of a cervical cancer control program.

12. Other Opportunities for Global Cancer Control

It is expected that other HPV-related cancers, anogenital cancers (anus, vulva, and vagina), and oropharyngeal cancer will decrease significantly from HPV vaccination, but, like with the cervix, it will take years if not decades before the impact will be observed.

Strategies to pool data from countries that have adopted HPV vaccination early and have good cancer registries (preferably with medical record linkage to vaccine status) will help accelerate the generation of evidence that HPV vaccination is a broadly protective, cancer-preventive vaccine and hopefully encourage its greater uptake.

Treatment of anal cancer precursors reduces anal cancer incidence [318]. There are recommendations for screening, by cytology and/or HPV testing, and management of positives, primarily targeting high-risk, HIV-infected individuals (men who have sex with men and transgender women) but also extending to intermediate-risk individuals [319]. Given the greater morbidity in treating precursors of anal cancer compared with cervical cancer and the lack of providers who can provide high-quality anoscopy, restricting to high-risk individuals is the most practical and likely to be the most cost-effective.

Targeting other oncogenic infections, such as Epstein–Barr virus (EBV), which causes nasopharyngeal cancer and lymphomas, hepatitis C virus (HCV), which causes liver cancer, and *h. pylori*, which causes non-cardia gastric cancer, is perhaps the next best opportunity to prevent/control a significant number of cancers globally. Active HCV can be detected using mRNA assays and treated with directly acting anti-viral medications to prevent liver cancer, but only 20% of liver cancers are due to HCV [320]. Nevertheless, a vaccine against HCV could simplify its global control. EBV vaccines are in development [321,322], but there is no identified nasopharyngeal precursor, and sampling the nasopharynx is more invasive than sampling the cervix. Whether a vaccine demonstrating that it prevents or treats EBV, or even prevents multiple sclerosis [323], is sufficient for regulatory approval instead of a cancer endpoint is unknown. Screening for EBV serum biomarkers for NPC control in high-risk populations is promising [324].

Gastric cancer [325] is one of the most common cancers, with an annual incidence of 1.1 million cases and an annual mortality of 0.77 million people, globally. Like cervical cancer, gastric cancer is characterized by order-of-magnitude differences in burden between high-burden and low-burden countries, like the U.S. Most of those gastric cases are non-cardia cancers caused by *H. pylori* infection. In the U.S., gastric cancer is a multiple disease with multiple causes, with *H. pylori*-related non-cardia cancer mostly affecting immigrant populations from high gastric cancer-burden countries [326–328]. Although population-level antibiotic treatment of *H. pylori* infection significantly reduces the carriage of *H. pylori* [329], *H. pylori* infection recurs soon after antibiotics are stopped [330], and the widespread use of antibiotics raises concerns about antibiotic stewardship in general and antibiotic resistance of *H. pylori* [331–334]. Yet, despite the overall global burden of and large health disparities in gastric cancer, research on developing alternative strategies for gastric cancer prevention and control is lagging [335]. Like with cervical cancer, a multi-prong strategy of targeted prophylaxis to prevent or treat early *H. pylori* infection, screening and interception of chronic *H. pylori* infection or possibly gastritis [336–338], and mitigation through early detection of gastric by endoscopy of high-risk populations might be considered now, but a biological (e.g., vaccine) against *H. pylori* would greatly facilitate gastric cancer control [339–341]. Novel delivery strategies for screening might improve coverage and cost-effectiveness, e.g., combining fecal screening for *H. pylori* antigen or DNA and colorectal cancer testing (FIT) to increase screening for both gastric and colorectal cancer [342–344], and targeting families of those known to have a *H. pylori* infection, since they likely share the same *H. pylori* infection, for screening and *H. pylori* treatment [345]. If an *H. pylori* vaccine is therapeutic, an *H. pylori* screen-and-vaccinate approach might be highly effective.

13. Final Comments

Cervical cancer is the cancer for which we have the greatest opportunity, through HPV-targeted interventions, to control and reduce the burden of a cancer worldwide. As discussed, there are several advancements that would accelerate this process, which are highlighted in Table 3. Still, even with current technologies, we could save millions of lives over the next decades.

Indeed, if we cannot do it for this cancer, what chance do we have to do it for any other cancer? Unfortunately, those with greater resources are the ones who are given preferential access to newer, more effective, HPV-targeted technologies, rather than equitable access for all, potentially exacerbating health inequities first introduced with Pap testing. We are now challenged to reverse the historical trends for these and virtually all health technologies and interventions and achieve universal access and delivery to "close the gap".

A comprehensive care program, from prophylaxis to palliation, must include the missing but necessary investments to build human and healthcare infrastructure capacities (including electronic health records) for delivery, as well as a global procurement strategy that makes access to these life-saving and live-improving interventions equitable. While the WHO's call to action for cervical cancer elimination as a public health problem is inspirational, a major human- and infrastructure-capacity-building investment must be made to realize it. Who is going to make that commitment?

The question of "How good is good enough?" also needs to be asked in relation to cervical cancer control. If the world's female population is vaccinated with a multivalent HPV vaccine at sufficiently high coverage, the incidence and mortality of cervical cancer will likely decrease almost an order of magnitude compared with today's rates and approach the age-standardized rate of 4 cervical cancers per 100,000 that WHO has set out as threshold for cervical cancer elimination as a public health problem. Although a combined strategy of HPV-based screening with HPV vaccination will accelerate the control of cervical cancer compared with HPV vaccination alone [15], its implementation is much more challenging because of the greater costs and human resource and logistical requirements, and, on a population level, fewer benefits and more harms. HPV vaccination is being implemented more rapidly than HPV testing because vaccination is a "simpler" process, i.e., one shot and one visit, vaccines are cheaper than HPV tests, and nearly every country has some infrastructure and expertise for vaccination; most if not all of the 194 WHO member states have at least diphtheria–tetanus–pertussis, hepatitis B, *Haemophilus influenzae* type b, measles-containing, and polio vaccines, and more than 60% have HPV vaccines, included in their routine vaccination schedules [346]. Several countries in Latin America started vaccination more than a decade ago, and they are still struggling to implement HPV screen-and-treat. In the absence of those investments needed for screening, interventions that may be best buys and the easiest to implement might be those at the beginning and end of life through prophylactic HPV vaccination in young childhood and palliation, including access to narcotic drugs for pain control, for incurable cervical cancer, respectively.

Unfortunately, the roll-out of HPV vaccination in LMICs has been much slower than desirable, and relatively few women living in LMICs have received HPV vaccination since it was first available almost two decades ago. As a consequence, there was a missed opportunity to HPV vaccinate approximately 1 billion preteen women over the last ~15 years, which could have averted approximately 10 million cases of cervical cancer over the next 30 years.

Importantly, while cervical cancer is uniquely preventable, its prevention must be placed in the context of local needs and resources: it is not a leading cause of death worldwide or in any World Bank classification of economies or continents [347]. Meanwhile, other preventable causes of death, such as heart disease and diabetes, are far more common causes of mortality [347,348]. Lack of access to clean water and associated diarrheal diseases kills more than an estimated 1.2 million people worldwide, many of whom are children living in LMICs [347,349]. Therefore, local needs and priorities should drive resource allocation to cervical cancer programs.

An investment in cervical cancer prevention and control could be catalytic if made with an eye toward addressing the broad set of health needs and inequities experienced by resource-constrained populations. As noted, the high cervical cancer burden in regions within HICs and LMICs across the world is a signpost for cancer and other health disparities [185]. We need to consider women as a whole being, not just their cervix, and their family and community if we are to move towards health equity globally. Reducing maternal mortality, e.g., cervical cancer-related mortality, reduces intergenerational consequences of those deaths, including orphaning of children and childhood death [350,351].

Such an investment would build the human, health system, and technical capacities to address the cluster of chronic and non-communicable diseases that still differentially burden lower-resourced populations [186]. This includes improved health systems and the introduction of electronic health records [352] to track and guide the care of patients, human capacity in medicine and public health to deliver care, molecular diagnostics, palliative care, etc. Just as the initiation of the 20th-century space program undoubtedly led to the technological revolution in the 21st century, an investment in cervical cancer prevention and control in the 21st century could lead to a health revolution in LMICs and HICs in the 22nd century. The World Health Organization (WHO) has a call to action. We have talked the talk—will we walk the walk?

Funding: Dr. Castle is a U.S. National Cancer Institute employee.

Acknowledgments: I thank Jose Jeronimo, Kathryn Kundrod, and Maria Demarco of the U.S. National Cancer Institute, for their feedback and thoughtful suggestions.

Conflicts of Interest: The author declares no conflict of interest. Disclaimer: The views and interpretations presented in this manuscript are those of Dr. Castle alone and do not represent those of NCI, NIH, DHHS, or the U.S. government. Disclosures: Dr. Castle has received HPV tests and assays for research at reduced or no cost from Cepheid and Atila Biosystems.

References

1. Bray, F.; Laversanne, M.; Sung, H.; Ferlay, J.; Siegel, R.L.; Soerjomataram, I.; Jemal, A. Global cancer statistics 2022: GLOBOCAN estimates of incidence and mortality worldwide for 36 cancers in 185 countries. *CA Cancer J. Clin.* **2024**, *74*, 229–263. [CrossRef] [PubMed]
2. Cohen, C.M.; Wentzensen, N.; Castle, P.E.; Schiffman, M.; Zuna, R.; Arend, R.C.; Clarke, M.A. Racial and Ethnic Disparities in Cervical Cancer Incidence, Survival, and Mortality by Histologic Subtype. *J. Clin. Oncol.* **2023**, *41*, 1059–1068. [CrossRef]
3. Scarinci, I.C.; Garcia, F.A.; Kobetz, E.; Partridge, E.E.; Brandt, H.M.; Bell, M.C.; Dignan, M.; Ma, G.X.; Daye, J.L.; Castle, P.E. Cervical cancer prevention: New tools and old barriers. *Cancer* **2010**, *116*, 2531–2542. [CrossRef]
4. Diaz, A.; Vo, B.; Baade, P.D.; Matthews, V.; Nattabi, B.; Bailie, J.; Whop, L.J.; Bailie, R.; Garvey, G. Service Level Factors Associated with Cervical Screening in Aboriginal and Torres Strait Islander Primary Health Care Centres in Australia. *Int. J. Environ. Res. Public. Health* **2019**, *16*, 3630. [CrossRef] [PubMed]
5. Exarchakou, A.; Rachet, B.; Belot, A.; Maringe, C.; Coleman, M.P. Impact of national cancer policies on cancer survival trends and socioeconomic inequalities in England, 1996–2013: Population based study. *BMJ* **2018**, *360*, k764. [CrossRef]
6. Goodwin, B.C.; Rowe, A.K.; Crawford-Williams, F.; Baade, P.; Chambers, S.K.; Ralph, N.; Aitken, J.F. Geographical Disparities in Screening and Cancer-Related Health Behaviour. *Int. J. Environ. Res. Public. Health* **2020**, *17*, 1246. [CrossRef] [PubMed]
7. Leinonen, M.K.; Campbell, S.; Klungsøyr, O.; Lönnberg, S.; Hansen, B.T.; Nygård, M. Personal and provider level factors influence participation to cervical cancer screening: A retrospective register-based study of 1.3 million women in Norway. *Prev. Med.* **2017**, *94*, 31–39. [CrossRef] [PubMed]
8. MacDonald, E.J.; Geller, S.; Sibanda, N.; Stevenson, K.; Denmead, L.; Adcock, A.; Cram, F.; Hibma, M.; Sykes, P.; Lawton, B. Reaching under-screened/never-screened indigenous peoples with human papilloma virus self-testing: A community-based cluster randomised controlled trial. *Aust. New Zealand J. Obstet. Gynaecol.* **2021**, *61*, 135–141. [CrossRef]
9. Brzoska, P.; Aksakal, T.; Yilmaz-Aslan, Y. Utilization of cervical cancer screening among migrants and non-migrants in Germany: Results from a large-scale population survey. *BMC Public Health* **2020**, *20*, 5. [CrossRef]
10. Vaccarella, S.; Georges, D.; Bray, F.; Ginsburg, O.; Charvat, H.; Martikainen, P.; Brønnum-Hansen, H.; Deboosere, P.; Bopp, M.; Leinsalu, M.; et al. Socioeconomic inequalities in cancer mortality between and within countries in Europe: A population-based study. *Lancet Reg. Health Eur.* **2023**, *25*, 100551. [CrossRef] [PubMed]
11. World Bank Group. GDP per Capita. Available online: https://data.worldbank.org/indicator/NY.GDP.PCAP.CD (accessed on 20 August 2024).
12. Walboomers, J.M.; Jacobs, M.V.; Manos, M.M.; Bosch, F.X.; Kummer, J.A.; Shah, K.V.; Snijders, P.J.; Peto, J.; Meijer, C.J.; Muñoz, N. Human papillomavirus is a necessary cause of invasive cervical cancer worldwide. *J. Pathol.* **1999**, *189*, 12–19. [CrossRef]
13. World Health Organization. Cervical Cancer Elimination Initiative. Available online: https://www.who.int/initiatives/cervical-cancer-elimination-initiative (accessed on 1 January 2024).
14. Castle, P.E.; Faupel-Badger, J.M.; Umar, A.; Rebbeck, T.R. A Proposed Framework and Lexicon for Cancer Prevention. *Cancer Discov.* **2024**, *14*, 594–599. [CrossRef] [PubMed]

15. Simms, K.T.; Steinberg, J.; Caruana, M.; Smith, M.A.; Lew, J.B.; Soerjomataram, I.; Castle, P.E.; Bray, F.; Canfell, K. Impact of scaled up human papillomavirus vaccination and cervical screening and the potential for global elimination of cervical cancer in 181 countries, 2020–2099: A modelling study. *Lancet Oncol.* **2019**, *20*, 394–407. [CrossRef] [PubMed]
16. Arroyo Mühr, L.S.; Gini, A.; Yilmaz, E.; Hassan, S.S.; Lagheden, C.; Hultin, E.; Garcia Serrano, A.; Ure, A.E.; Andersson, H.; Merino, R.; et al. Concomitant human papillomavirus (HPV) vaccination and screening for elimination of HPV and cervical cancer. *Nat. Commun.* **2024**, *15*, 3679. [CrossRef] [PubMed]
17. De Palo, G. Cervical precancer and cancer, past, present and future. *Eur. J. Gynaecol. Oncol.* **2004**, *25*, 269–278.
18. Gasparini, R.; Panatto, D. Cervical cancer: From Hippocrates through Rigoni-Stern to zur Hausen. *Vaccine* **2009**, *27* (Suppl. 1), A4–A5. [CrossRef]
19. Mammas, I.N.; Spandidos, D.A. Four historic legends in human papillomaviruses research. *J. BUON* **2015**, *20*, 658–661.
20. Papanicolaou, G.N.; Traut, H.F. The diagnostic value of vaginal smears in carcinoma of the uterus. *Am. J. Obstet. Gynecol.* **1941**, *42*, 193–206. [CrossRef]
21. Papanicolaou, G.N. A New Procedure for Staining Vaginal Smears. *Science* **1942**, *95*, 438–439. [CrossRef]
22. Ayre, J.E. Selective cytology smear for diagnosis of cancer. *Am. J. Obstet. Gynecol.* **1947**, *53*, 609–617. [CrossRef]
23. Davey, D.D. American Cancer Society signals transition in cervical cancer screening from cytology to HPV tests. *Cancer Cytopathol.* **2021**, *129*, 259–261. [CrossRef] [PubMed]
24. zur Hausen, H. Human papillomaviruses and their possible role in squamous cell carcinomas. *Curr. Top. Microbiol. Immunol.* **1977**, *78*, 1–30. [CrossRef] [PubMed]
25. Dürst, M.; Gissmann, L.; Ikenberg, H.; zur Hausen, H. A papillomavirus DNA from a cervical carcinoma and its prevalence in cancer biopsy samples from different geographic regions. *Proc. Natl. Acad. Sci. USA* **1983**, *80*, 3812–3815. [CrossRef]
26. Bouvard, V.; Wentzensen, N.; Mackie, A.; Berkhof, J.; Brotherton, J.; Giorgi-Rossi, P.; Kupets, R.; Smith, R.; Arrossi, S.; Bendahhou, K.; et al. The IARC Perspective on Cervical Cancer Screening. *N. Engl. J. Med.* **2021**, *385*, 1908–1918. [CrossRef]
27. World Health Organization. WHO Updates Recommendations on HPV Vaccination Schedule. Available online: https://www.who.int/news/item/20-12-2022-WHO-updates-recommendations-on-HPV-vaccination-schedule#:~:text=WHO%20now%20recommends:,women%20older%20than%2021%20years (accessed on 13 January 2024).
28. de Sanjose, S.; Quint, W.G.; Alemany, L.; Geraets, D.T.; Klaustermeier, J.E.; Lloveras, B.; Tous, S.; Felix, A.; Bravo, L.E.; Shin, H.R.; et al. Human papillomavirus genotype attribution in invasive cervical cancer: A retrospective cross-sectional worldwide study. *Lancet Oncol.* **2010**, *11*, 1048–1056. [CrossRef] [PubMed]
29. Schiffman, M.; Clifford, G.; Buonaguro, F.M. Classification of weakly carcinogenic human papillomavirus types: Addressing the limits of epidemiology at the borderline. *Infect. Agent. Cancer* **2009**, *4*, 8. [CrossRef]
30. Human Papillomaviruses. In *IARC Working Group on the Evaluation of Carcinogenic Risks to Humans, and World Health Organization*; International Agency for Research on Cancer: Lyon, France, 2007.
31. Geraets, D.; Alemany, L.; Guimera, N.; de Sanjose, S.; de Koning, M.; Molijn, A.; Jenkins, D.; Bosch, X.; Quint, W. Detection of rare and possibly carcinogenic human papillomavirus genotypes as single infections in invasive cervical cancer. *J. Pathol.* **2012**, *228*, 534–543. [CrossRef]
32. Guan, P.; Howell-Jones, R.; Li, N.; Bruni, L.; de Sanjosé, S.; Franceschi, S.; Clifford, G.M. Human papillomavirus types in 115,789 HPV-positive women: A meta-analysis from cervical infection to cancer. *Int. J. Cancer* **2012**, *131*, 2349–2359. [CrossRef]
33. Schiffman, M.; Khan, M.J.; Solomon, D.; Herrero, R.; Wacholder, S.; Hildesheim, A.; Rodriguez, A.C.; Bratti, M.C.; Wheeler, C.M.; Burk, R.D. A study of the impact of adding HPV types to cervical cancer screening and triage tests. *J. Natl. Cancer Inst.* **2005**, *97*, 147–150. [CrossRef]
34. Bosch, F.X.; Broker, T.R.; Forman, D.; Moscicki, A.B.; Gillison, M.L.; Doorbar, J.; Stern, P.L.; Stanley, M.; Arbyn, M.; Poljak, M.; et al. Comprehensive control of human papillomavirus infections and related diseases. *Vaccine* **2013**, *31* (Suppl. 6), G1–G31. [CrossRef]
35. Serrano, B.; Brotons, M.; Bosch, F.X.; Bruni, L. Epidemiology and burden of HPV-related disease. *Best. Pract. Res. Clin. Obstet. Gynaecol.* **2018**, *47*, 14–26. [CrossRef] [PubMed]
36. Forman, D.; de Martel, C.; Lacey, C.J.; Soerjomataram, I.; Lortet-Tieulent, J.; Bruni, L.; Vignat, J.; Ferlay, J.; Bray, F.; Plummer, M.; et al. Global burden of human papillomavirus and related diseases. *Vaccine* **2012**, *30* (Suppl. 5), F12–F23. [CrossRef]
37. Castle, P.E.; Jeronimo, J.; Schiffman, M.; Herrero, R.; Rodríguez, A.C.; Bratti, M.C.; Hildesheim, A.; Wacholder, S.; Long, L.R.; Neve, L.; et al. Age-related changes of the cervix influence human papillomavirus type distribution. *Cancer Res.* **2006**, *66*, 1218–1224. [CrossRef]
38. Castle, P.E.; Rodriguez, A.C.; Porras, C.; Herrero, R.; Schiffman, M.; Gonzalez, P.; Hildesheim, A.; Burk, R.D. A comparison of cervical and vaginal human papillomavirus. *Sex. Transm. Dis.* **2007**, *34*, 849–855. [CrossRef]
39. Castle, P.E.; Schiffman, M.; Bratti, M.C.; Hildesheim, A.; Herrero, R.; Hutchinson, M.L.; Rodriguez, A.C.; Wacholder, S.; Sherman, M.E.; Kendall, H.; et al. A population-based study of vaginal human papillomavirus infection in hysterectomized women. *J. Infect. Dis.* **2004**, *190*, 458–467. [CrossRef] [PubMed]
40. Castle, P.E.; Schiffman, M.; Glass, A.G.; Rush, B.B.; Scott, D.R.; Wacholder, S.; Dunn, A.; Burk, R.D. Human papillomavirus prevalence in women who have and have not undergone hysterectomies. *J. Infect. Dis.* **2006**, *194*, 1702–1705. [CrossRef]
41. Egawa, N.; Egawa, K.; Griffin, H.; Doorbar, J. Human Papillomaviruses; Epithelial Tropisms, and the Development of Neoplasia. *Viruses* **2015**, *7*, 3863–3890. [CrossRef] [PubMed]

42. Befano, B.; Campos, N.G.; Egemen, D.; Herrero, R.; Schiffman, M.; Porras, C.; Lowy, D.R.; Rodriguez, A.C.; Schiller, J.T.; Ocampo, R.; et al. Estimating human papillomavirus vaccine efficacy from a single-arm trial: Proof-of-principle in the Costa Rica Vaccine Trial. *J. Natl. Cancer Inst.* **2023**, *115*, 788–795. [CrossRef] [PubMed]
43. de Martel, C.; Plummer, M.; Vignat, J.; Franceschi, S. Worldwide burden of cancer attributable to HPV by site, country and HPV type. *Int. J. Cancer* **2017**, *141*, 664–670. [CrossRef]
44. Vidal, A.C.; Murphy, S.K.; Hernandez, B.Y.; Vasquez, B.; Bartlett, J.A.; Oneko, O.; Mlay, P.; Obure, J.; Overcash, F.; Smith, J.S.; et al. Distribution of HPV genotypes in cervical intraepithelial lesions and cervical cancer in Tanzanian women. *Infect. Agent. Cancer* **2011**, *6*, 20. [CrossRef]
45. Denny, L.; Adewole, I.; Anorlu, R.; Dreyer, G.; Moodley, M.; Smith, T.; Snyman, L.; Wiredu, E.; Molijn, A.; Quint, W.; et al. Human papillomavirus prevalence and type distribution in invasive cervical cancer in sub-Saharan Africa. *Int. J. Cancer* **2014**, *134*, 1389–1398. [CrossRef]
46. Pinheiro, M.; Gage, J.C.; Clifford, G.M.; Demarco, M.; Cheung, L.C.; Chen, Z.; Yeager, M.; Cullen, M.; Boland, J.F.; Chen, X.; et al. Association of HPV35 with cervical carcinogenesis among women of African ancestry: Evidence of viral-host interaction with implications for disease intervention. *Int. J. Cancer* **2020**, *147*, 2677–2686. [CrossRef]
47. Siriaunkgul, S.; Suwiwat, S.; Settakorn, J.; Khunamornpong, S.; Tungsinmunkong, K.; Boonthum, A.; Chaisuksunt, V.; Lekawanvijit, S.; Srisomboon, J.; Thorner, P.S. HPV genotyping in cervical cancer in Northern Thailand: Adapting the linear array HPV assay for use on paraffin-embedded tissue. *Gynecol. Oncol.* **2008**, *108*, 555–560. [CrossRef] [PubMed]
48. Chen, H.C.; You, S.L.; Hsieh, C.Y.; Schiffman, M.; Lin, C.Y.; Pan, M.H.; Chou, Y.C.; Liaw, K.L.; Hsing, A.W.; Chen, C.J. Prevalence of genotype-specific human papillomavirus infection and cervical neoplasia in Taiwan: A community-based survey of 10,602 women. *Int. J. Cancer* **2011**, *128*, 1192–1203. [CrossRef]
49. Chan, P.K.; Cheung, T.H.; Li, W.H.; Yu, M.Y.; Chan, M.Y.; Yim, S.F.; Ho, W.C.; Yeung, A.C.; Ho, K.M.; Ng, H.K. Attribution of human papillomavirus types to cervical intraepithelial neoplasia and invasive cancers in Southern China. *Int. J. Cancer* **2012**, *131*, 692–705. [CrossRef]
50. Merck. Merck Announces Plans to Conduct Clinical Trials of a Novel Investigational Multi-Valent Human Papillomavirus (HPV) Vaccine and Single-Dose Regimen for GARDASIL®9. 2024. Available online: https://www.merck.com/news/merck-announces-plans-to-conduct-clinical-trials-of-a-novel-investigational-multi-valent-human-papillomavirus-hpv-vaccine-and-single-dose-regimen-for-gardasil-9/ (accessed on 21 August 2024).
51. The Cancer Genome Atlas Research Network. Integrated genomic and molecular characterization of cervical cancer. *Nature* **2017**, *543*, 378–384. [CrossRef] [PubMed]
52. Pendergrass, P.B.; Belovicz, M.W.; Reeves, C.A. Surface area of the human vagina as measured from vinyl polysiloxane casts. *Gynecol. Obstet. Invest.* **2003**, *55*, 110–113. [CrossRef] [PubMed]
53. World Health Organization. Chapter 1: An introduction to the anatomy of the uterine cervix. In *Colposcopy and Treatment of Cervical Intraepithelial Neoplasia: A Beginners' Manual*; Sellors, J.W., Sankaranarayanan, R., Eds.; WHO: Geneva, Switzerland, 2003.
54. Doorbar, J.; Griffin, H. Refining our understanding of cervical neoplasia and its cellular origins. *Papillomavirus Res.* **2019**, *7*, 176–179. [CrossRef]
55. Schiffman, M.; Castle, P.E.; Jeronimo, J.; Rodriguez, A.C.; Wacholder, S. Human papillomavirus and cervical cancer. *Lancet* **2007**, *370*, 890–907. [CrossRef]
56. Brown, D.R.; Shew, M.L.; Qadadri, B.; Neptune, N.; Vargas, M.; Tu, W.; Juliar, B.E.; Breen, T.E.; Fortenberry, J.D. A longitudinal study of genital human papillomavirus infection in a cohort of closely followed adolescent women. *J. Infect. Dis.* **2005**, *191*, 182–192. [CrossRef]
57. Ho, G.Y.; Bierman, R.; Beardsley, L.; Chang, C.J.; Burk, R.D. Natural history of cervicovaginal papillomavirus infection in young women. *N. Engl. J. Med.* **1998**, *338*, 423–428. [CrossRef] [PubMed]
58. Sun, X.W.; Kuhn, L.; Ellerbrock, T.V.; Chiasson, M.A.; Bush, T.J.; Wright, T.C., Jr. Human papillomavirus infection in women infected with the human immunodeficiency virus. *N. Engl. J. Med.* **1997**, *337*, 1343–1349. [CrossRef]
59. Syrjänen, S.; Shabalova, I.; Petrovichev, N.; Podistov, J.; Ivanchenko, O.; Zakharenko, S.; Nerovjna, R.; Kljukina, L.; Branovskaja, M.; Juschenko, A.; et al. Age-specific incidence and clearance of high-risk human papillomavirus infections in women in the former Soviet Union. *Int. J. STD AIDS* **2005**, *16*, 217–223. [CrossRef] [PubMed]
60. Winer, R.L.; Lee, S.K.; Hughes, J.P.; Adam, D.E.; Kiviat, N.B.; Koutsky, L.A. Genital human papillomavirus infection: Incidence and risk factors in a cohort of female university students. *Am. J. Epidemiol.* **2003**, *157*, 218–226. [CrossRef] [PubMed]
61. Woodman, C.B.; Collins, S.; Winter, H.; Bailey, A.; Ellis, J.; Prior, P.; Yates, M.; Rollason, T.P.; Young, L.S. Natural history of cervical human papillomavirus infection in young women: A longitudinal cohort study. *Lancet* **2001**, *357*, 1831–1836. [CrossRef] [PubMed]
62. Chesson, H.W.; Dunne, E.F.; Hariri, S.; Markowitz, L.E. The estimated lifetime probability of acquiring human papillomavirus in the United States. *Sex. Transm. Dis.* **2014**, *41*, 660–664. [CrossRef]
63. Castle, P.E.; Rodríguez, A.C.; Burk, R.D.; Herrero, R.; Wacholder, S.; Alfaro, M.; Morales, J.; Guillen, D.; Sherman, M.E.; Solomon, D.; et al. Short term persistence of human papillomavirus and risk of cervical precancer and cancer: Population based cohort study. *BMJ* **2009**, *339*, b2569. [CrossRef]
64. Koshiol, J.; Lindsay, L.; Pimenta, J.M.; Poole, C.; Jenkins, D.; Smith, J.S. Persistent human papillomavirus infection and cervical neoplasia: A systematic review and meta-analysis. *Am. J. Epidemiol.* **2008**, *168*, 123–137. [CrossRef]

65. Kjær, S.K.; Frederiksen, K.; Munk, C.; Iftner, T. Long-term absolute risk of cervical intraepithelial neoplasia grade 3 or worse following human papillomavirus infection: Role of persistence. *J. Natl. Cancer Inst.* **2010**, *102*, 1478–1488. [CrossRef]
66. Tainio, K.; Athanasiou, A.; Tikkinen, K.A.O.; Aaltonen, R.; Cárdenas, J.; Hernándes; Glazer-Livson, S.; Jakobsson, M.; Joronen, K.; Kiviharju, M.; et al. Clinical course of untreated cervical intraepithelial neoplasia grade 2 under active surveillance: Systematic review and meta-analysis. *BMJ* **2018**, *360*, k499. [CrossRef]
67. Castle, P.E.; Wentzensen, N. Clarifying the Equivocal Diagnosis of Cervical Intraepithelial Neoplasia 2: Still a Work in Progress. *J. Clin. Oncol.* **2023**, *41*, 419–420. [CrossRef]
68. Lycke, K.D.; Kahlert, J.; Damgaard, R.K.; Eriksen, D.O.; Bennetsen, M.H.; Gravitt, P.E.; Petersen, L.K.; Hammer, A. Clinical course of cervical intraepithelial neoplasia grade 2: A population-based cohort study. *Am. J. Obstet. Gynecol.* **2023**, *229*, e651–e656. [CrossRef]
69. Burger, E.A.; de Kok, I.; Groene, E.; Killen, J.; Canfell, K.; Kulasingam, S.; Kuntz, K.M.; Matthijsse, S.; Regan, C.; Simms, K.T.; et al. Estimating the Natural History of Cervical Carcinogenesis Using Simulation Models: A CISNET Comparative Analysis. *J. Natl. Cancer Inst.* **2020**, *112*, 955–963. [CrossRef]
70. McCredie, M.R.; Sharples, K.J.; Paul, C.; Baranyai, J.; Medley, G.; Jones, R.W.; Skegg, D.C. Natural history of cervical neoplasia and risk of invasive cancer in women with cervical intraepithelial neoplasia 3: A retrospective cohort study. *Lancet Oncol.* **2008**, *9*, 425–434. [CrossRef]
71. Schiffman, M.; Rodríguez, A.C. Heterogeneity in CIN3 diagnosis. *Lancet Oncol.* **2008**, *9*, 404–406. [CrossRef]
72. Plummer, M.; Peto, J.; Franceschi, S. Time since first sexual intercourse and the risk of cervical cancer. *Int. J. Cancer* **2012**, *130*, 2638–2644. [CrossRef] [PubMed]
73. Friborg, J.; Koch, A.; Wohlfahrt, J.; Storm, H.H.; Melbye, M. Cancer in Greenlandic Inuit 1973–1997: A cohort study. *Int. J. Cancer* **2003**, *107*, 1017–1022. [CrossRef]
74. Yang, M.; Du, J.; Lu, H.; Xiang, F.; Mei, H.; Xiao, H. Global trends and age-specific incidence and mortality of cervical cancer from 1990 to 2019: An international comparative study based on the Global Burden of Disease. *BMJ Open* **2022**, *12*, e055470. [CrossRef]
75. Winer, R.L.; Hughes, J.P.; Feng, Q.; O'Reilly, S.; Kiviat, N.B.; Holmes, K.K.; Koutsky, L.A. Condom use and the risk of genital human papillomavirus infection in young women. *N. Engl. J. Med.* **2006**, *354*, 2645–2654. [CrossRef] [PubMed]
76. Lam, J.U.; Rebolj, M.; Dugué, P.A.; Bonde, J.; von Euler-Chelpin, M.; Lynge, E. Condom use in prevention of Human Papillomavirus infections and cervical neoplasia: Systematic review of longitudinal studies. *J. Med. Screen.* **2014**, *21*, 38–50. [CrossRef] [PubMed]
77. Tobian, A.A.; Serwadda, D.; Quinn, T.C.; Kigozi, G.; Gravitt, P.E.; Laeyendecker, O.; Charvat, B.; Ssempijja, V.; Riedesel, M.; Oliver, A.E.; et al. Male circumcision for the prevention of HSV-2 and HPV infections and syphilis. *N. Engl. J. Med.* **2009**, *360*, 1298–1309. [CrossRef]
78. Shapiro, S.B.; Laurie, C.; El-Zein, M.; Franco, E.L. Association between male circumcision and human papillomavirus infection in males and females: A systematic review, meta-analysis, and meta-regression. *Clin. Microbiol. Infect.* **2023**, *29*, 968–978. [CrossRef] [PubMed]
79. Laurie, C.; El-Zein, M.; Botting-Provost, S.; Tota, J.E.; Tellier, P.P.; Coutlée, F.; Burchell, A.N.; Franco, E.L. Efficacy and safety of a self-applied carrageenan-based gel to prevent human papillomavirus infection in sexually active young women (CATCH study): An exploratory phase IIB randomised, placebo-controlled trial. *EClinicalMedicine* **2023**, *60*, 102038. [CrossRef]
80. Laurie, C.; El-Zein, M.; Franco, E.L. Safety of carrageenan-based gels as preventive microbicides: A narrative review. *Sex. Transm. Infect.* **2024**, *100*, 388–394. [CrossRef]
81. Grulich, A.E.; van Leeuwen, M.T.; Falster, M.O.; Vajdic, C.M. Incidence of cancers in people with HIV/AIDS compared with immunosuppressed transplant recipients: A meta-analysis. *Lancet* **2007**, *370*, 59–67. [CrossRef] [PubMed]
82. Yuan, T.; Hu, Y.; Zhou, X.; Yang, L.; Wang, H.; Li, L.; Wang, J.; Qian, H.Z.; Clifford, G.M.; Zou, H. Incidence and mortality of non-AIDS-defining cancers among people living with HIV: A systematic review and meta-analysis. *EClinicalMedicine* **2022**, *52*, 101613. [CrossRef]
83. Jin, F.; Vajdic, C.M.; Poynten, I.M.; McGee-Avila, J.K.; Castle, P.E.; Grulich, A.E. Cancer risk in people living with HIV and solid organ transplant recipients: A systematic review and meta-analysis. *Lancet Oncol.* **2024**, *25*, 933–944. [CrossRef] [PubMed]
84. Ibrahim Khalil, A.; Zhang, L.; Muwonge, R.; Sauvaget, C.; Basu, P. Efficacy and safety of therapeutic HPV vaccines to treat CIN 2/CIN 3 lesions: A systematic review and meta-analysis of phase II/III clinical trials. *BMJ Open* **2023**, *13*, e069616. [CrossRef]
85. Santesso, N.; Mustafa, R.A.; Wiercioch, W.; Kehar, R.; Gandhi, S.; Chen, Y.; Cheung, A.; Hopkins, J.; Khatib, R.; Ma, B.; et al. Systematic reviews and meta-analyses of benefits and harms of cryotherapy, LEEP, and cold knife conization to treat cervical intraepithelial neoplasia. *Int. J. Gynaecol. Obstet.* **2016**, *132*, 266–271. [CrossRef]
86. Prudden, H.J.; Achilles, S.L.; Schocken, C.; Broutet, N.; Canfell, K.; Akaba, H.; Basu, P.; Bhatla, N.; Chirenje, Z.M.; Delany-Moretlwe, S.; et al. Understanding the public health value and defining preferred product characteristics for therapeutic human papillomavirus (HPV) vaccines: World Health Organization consultations, October 2021–March 2022. *Vaccine* **2022**, *40*, 5843–5855. [CrossRef]
87. Doorbar, J. The human Papillomavirus twilight zone—Latency, immune control and subclinical infection. *Tumour Virus Res.* **2023**, *16*, 200268. [CrossRef] [PubMed]
88. Gravitt, P.E.; Winer, R.L. Natural History of HPV Infection across the Lifespan: Role of Viral Latency. *Viruses* **2017**, *9*, 267. [CrossRef] [PubMed]

89. Schiller, J.T.; Lowy, D.R. Understanding and learning from the success of prophylactic human papillomavirus vaccines. *Nat. Rev. Microbiol.* 2012, *10*, 681–692. [CrossRef] [PubMed]
90. Beachler, D.C.; Jenkins, G.; Safaeian, M.; Kreimer, A.R.; Wentzensen, N. Natural Acquired Immunity Against Subsequent Genital Human Papillomavirus Infection: A Systematic Review and Meta-analysis. *J. Infect. Dis.* 2016, *213*, 1444–1454. [CrossRef]
91. Yokoji, K.; Giguère, K.; Malagón, T.; Rönn, M.M.; Mayaud, P.; Kelly, H.; Delany-Moretlwe, S.; Drolet, M.; Brisson, M.; Boily, M.C.; et al. Association of naturally acquired type-specific HPV antibodies and subsequent HPV re-detection: Systematic review and meta-analysis. *Infect. Agent. Cancer* 2023, *18*, 70. [CrossRef]
92. Tsang, S.H.; Sampson, J.N.; Schussler, J.; Porras, C.; Wagner, S.; Boland, J.; Cortes, B.; Lowy, D.R.; Schiller, J.T.; Schiffman, M.; et al. Durability of Cross-Protection by Different Schedules of the Bivalent HPV Vaccine: The CVT Trial. *J. Natl. Cancer Inst.* 2020, *112*, 1030–1037. [CrossRef]
93. Tota, J.E.; Struyf, F.; Sampson, J.N.; Gonzalez, P.; Ryser, M.; Herrero, R.; Schussler, J.; Karkada, N.; Rodriguez, A.C.; Folschweiller, N.; et al. Efficacy of the AS04-Adjuvanted HPV16/18 Vaccine: Pooled Analysis of the Costa Rica Vaccine and PATRICIA Randomized Controlled Trials. *J. Natl. Cancer Inst.* 2020, *112*, 818–828. [CrossRef]
94. Brown, D.R.; Joura, E.A.; Yen, G.P.; Kothari, S.; Luxembourg, A.; Saah, A.; Walia, A.; Perez, G.; Khoury, H.; Badgley, D.; et al. Systematic literature review of cross-protective effect of HPV vaccines based on data from randomized clinical trials and real-world evidence. *Vaccine* 2021, *39*, 2224–2236. [CrossRef] [PubMed]
95. Joura, E.A.; Giuliano, A.R.; Iversen, O.E.; Bouchard, C.; Mao, C.; Mehlsen, J.; Moreira, E.D., Jr.; Ngan, Y.; Petersen, L.K.; Lazcano-Ponce, E.; et al. A 9-valent HPV vaccine against infection and intraepithelial neoplasia in women. *N. Engl. J. Med.* 2015, *372*, 711–723. [CrossRef]
96. Sharma, H.; Parekh, S.; Pujari, P.; Shewale, S.; Desai, S.; Bhatla, N.; Joshi, S.; Pimple, S.; Kawade, A.; Balasubramani, L.; et al. Immunogenicity and safety of a new quadrivalent HPV vaccine in girls and boys aged 9-14 years versus an established quadrivalent HPV vaccine in women aged 15–26 years in India: A randomised, active-controlled, multicentre, phase 2/3 trial. *Lancet Oncol.* 2023, *24*, 1321–1333. [CrossRef]
97. Zaman, K.; Schuind, A.E.; Adjei, S.; Antony, K.; Aponte, J.J.; Buabeng, P.B.; Qadri, F.; Kemp, T.J.; Hossain, L.; Pinto, L.A.; et al. Safety and immunogenicity of Innovax bivalent human papillomavirus vaccine in girls 9–14 years of age: Interim analysis from a phase 3 clinical trial. *Vaccine* 2024, *42*, 2290–2298. [CrossRef] [PubMed]
98. Zhao, F.H.; Wu, T.; Hu, Y.M.; Wei, L.H.; Li, M.Q.; Huang, W.J.; Chen, W.; Huang, S.J.; Pan, Q.J.; Zhang, X.; et al. Efficacy, safety, and immunogenicity of an Escherichia coli-produced Human Papillomavirus (16 and 18) L1 virus-like-particle vaccine: End-of-study analysis of a phase 3, double-blind, randomised, controlled trial. *Lancet Infect. Dis.* 2022, *22*, 1756–1768. [CrossRef]
99. Zhu, F.C.; Zhong, G.H.; Huang, W.J.; Chu, K.; Zhang, L.; Bi, Z.F.; Zhu, K.X.; Chen, Q.; Zheng, T.Q.; Zhang, M.L.; et al. Head-to-head immunogenicity comparison of an Escherichia coli-produced 9-valent human papillomavirus vaccine and Gardasil 9 in women aged 18–26 years in China: A randomised blinded clinical trial. *Lancet Infect. Dis.* 2023, *23*, 1313–1322. [CrossRef]
100. Schiller, J.T.; Castellsagué, X.; Garland, S.M. A review of clinical trials of human papillomavirus prophylactic vaccines. *Vaccine* 2012, *30* (Suppl. 5), F123–F138. [CrossRef] [PubMed]
101. Lei, J.; Ploner, A.; Elfström, K.M.; Wang, J.; Roth, A.; Fang, F.; Sundström, K.; Dillner, J.; Sparén, P. HPV Vaccination and the Risk of Invasive Cervical Cancer. *N. Engl. J. Med.* 2020, *383*, 1340–1348. [CrossRef]
102. Luostarinen, T.; Apter, D.; Dillner, J.; Eriksson, T.; Harjula, K.; Natunen, K.; Paavonen, J.; Pukkala, E.; Lehtinen, M. Vaccination protects against invasive HPV-associated cancers. *Int. J. Cancer* 2018, *142*, 2186–2187. [CrossRef] [PubMed]
103. Kjaer, S.K.; Dehlendorff, C.; Belmonte, F.; Baandrup, L. Real-World Effectiveness of Human Papillomavirus Vaccination Against Cervical Cancer. *J. Natl. Cancer Inst.* 2021, *113*, 1329–1335. [CrossRef]
104. Falcaro, M.; Castañon, A.; Ndlela, B.; Checchi, M.; Soldan, K.; Lopez-Bernal, J.; Elliss-Brookes, L.; Sasieni, P. The effects of the national HPV vaccination programme in England, UK, on cervical cancer and grade 3 cervical intraepithelial neoplasia incidence: A register-based observational study. *Lancet* 2021, *398*, 2084–2092. [CrossRef]
105. Palmer, T.J.; Kavanagh, K.; Cuschieri, K.; Cameron, R.; Graham, C.; Wilson, A.; Roy, K. Invasive cervical cancer incidence following bivalent human papillomavirus vaccination: A population-based observational study of age at immunization, dose, and deprivation. *J. Natl. Cancer Inst.* 2024, *116*, 857–865. [CrossRef]
106. Villa, A.; Patton, L.L.; Giuliano, A.R.; Estrich, C.G.; Pahlke, S.C.; O'Brien, K.K.; Lipman, R.D.; Araujo, M.W.B. Summary of the evidence on the safety, efficacy, and effectiveness of human papillomavirus vaccines: Umbrella review of systematic reviews. *J. Am. Dent. Assoc.* 2020, *151*, 245–254.e224. [CrossRef]
107. Willame, C.; Gadroen, K.; Bramer, W.; Weibel, D.; Sturkenboom, M. Systematic Review and Meta-analysis of Postlicensure Observational Studies on Human Papillomavirus Vaccination and Autoimmune and Other Rare Adverse Events. *Pediatr. Infect. Dis. J.* 2020, *39*, 287–293. [CrossRef] [PubMed]
108. Scheller, N.M.; Pasternak, B.; Mølgaard-Nielsen, D.; Svanström, H.; Hviid, A. Quadrivalent HPV Vaccination and the Risk of Adverse Pregnancy Outcomes. *N. Engl. J. Med.* 2017, *376*, 1223–1233. [CrossRef] [PubMed]
109. Porras, C.; Tsang, S.H.; Herrero, R.; Guillén, D.; Darragh, T.M.; Stoler, M.H.; Hildesheim, A.; Wagner, S.; Boland, J.; Lowy, D.R.; et al. Efficacy of the bivalent HPV vaccine against HPV 16/18-associated precancer: Long-term follow-up results from the Costa Rica Vaccine Trial. *Lancet Oncol.* 2020, *21*, 1643–1652. [CrossRef]

110. Basu, P.; Malvi, S.G.; Joshi, S.; Bhatla, N.; Muwonge, R.; Lucas, E.; Verma, Y.; Esmy, P.O.; Poli, U.R.R.; Shah, A.; et al. Vaccine efficacy against persistent human papillomavirus (HPV) 16/18 infection at 10 years after one, two, and three doses of quadrivalent HPV vaccine in girls in India: A multicentre, prospective, cohort study. *Lancet Oncol.* **2021**, *22*, 1518–1529. [CrossRef]
111. Baisley, K.; Kemp, T.J.; Kreimer, A.R.; Basu, P.; Changalucha, J.; Hildesheim, A.; Porras, C.; Whitworth, H.; Herrero, R.; Lacey, C.J.; et al. Comparing one dose of HPV vaccine in girls aged 9-14 years in Tanzania (DoRIS) with one dose of HPV vaccine in historical cohorts: An immunobridging analysis of a randomised controlled trial. *Lancet Glob. Health* **2022**, *10*, e1485–e1493. [CrossRef] [PubMed]
112. Barnabas, R.V.; Brown, E.R.; Onono, M.A.; Bukusi, E.A.; Njoroge, B.; Winer, R.L.; Galloway, D.A.; Pinder, L.F.; Donnell, D.; I, N.W.; et al. Durability of single-dose HPV vaccination in young Kenyan women: Randomized controlled trial 3-year results. *Nat. Med.* **2023**, *29*, 3224–3232. [CrossRef] [PubMed]
113. Kreimer, A.R.; Cernuschi, T.; Rees, H.; Brotherton, J.M.L.; Porras, C.; Schiller, J. Public health opportunities resulting from sufficient HPV vaccine supply and a single-dose vaccination schedule. *J. Natl. Cancer Inst.* **2023**, *115*, 246–249. [CrossRef]
114. Kreimer, A.R.; Sampson, J.N.; Porras, C.; Schiller, J.T.; Kemp, T.; Herrero, R.; Wagner, S.; Boland, J.; Schussler, J.; Lowy, D.R.; et al. Evaluation of Durability of a Single Dose of the Bivalent HPV Vaccine: The CVT Trial. *J. Natl. Cancer Inst.* **2020**, *112*, 1038–1046. [CrossRef] [PubMed]
115. Kreimer, A.R.; Struyf, F.; Del Rosario-Raymundo, M.R.; Hildesheim, A.; Skinner, S.R.; Wacholder, S.; Garland, S.M.; Herrero, R.; David, M.P.; Wheeler, C.M.; et al. Efficacy of fewer than three doses of an HPV-16/18 AS04-adjuvanted vaccine: Combined analysis of data from the Costa Rica Vaccine and PATRICIA Trials. *Lancet Oncol.* **2015**, *16*, 775–786. [CrossRef]
116. Castle, P.E.; Einstein, M.H.; Sahasrabuddhe, V.V. Cervical cancer prevention and control in women living with human immunodeficiency virus. *CA Cancer J. Clin.* **2021**, *71*, 505–526. [CrossRef] [PubMed]
117. Staadegaard, L.; Rönn, M.M.; Soni, N.; Bellerose, M.E.; Bloem, P.; Brisson, M.; Maheu-Giroux, M.; Barnabas, R.V.; Drolet, M.; Mayaud, P.; et al. Immunogenicity, safety, and efficacy of the HPV vaccines among people living with HIV: A systematic review and meta-analysis. *EClinicalMedicine* **2022**, *52*, 101585. [CrossRef] [PubMed]
118. Zizza, A.; Banchelli, F.; Guido, M.; Marotta, C.; Di Gennaro, F.; Mazzucco, W.; Pistotti, V.; D'Amico, R. Efficacy and safety of human papillomavirus vaccination in HIV-infected patients: A systematic review and meta-analysis. *Sci. Rep.* **2021**, *11*, 4954. [CrossRef] [PubMed]
119. Curry, S.J.; Krist, A.H.; Owens, D.K.; Barry, M.J.; Caughey, A.B.; Davidson, K.W.; Doubeni, C.A.; Epling, J.W., Jr.; Kemper, A.R.; Kubik, M.; et al. Screening for Cervical Cancer: US Preventive Services Task Force Recommendation Statement. *JAMA* **2018**, *320*, 674–686. [CrossRef] [PubMed]
120. Fontham, E.T.H.; Wolf, A.M.D.; Church, T.R.; Etzioni, R.; Flowers, C.R.; Herzig, A.; Guerra, C.E.; Oeffinger, K.C.; Shih, Y.T.; Walter, L.C.; et al. Cervical cancer screening for individuals at average risk: 2020 guideline update from the American Cancer Society. *CA Cancer J. Clin.* **2020**, *70*, 321–346. [CrossRef]
121. Perkins, R.B.; Wentzensen, N.; Guido, R.S.; Schiffman, M. Cervical Cancer Screening: A Review. *JAMA* **2023**, *330*, 547–558. [CrossRef]
122. Koliopoulos, G.; Nyaga, V.N.; Santesso, N.; Bryant, A.; Martin-Hirsch, P.P.; Mustafa, R.A.; Schünemann, H.; Paraskevaidis, E.; Arbyn, M. Cytology versus HPV testing for cervical cancer screening in the general population. *Cochrane Database Syst. Rev.* **2017**, *8*, Cd008587. [CrossRef] [PubMed]
123. Ronco, G.; Dillner, J.; Elfström, K.M.; Tunesi, S.; Snijders, P.J.; Arbyn, M.; Kitchener, H.; Segnan, N.; Gilham, C.; Giorgi-Rossi, P.; et al. Efficacy of HPV-based screening for prevention of invasive cervical cancer: Follow-up of four European randomised controlled trials. *Lancet* **2014**, *383*, 524–532. [CrossRef]
124. Sankaranarayanan, R.; Nene, B.M.; Shastri, S.S.; Jayant, K.; Muwonge, R.; Budukh, A.M.; Hingmire, S.; Malvi, S.G.; Thorat, R.; Kothari, A.; et al. HPV screening for cervical cancer in rural India. *N. Engl. J. Med.* **2009**, *360*, 1385–1394. [CrossRef]
125. Dillner, J.; Rebolj, M.; Birembaut, P.; Petry, K.U.; Szarewski, A.; Munk, C.; de Sanjose, S.; Naucler, P.; Lloveras, B.; Kjaer, S.; et al. Long term predictive values of cytology and human papillomavirus testing in cervical cancer screening: Joint European cohort study. *BMJ* **2008**, *337*, a1754. [CrossRef]
126. Gage, J.C.; Schiffman, M.; Katki, H.A.; Castle, P.E.; Fetterman, B.; Wentzensen, N.; Poitras, N.E.; Lorey, T.; Cheung, L.C.; Kinney, W.K. Reassurance against future risk of precancer and cancer conferred by a negative human papillomavirus test. *J. Natl. Cancer Inst.* **2014**, *106*, dju153. [CrossRef]
127. Arbyn, M.; Castle, P.E.; Schiffman, M.; Wentzensen, N.; Heckman-Stoddard, B.; Sahasrabuddhe, V.V. Meta-analysis of agreement/concordance statistics in studies comparing self- vs clinician-collected samples for HPV testing in cervical cancer screening. *Int. J. Cancer* **2022**, *151*, 308–312. [CrossRef] [PubMed]
128. Arbyn, M.; Smith, S.B.; Temin, S.; Sultana, F.; Castle, P. Detecting cervical precancer and reaching underscreened women by using HPV testing on self samples: Updated meta-analyses. *BMJ* **2018**, *363*, k4823. [CrossRef] [PubMed]
129. Costa, S.; Verberckmoes, B.; Castle, P.E.; Arbyn, M. Offering HPV self-sampling kits: An updated meta-analysis of the effectiveness of strategies to increase participation in cervical cancer screening. *Br. J. Cancer* **2023**, *128*, 805–813. [CrossRef] [PubMed]
130. Nishimura, H.; Yeh, P.T.; Oguntade, H.; Kennedy, C.E.; Narasimhan, M. HPV self-sampling for cervical cancer screening: A systematic review of values and preferences. *BMJ Glob. Health* **2021**, *6*, e003743. [CrossRef]
131. Camara, H.; Zhang, Y.; Lafferty, L.; Vallely, A.J.; Guy, R.; Kelly-Hanku, A. Self-collection for HPV-based cervical screening: A qualitative evidence meta-synthesis. *BMC Public Health* **2021**, *21*, 1503. [CrossRef]

132. Morgan, K.; Azzani, M.; Khaing, S.L.; Wong, Y.L.; Su, T.T. Acceptability of Women Self-Sampling versus Clinician-Collected Samples for HPV DNA Testing: A Systematic Review. *J. Low. Genit. Tract. Dis.* **2019**, *23*, 193–199. [CrossRef]
133. Pils, S.; Mlakar, J.; Poljak, M.; Domjanič, G.G.; Kaufmann, U.; Springer, S.; Salat, A.; Langthaler, E.; Joura, E.A. HPV screening in the urine of transpeople—A prevalence study. *EClinicalMedicine* **2022**, *54*, 101702. [CrossRef]
134. Cho, H.W.; Shim, S.R.; Lee, J.K.; Hong, J.H. Accuracy of human papillomavirus tests on self-collected urine versus clinician-collected samples for the detection of cervical precancer: A systematic review and meta-analysis. *J. Gynecol. Oncol.* **2022**, *33*, e4. [CrossRef]
135. Shin, H.Y.; Lee, B.; Hwang, S.H.; Lee, D.O.; Sung, N.Y.; Park, J.Y.; Jun, J.K. Evaluation of satisfaction with three different cervical cancer screening modalities: Clinician-collected Pap test vs. HPV test by self-sampling vs. HPV test by urine sampling. *J. Gynecol. Oncol.* **2019**, *30*, e76. [CrossRef]
136. Sargent, A.; Fletcher, S.; Bray, K.; Kitchener, H.C.; Crosbie, E.J. Cross-sectional study of HPV testing in self-sampled urine and comparison with matched vaginal and cervical samples in women attending colposcopy for the management of abnormal cervical screening. *BMJ Open* **2019**, *9*, e025388. [CrossRef]
137. Ørnskov, D.; Jochumsen, K.; Steiner, P.H.; Grunnet, I.M.; Lykkebo, A.W.; Waldstrøm, M. Clinical performance and acceptability of self-collected vaginal and urine samples compared with clinician-taken cervical samples for HPV testing among women referred for colposcopy. A cross-sectional study. *BMJ Open* **2021**, *11*, e041512. [CrossRef]
138. Rohner, E.; McGuire, F.H.; Liu, Y.; Li, Q.; Miele, K.; Desai, S.A.; Schmitt, J.W.; Knittel, A.; Nelson, J.A.E.; Edelman, C.; et al. Racial and Ethnic Differences in Acceptability of Urine and Cervico-Vaginal Sample Self-Collection for HPV-Based Cervical Cancer Screening. *J. Womens Health* **2020**, *29*, 971–979. [CrossRef]
139. Castle, P.E.; Solomon, D.; Schiffman, M.; Wheeler, C.M. Human papillomavirus type 16 infections and 2-year absolute risk of cervical precancer in women with equivocal or mild cytologic abnormalities. *J. Natl. Cancer Inst.* **2005**, *97*, 1066–1071. [CrossRef]
140. Castle, P.E.; Stoler, M.H.; Wright, T.C., Jr.; Sharma, A.; Wright, T.L.; Behrens, C.M. Performance of carcinogenic human papillomavirus (HPV) testing and HPV16 or HPV18 genotyping for cervical cancer screening of women aged 25 years and older: A subanalysis of the ATHENA study. *Lancet Oncol.* **2011**, *12*, 880–890. [CrossRef] [PubMed]
141. Khan, M.J.; Castle, P.E.; Lorincz, A.T.; Wacholder, S.; Sherman, M.; Scott, D.R.; Rush, B.B.; Glass, A.G.; Schiffman, M. The elevated 10-year risk of cervical precancer and cancer in women with human papillomavirus (HPV) type 16 or 18 and the possible utility of type-specific HPV testing in clinical practice. *J. Natl. Cancer Inst.* **2005**, *97*, 1072–1079. [CrossRef] [PubMed]
142. Stoler, M.H.; Parvu, V.; Yanson, K.; Andrews, J.; Vaughan, L. Risk stratification of HPV-positive results using extended genotyping and cytology: Data from the baseline phase of the Onclarity trial. *Gynecol. Oncol.* **2023**, *174*, 68–75. [CrossRef] [PubMed]
143. Stoler, M.H.; Wright, T.C., Jr.; Parvu, V.; Yanson, K.; Cooper, C.K.; Andrews, J.A. Detection of high-grade cervical neoplasia using extended genotyping: Performance data from the longitudinal phase of the Onclarity trial. *Gynecol. Oncol.* **2023**, *170*, 143–152. [CrossRef]
144. Wheeler, C.M.; Torrez-Martinez, N.E.; Torres-Chavolla, E.; Parvu, V.; Andrews, J.C.; Du, R.; Robertson, M.; Joste, N.E.; Cuzick, J. Comparing the performance of 2 human papillomavirus assays for a new use indication: A real-world evidence-based evaluation in the United States. *Am. J. Obstet. Gynecol.* **2024**, *230*, e241–e243. [CrossRef]
145. Clarke, M.A.; Wentzensen, N.; Perkins, R.B.; Garcia, F.; Arrindell, D.; Chelmow, D.; Cheung, L.C.; Darragh, T.M.; Egemen, D.; Guido, R.; et al. Recommendations for Use of p16/Ki67 Dual Stain for Management of Individuals Testing Positive for Human Papillomavirus. *J. Low. Genit. Tract. Dis.* **2024**, *28*, 124–130. [CrossRef]
146. Wentzensen, N.; Clarke, M.A.; Bremer, R.; Poitras, N.; Tokugawa, D.; Goldhoff, P.E.; Castle, P.E.; Schiffman, M.; Kingery, J.D.; Grewal, K.K.; et al. Clinical Evaluation of Human Papillomavirus Screening With p16/Ki-67 Dual Stain Triage in a Large Organized Cervical Cancer Screening Program. *JAMA Intern. Med.* **2019**, *179*, 881–888. [CrossRef]
147. Wright, T.C., Jr.; Stoler, M.H.; Ranger-Moore, J.; Fang, Q.; Volkir, P.; Safaeian, M.; Ridder, R. Clinical validation of p16/Ki-67 dual-stained cytology triage of HPV-positive women: Results from the IMPACT trial. *Int. J. Cancer* **2022**, *150*, 461–471. [CrossRef]
148. von Knebel Doeberitz, M.; Prigge, E.S. Role of DNA methylation in HPV associated lesions. *Papillomavirus Res.* **2019**, *7*, 180–183. [CrossRef] [PubMed]
149. Bowden, S.J.; Kalliala, I.; Veroniki, A.A.; Arbyn, M.; Mitra, A.; Lathouras, K.; Mirabello, L.; Chadeau-Hyam, M.; Paraskevaidis, E.; Flanagan, J.M.; et al. The use of human papillomavirus DNA methylation in cervical intraepithelial neoplasia: A systematic review and meta-analysis. *EBioMedicine* **2019**, *50*, 246–259. [CrossRef]
150. Kelly, H.; Benavente, Y.; Pavon, M.A.; De Sanjose, S.; Mayaud, P.; Lorincz, A.T. Performance of DNA methylation assays for detection of high-grade cervical intraepithelial neoplasia (CIN2+): A systematic review and meta-analysis. *Br. J. Cancer* **2019**, *121*, 954–965. [CrossRef] [PubMed]
151. Taghavi, K.; Zhao, F.; Downham, L.; Baena, A.; Basu, P. Molecular triaging options for women testing HPV positive with self-collected samples. *Front. Oncol.* **2023**, *13*, 1243888. [CrossRef] [PubMed]
152. Liu, Y.; Siejka-Zielińska, P.; Velikova, G.; Bi, Y.; Yuan, F.; Tomkova, M.; Bai, C.; Chen, L.; Schuster-Böckler, B.; Song, C.X. Bisulfite-free direct detection of 5-methylcytosine and 5-hydroxymethylcytosine at base resolution. *Nat. Biotechnol.* **2019**, *37*, 424–429. [CrossRef]
153. Vaisvila, R.; Ponnaluri, V.K.C.; Sun, Z.; Langhorst, B.W.; Saleh, L.; Guan, S.; Dai, N.; Campbell, M.A.; Sexton, B.S.; Marks, K.; et al. Enzymatic methyl sequencing detects DNA methylation at single-base resolution from picograms of DNA. *Genome Res.* **2021**, *31*, 1280–1289. [CrossRef] [PubMed]

154. Schreiberhuber, L.; Barrett, J.E.; Wang, J.; Redl, E.; Herzog, C.; Vavourakis, C.D.; Sundström, K.; Dillner, J.; Widschwendter, M. Cervical cancer screening using DNA methylation triage in a real-world population. *Nat. Med.* **2024**, *30*, 2251–2257. [CrossRef]
155. de Sanjosé, S.; Perkins, R.B.; Campos, N.; Inturrisi, F.; Egemen, D.; Befano, B.; Rodriguez, A.C.; Jerónimo, J.; Cheung, L.C.; Desai, K.; et al. Design of the HPV-automated visual evaluation (PAVE) study: Validating a novel cervical screening strategy. *eLife* **2024**, *12*, RP91469. [CrossRef]
156. Xue, P.; Wang, J.; Qin, D.; Yan, H.; Qu, Y.; Seery, S.; Jiang, Y.; Qiao, Y. Deep learning in image-based breast and cervical cancer detection: A systematic review and meta-analysis. *NPJ Digit. Med.* **2022**, *5*, 19. [CrossRef]
157. Parham, G.P.; Egemen, D.; Befano, B.; Mwanahamuntu, M.H.; Rodriguez, A.C.; Antani, S.; Chisele, S.; Munalula, M.K.; Kaunga, F.; Musonda, F.; et al. Validation in Zambia of a cervical screening strategy including HPV genotyping and artificial intelligence (AI)-based automated visual evaluation. *Infect. Agent. Cancer* **2023**, *18*, 61. [CrossRef] [PubMed]
158. Schiffman, M.; Doorbar, J.; Wentzensen, N.; de Sanjosé, S.; Fakhry, C.; Monk, B.J.; Stanley, M.A.; Franceschi, S. Carcinogenic human papillomavirus infection. *Nat. Rev. Dis. Primers* **2016**, *2*, 16086. [CrossRef] [PubMed]
159. Doorbar, J.; Quint, W.; Banks, L.; Bravo, I.G.; Stoler, M.; Broker, T.R.; Stanley, M.A. The biology and life-cycle of human papillomaviruses. *Vaccine* **2012**, *30* (Suppl. 5), F55–F70. [CrossRef]
160. Iftner, T.; Neis, K.J.; Castanon, A.; Landy, R.; Holz, B.; Woll-Herrmann, A.; Iftner, A.; Staebler, A.; Wallwiener, D.; Hann von Weyhern, C.; et al. Longitudinal Clinical Performance of the RNA-Based Aptima Human Papillomavirus (AHPV) Assay in Comparison to the DNA-Based Hybrid Capture 2 HPV Test in Two Consecutive Screening Rounds with a 6-Year Interval in Germany. *J. Clin. Microbiol.* **2019**, *57*, e01177-18. [CrossRef]
161. Iftner, T.; Becker, S.; Neis, K.J.; Castanon, A.; Iftner, A.; Holz, B.; Staebler, A.; Henes, M.; Rall, K.; Haedicke, J.; et al. Head-to-Head Comparison of the RNA-Based Aptima Human Papillomavirus (HPV) Assay and the DNA-Based Hybrid Capture 2 HPV Test in a Routine Screening Population of Women Aged 30 to 60 Years in Germany. *J. Clin. Microbiol.* **2015**, *53*, 2509–2516. [CrossRef] [PubMed]
162. Qiao, Y.L.; Jeronimo, J.; Zhao, F.H.; Schweizer, J.; Chen, W.; Valdez, M.; Lu, P.; Zhang, X.; Kang, L.N.; Bansil, P.; et al. Lower cost strategies for triage of human papillomavirus DNA-positive women. *Int. J. Cancer* **2014**, *134*, 2891–2901. [CrossRef]
163. Castle, P.E.; Sideri, M.; Jeronimo, J.; Solomon, D.; Schiffman, M. Risk assessment to guide the prevention of cervical cancer. *J. Low. Genit. Tract. Dis.* **2008**, *12*, 1–7. [CrossRef]
164. Perkins, R.B.; Guido, R.S.; Castle, P.E.; Chelmow, D.; Einstein, M.H.; Garcia, F.; Huh, W.K.; Kim, J.J.; Moscicki, A.B.; Nayar, R.; et al. 2019 ASCCP Risk-Based Management Consensus Guidelines for Abnormal Cervical Cancer Screening Tests and Cancer Precursors. *J. Low. Genit. Tract. Dis.* **2020**, *24*, 102–131. [CrossRef]
165. Schiffman, M.; Wentzensen, N.; Perkins, R.B.; Guido, R.S. An Introduction to the 2019 ASCCP Risk-Based Management Consensus Guidelines. *J. Low. Genit. Tract. Dis.* **2020**, *24*, 87–89. [CrossRef]
166. Burger, E.A.; Kim, J.J.; Sy, S.; Castle, P.E. Age of Acquiring Causal Human Papillomavirus (HPV) Infections: Leveraging Simulation Models to Explore the Natural History of HPV-induced Cervical Cancer. *Clin. Infect. Dis.* **2017**, *65*, 893–899. [CrossRef]
167. Schiffman, M.; Castle, P.E. The promise of global cervical-cancer prevention. *N. Engl. J. Med.* **2005**, *353*, 2101–2104. [CrossRef]
168. Wheeler, C.M.; Hunt, W.C.; Joste, N.E.; Key, C.R.; Quint, W.G.; Castle, P.E. Human papillomavirus genotype distributions: Implications for vaccination and cancer screening in the United States. *J. Natl. Cancer Inst.* **2009**, *101*, 475–487. [CrossRef] [PubMed]
169. Adcock, R.; Cuzick, J.; Hunt, W.C.; McDonald, R.M.; Wheeler, C.M. Role of HPV Genotype, Multiple Infections, and Viral Load on the Risk of High-Grade Cervical Neoplasia. *Cancer Epidemiol. Biomarkers Prev.* **2019**, *28*, 1816–1824. [CrossRef]
170. Clifford, G.M.; Tully, S.; Franceschi, S. Carcinogenicity of Human Papillomavirus (HPV) Types in HIV-Positive Women: A Meta-Analysis From HPV Infection to Cervical Cancer. *Clin. Infect. Dis.* **2017**, *64*, 1228–1235. [CrossRef]
171. Dovey de la Cour, C.; Guleria, S.; Nygård, M.; Trygvadóttir, L.; Sigurdsson, K.; Liaw, K.L.; Hortlund, M.; Lagheden, C.; Hansen, B.T.; Munk, C.; et al. Human papillomavirus types in cervical high-grade lesions or cancer among Nordic women-Potential for prevention. *Cancer Med.* **2019**, *8*, 839–849. [CrossRef] [PubMed]
172. Castle, P.E.; Schiffman, M.; Wheeler, C.M.; Wentzensen, N.; Gravitt, P.E. Impact of improved classification on the association of human papillomavirus with cervical precancer. *Am. J. Epidemiol.* **2010**, *171*, 155–163. [CrossRef] [PubMed]
173. Tsoumpou, I.; Arbyn, M.; Kyrgiou, M.; Wentzensen, N.; Koliopoulos, G.; Martin-Hirsch, P.; Malamou-Mitsi, V.; Paraskevaidis, E. p16(INK4a) immunostaining in cytological and histological specimens from the uterine cervix: A systematic review and meta-analysis. *Cancer Treat. Rev.* **2009**, *35*, 210–220. [CrossRef]
174. Castle, P.E.; Pierz, A.J.; Adcock, R.; Aslam, S.; Basu, P.S.; Belinson, J.L.; Cuzick, J.; El-Zein, M.; Ferreccio, C.; Firnhaber, C.; et al. A Pooled Analysis to Compare the Clinical Characteristics of Human Papillomavirus-positive and -Negative Cervical Precancers. *Cancer Prev. Res.* **2020**, *13*, 829–840. [CrossRef]
175. Castle, P.E.; Schiffman, M.; Wheeler, C.M.; Solomon, D. Evidence for frequent regression of cervical intraepithelial neoplasia-grade 2. *Obstet. Gynecol.* **2009**, *113*, 18–25. [CrossRef]
176. Castle, P.E.; Stoler, M.H.; Solomon, D.; Schiffman, M. The relationship of community biopsy-diagnosed cervical intraepithelial neoplasia grade 2 to the quality control pathology-reviewed diagnoses: An ALTS report. *Am. J. Clin. Pathol.* **2007**, *127*, 805–815. [CrossRef]
177. Cogliano, V.; Baan, R.; Straif, K.; Grosse, Y.; Secretan, B.; El Ghissassi, F. Carcinogenicity of human papillomaviruses. *Lancet Oncol.* **2005**, *6*, 204. [CrossRef] [PubMed]

178. Palmer, M.; Katanoda, K.; Saito, E.; Acuti Martellucci, C.; Tanaka, S.; Ikeda, S.; Sakamoto, H.; Machelek, D.; Ml Brotherton, J.; Hocking, J.S. Genotype prevalence and age distribution of human papillomavirus from infection to cervical cancer in Japanese women: A systematic review and meta-analysis. *Vaccine* **2022**, *40*, 5971–5996. [CrossRef]
179. Wentzensen, N.; Wacholder, S. From differences in means between cases and controls to risk stratification: A business plan for biomarker development. *Cancer Discov.* **2013**, *3*, 148–157. [CrossRef]
180. Castle, P.E.; Kinney, W.K.; Chen, L.; Kim, J.J.; Jenison, S.; Rossi, G.; Kang, H.; Cuzick, J.; Wheeler, C.M. Adherence to National Guidelines on Cervical Screening: A Population-Based Evaluation from a Statewide Registry. *J. Natl. Cancer Inst.* **2021**, *114*, 626–630. [CrossRef] [PubMed]
181. Wright, J.D.; Chen, L.; Tergas, A.I.; Melamed, A.; St Clair, C.M.; Hou, J.Y.; Khoury-Collado, F.; Gockley, A.; Accordino, M.; Hershman, D.L. Overuse of Cervical Cancer Screening Tests Among Women With Average Risk in the United States From 2013 to 2014. *JAMA Netw. Open* **2021**, *4*, e218373. [CrossRef] [PubMed]
182. Salingaros, S.; Shieh, Y.; Finkel, M.L.; Polaneczky, M.; Korenstein, D.; Marti, J.L. Public cervical cancer screening recommendations from US cancer centers: Assessing adherence to national guidelines. *J. Med. Screen.* **2024**, *31*, 201–204. [CrossRef]
183. Habbema, D.; De Kok, I.M.; Brown, M.L. Cervical cancer screening in the United States and the Netherlands: A tale of two countries. *Milbank Q.* **2012**, *90*, 5–37. [CrossRef] [PubMed]
184. Habbema, D.; Weinmann, S.; Arbyn, M.; Kamineni, A.; Williams, A.E.; de Kok, I.M.; van Kemenade, F.; Field, T.S.; van Rosmalen, J.; Brown, M.L. Harms of cervical cancer screening in the United States and the Netherlands. *Int. J. Cancer* **2017**, *140*, 1215–1222. [CrossRef] [PubMed]
185. Freeman, H.P.; Wingrove, B.K. *Excess Cervical Cancer Mortality: A Marker for Low Access to Health Care in Poor Communities*; National Cancer Institute: Bethesda, MD, USA, 2005.
186. Castle, P.E. Charting the Future of Cancer Health Disparities Research-Letter. *Cancer Res.* **2018**, *78*, 1883–1885. [CrossRef]
187. Moss, J.L.; Pinto, C.N.; Srinivasan, S.; Cronin, K.A.; Croyle, R.T. Enduring Cancer Disparities by Persistent Poverty, Rurality, and Race: 1990–1992 to 2014–2018. *J. Natl. Cancer Inst.* **2022**, *114*, 829–836. [CrossRef]
188. Human papillomavirus vaccination coverage among adolescent girls, 2007–2012, and postlicensure vaccine safety monitoring, 2006–2013—United States. *MMWR Morb. Mortal. Wkly. Rep.* **2013**, *62*, 591–595.
189. Pingali, C.; Yankey, D.; Elam-Evans, L.D.; Markowitz, L.E.; Valier, M.R.; Fredua, B.; Crowe, S.J.; DeSisto, C.L.; Stokley, S.; Singleton, J.A. Vaccination Coverage Among Adolescents Aged 13–17 Years—National Immunization Survey-Teen, United States, 2022. *MMWR Morb. Mortal. Wkly. Rep.* **2023**, *72*, 912–919. [CrossRef]
190. Barbaro, B.; Brotherton, J.M. Assessing HPV vaccine coverage in Australia by geography and socioeconomic status: Are we protecting those most at risk? *Aust. New Zealand J. Public Health* **2014**, *38*, 419–423. [CrossRef]
191. Cancer Australia. National Cancer Control Indicators: HPV Vaccination Uptake. Available online: https://ncci.canceraustralia.gov.au/prevention/hpv-vaccination-uptake/hpv-vaccination-uptake# (accessed on 21 August 2024).
192. Australian Government. Cancer Australia: Cervical Cancer. Available online: https://www.canceraustralia.gov.au/cancer-types/cervical-cancer/statistics#:~:text=In%202022,%20it%20is%20estimated,by%20the%20age%20of%2085.&text=In%202018,%20the%20age-standardised,7.3%20cases%20per%20100,000%20females. (accessed on 19 August 2024).
193. Immunize.org. Vaccine-Specific Requirements: State Laws and Requirements by Vaccine. Available online: https://www.immunize.org/official-guidance/state-policies/requirements/ (accessed on 12 July 2024).
194. Centers for Disease Control and Prevention (National Center for Health Statistics). Table VaxCh. Vaccination coverage for selected diseases by age 24 months, by race and Hispanic origin, poverty level, and location of residence: United States, birth years 2010–2016 (2020–2021). Available online: https://www.cdc.gov/nchs/data/hus/2020-2021/VaxCh.pdf (accessed on 12 July 2024).
195. Holman, D.M.; Benard, V.; Roland, K.B.; Watson, M.; Liddon, N.; Stokley, S. Barriers to human papillomavirus vaccination among US adolescents: A systematic review of the literature. *JAMA Pediatr.* **2014**, *168*, 76–82. [CrossRef] [PubMed]
196. Ferrer, H.B.; Trotter, C.; Hickman, M.; Audrey, S. Barriers and facilitators to HPV vaccination of young women in high-income countries: A qualitative systematic review and evidence synthesis. *BMC Public Health* **2014**, *14*, 700. [CrossRef] [PubMed]
197. Kasting, M.L.; Shapiro, G.K.; Rosberger, Z.; Kahn, J.A.; Zimet, G.D. Tempest in a teapot: A systematic review of HPV vaccination and risk compensation research. *Hum. Vaccin. Immunother.* **2016**, *12*, 1435–1450. [CrossRef]
198. Madhivanan, P.; Pierre-Victor, D.; Mukherjee, S.; Bhoite, P.; Powell, B.; Jean-Baptiste, N.; Clarke, R.; Avent, T.; Krupp, K. Human Papillomavirus Vaccination and Sexual Disinhibition in Females: A Systematic Review. *Am. J. Prev. Med.* **2016**, *51*, 373–383. [CrossRef]
199. Cartmell, K.B.; Mzik, C.R.; Sundstrom, B.L.; Luque, J.S.; White, A.; Young-Pierce, J. HPV Vaccination Communication Messages, Messengers, and Messaging Strategies. *J. Cancer Educ.* **2019**, *34*, 1014–1023. [CrossRef]
200. Gilkey, M.B.; Zhou, M.; McRee, A.L.; Kornides, M.L.; Bridges, J.F.P. Parents' Views on the Best and Worst Reasons for Guideline-Consistent HPV Vaccination. *Cancer Epidemiol. Biomarkers Prev.* **2018**, *27*, 762–767. [CrossRef]
201. Lama, Y.; Qin, Y.; Nan, X.; Knott, C.; Adebamowo, C.; Ntiri, S.O.; Wang, M.Q. Human Papillomavirus Vaccine Acceptability and Campaign Message Preferences Among African American Parents: A Qualitative Study. *J. Cancer Educ.* **2022**, *37*, 1691–1701. [CrossRef]

202. Donovan, B.; Franklin, N.; Guy, R.; Grulich, A.E.; Regan, D.G.; Ali, H.; Wand, H.; Fairley, C.K. Quadrivalent human papillomavirus vaccination and trends in genital warts in Australia: Analysis of national sentinel surveillance data. *Lancet Infect. Dis.* **2011**, *11*, 39–44. [CrossRef]
203. Burger, E.A.; Sy, S.; Nygård, M.; Kristiansen, I.S.; Kim, J.J. Prevention of HPV-related cancers in Norway: Cost-effectiveness of expanding the HPV vaccination program to include pre-adolescent boys. *PLoS ONE* **2014**, *9*, e89974. [CrossRef] [PubMed]
204. Foerster, V.; Khangura, S.; Severn, M. CADTH Rapid Response Reports. In *HPV Vaccination in Men: A Review of Clinical Effectiveness, Cost-Effectiveness, and Guidelines*; Canadian Agency for Drugs and Technologies in Health: Ottawa, ON, USA, 2017.
205. Linertová, R.; Guirado-Fuentes, C.; Mar Medina, J.; Imaz-Iglesia, I.; Rodríguez-Rodríguez, L.; Carmona-Rodríguez, M. Cost-effectiveness of extending the HPV vaccination to boys: A systematic review. *J. Epidemiol. Community Health* **2021**, *75*, 910–916. [CrossRef]
206. Ng, S.S.; Hutubessy, R.; Chaiyakunapruk, N. Systematic review of cost-effectiveness studies of human papillomavirus (HPV) vaccination: 9-Valent vaccine, gender-neutral and multiple age cohort vaccination. *Vaccine* **2018**, *36*, 2529–2544. [CrossRef] [PubMed]
207. Wolff, E.; Elfström, K.M.; Haugen Cange, H.; Larsson, S.; Englund, H.; Sparén, P.; Roth, A. Cost-effectiveness of sex-neutral HPV-vaccination in Sweden, accounting for herd-immunity and sexual behaviour. *Vaccine* **2018**, *36*, 5160–5165. [CrossRef] [PubMed]
208. Scarinci, I.C.; Li, Y.; Tucker, L.; Campos, N.G.; Kim, J.J.; Peral, S.; Castle, P.E. Given a choice between self-sampling at home for HPV testing and standard of care screening at the clinic, what do African American women choose? Findings from a group randomized controlled trial. *Prev. Med.* **2021**, *142*, 106358. [CrossRef] [PubMed]
209. Winer, R.L.; Lin, J.; Anderson, M.L.; Tiro, J.A.; Green, B.B.; Gao, H.; Meenan, R.T.; Hansen, K.; Sparks, A.; Buist, D.S.M. Strategies to Increase Cervical Cancer Screening With Mailed Human Papillomavirus Self-Sampling Kits: A Randomized Clinical Trial. *JAMA* **2023**, *330*, 1971–1981. [CrossRef]
210. Centers for Disease Control and Prevention. National Breast and Cervical Cancer Early Detection Program (NBCCEDP). 2023. Available online: https://www.cdc.gov/breast-cervical-cancer-screening/about/index.html (accessed on 21 August 2024).
211. 106th Congress. Breast and Cervical Cancer Prevention and Treatment Act (BCCPTA) (Public Law 106–354). 2000. Available online: https://www.congress.gov/106/plaws/publ354/PLAW-106publ354.pdf (accessed on 21 August 2024).
212. Tangka, F.; Kenny, K.; Miller, J.; Howard, D.H. The eligibility and reach of the national breast and cervical cancer early detection program after implementation of the affordable care act. *Cancer Causes Control* **2020**, *31*, 473–489. [CrossRef]
213. Shalowitz, D.I.; Vinograd, A.M.; Giuntoli, R.L., 2nd. Geographic access to gynecologic cancer care in the United States. *Gynecol. Oncol.* **2015**, *138*, 115–120. [CrossRef]
214. Ackroyd, S.A.; Shih, Y.T.; Kim, B.; Lee, N.K.; Halpern, M.T. A look at the gynecologic oncologist workforce—Are we meeting patient demand? *Gynecol. Oncol.* **2021**, *163*, 229–236. [CrossRef]
215. Allanson, E.R.; Zafar, S.N.; Anakwenze, C.P.; Schmeler, K.M.; Trimble, E.L.; Grover, S. The global burden of cervical cancer requiring surgery: Database estimates. *Infect. Agent. Cancer* **2024**, *19*, 5. [CrossRef]
216. Rayburn, W.F.; Klagholz, J.C.; Murray-Krezan, C.; Dowell, L.E.; Strunk, A.L. Distribution of American Congress of Obstetricians and Gynecologists fellows and junior fellows in practice in the United States. *Obstet. Gynecol.* **2012**, *119*, 1017–1022. [CrossRef]
217. Friedman, S.; Shaw, J.G.; Hamilton, A.B.; Vinekar, K.; Washington, D.L.; Mattocks, K.; Yano, E.M.; Phibbs, C.S.; Johnson, A.M.; Saechao, F.; et al. Gynecologist Supply Deserts Across the VA and in the Community. *J. Gen. Intern. Med.* **2022**, *37*, 690–697. [CrossRef] [PubMed]
218. Cleary, J.; Powell, R.A.; Munene, G.; Mwangi-Powell, F.N.; Luyirika, E.; Kiyange, F.; Merriman, A.; Scholten, W.; Radbruch, L.; Torode, J.; et al. Formulary availability and regulatory barriers to accessibility of opioids for cancer pain in Africa: A report from the Global Opioid Policy Initiative (GOPI). *Ann. Oncol.* **2013**, *24* (Suppl. 11), xi14–xi23. [CrossRef]
219. Kim, J.J.; Simms, K.T.; Killen, J.; Smith, M.A.; Burger, E.A.; Sy, S.; Regan, C.; Canfell, K. Human papillomavirus vaccination for adults aged 30 to 45 years in the United States: A cost-effectiveness analysis. *PLoS Med.* **2021**, *18*, e1003534. [CrossRef]
220. Chesson, H.W.; Meites, E.; Ekwueme, D.U.; Saraiya, M.; Markowitz, L.E. Cost-effectiveness of HPV vaccination for adults through age 45 years in the United States: Estimates from a simplified transmission model. *Vaccine* **2020**, *38*, 8032–8039. [CrossRef] [PubMed]
221. León-Maldonado, L.; Cabral, A.; Brown, B.; Ryan, G.W.; Maldonado, A.; Salmerón, J.; Allen-Leigh, B.; Lazcano-Ponce, E. Feasibility of a combined strategy of HPV vaccination and screening in Mexico: The FASTER-Tlalpan study experience. *Hum. Vaccin. Immunother.* **2019**, *15*, 1986–1994. [CrossRef] [PubMed]
222. Bosch, F.X.; Robles, C.; Díaz, M.; Arbyn, M.; Baussano, I.; Clavel, C.; Ronco, G.; Dillner, J.; Lehtinen, M.; Petry, K.U.; et al. HPV-FASTER: Broadening the scope for prevention of HPV-related cancer. *Nat. Rev. Clin. Oncol.* **2016**, *13*, 119–132. [CrossRef]
223. Bruni, L.; Saura-Lázaro, A.; Montoliu, A.; Brotons, M.; Alemany, L.; Diallo, M.S.; Afsar, O.Z.; LaMontagne, D.S.; Mosina, L.; Contreras, M.; et al. HPV vaccination introduction worldwide and WHO and UNICEF estimates of national HPV immunization coverage 2010–2019. *Prev. Med.* **2021**, *144*, 106399. [CrossRef]
224. GAVI. Human Papillomavirus Vaccine Support. Available online: https://www.gavi.org/types-support/vaccine-support/human-papillomavirus (accessed on 21 August 2024).
225. Pan American Health Organization (PAHO). PAHO Revolving Fund Vaccine Prices for 2023. Available online: https://www.paho.org/en/documents/paho-revolving-fund-vaccine-prices-2023 (accessed on 21 August 2024).

226. World Health Organization. *Redesigning Child and Adolescent Health Programmes*; WHO: Geneva, Switzerland, 2019.
227. Patton, G.C.; Coffey, C.; Cappa, C.; Currie, D.; Riley, L.; Gore, F.; Degenhardt, L.; Richardson, D.; Astone, N.; Sangowawa, A.O.; et al. Health of the world's adolescents: A synthesis of internationally comparable data. *Lancet* **2012**, *379*, 1665–1675. [CrossRef] [PubMed]
228. Resnick, M.D.; Catalano, R.F.; Sawyer, S.M.; Viner, R.; Patton, G.C. Seizing the opportunities of adolescent health. *Lancet* **2012**, *379*, 1564–1567. [CrossRef]
229. Sawyer, S.M.; Afifi, R.A.; Bearinger, L.H.; Blakemore, S.J.; Dick, B.; Ezeh, A.C.; Patton, G.C. Adolescence: A foundation for future health. *Lancet* **2012**, *379*, 1630–1640. [CrossRef] [PubMed]
230. Viner, R.M.; Ozer, E.M.; Denny, S.; Marmot, M.; Resnick, M.; Fatusi, A.; Currie, C. Adolescence and the social determinants of health. *Lancet* **2012**, *379*, 1641–1652. [CrossRef] [PubMed]
231. Sawyer, S.M.; Reavley, N.; Bonell, C.; Patton, G.C. Platforms for Delivering Adolescent Health Actions. In *Child and Adolescent Health and Development*; Bundy, D.A.P., Silva, N.D., Horton, S., Jamison, D.T., Patton, G.C., Eds.; The International Bank for Reconstruction and Development/The World Bank: Washington, DC, USA, 2017. [CrossRef]
232. Ross, D.A.; Mshana, G.; Guthold, R. Adolescent Health Series: The health of adolescents in sub-Saharan Africa: Challenges and opportunities. *Trop. Med. Int. Health* **2021**, *26*, 1326–1332. [CrossRef] [PubMed]
233. Population Reference Bureau (PRB). World population data sheet. Available online: https://interactives.prb.org/2021-wpds/ (accessed on 21 August 2024).
234. United Nations, Department of Economic and Social Affairs, Population Division. *World Population Prospects 2019*; United Nations: New York, NY, USA, 2019.
235. World Bank Group. Lower secondary completion rate, total (% of relevant age group). Available online: https://data.worldbank.org/indicator/SE.SEC.CMPT.LO.ZS (accessed on 19 April 2024).
236. World Health Organization. Essential Programme on Immunization. Available online: https://www.who.int/teams/immunization-vaccines-and-biologicals/essential-programme-on-immunization (accessed on 19 April 2024).
237. World Health Organization. WHO recommendations for routine immunization—summary tables. Available online: https://www.who.int/teams/immunization-vaccines-and-biologicals/policies/who-recommendations-for-routine-immunization--summary-tables (accessed on 19 April 2024).
238. UNICEF; World Health Organization. *Progress Towards Global Immunization Goals—2019*; UNICEF: New York, NY, USA, 2020.
239. Our World in Data. Vaccination. Available online: https://ourworldindata.org/vaccination (accessed on 22 April 2024).
240. UNICEF. Immunization Country Profiles. Available online: https://data.unicef.org/resources/immunization-country-profiles/ (accessed on 22 April 2024).
241. Bobo, F.T.; Asante, A.; Woldie, M.; Dawson, A.; Hayen, A. Child vaccination in sub-Saharan Africa: Increasing coverage addresses inequalities. *Vaccine* **2022**, *40*, 141–150. [CrossRef]
242. Vanderslott, S.; Marks, T. Charting mandatory childhood vaccination policies worldwide. *Vaccine* **2021**, *39*, 4054–4062. [CrossRef]
243. Schwarz, T.F.; Galaj, A.; Spaczynski, M.; Wysocki, J.; Kaufmann, A.M.; Poncelet, S.; Suryakiran, P.V.; Folschweiller, N.; Thomas, F.; Lin, L.; et al. Ten-year immune persistence and safety of the HPV-16/18 AS04-adjuvanted vaccine in females vaccinated at 15–55 years of age. *Cancer Med.* **2017**, *6*, 2723–2731. [CrossRef]
244. Schwarz, T.F.; Huang, L.M.; Valencia, A.; Panzer, F.; Chiu, C.H.; Decreux, A.; Poncelet, S.; Karkada, N.; Folschweiller, N.; Lin, L.; et al. A ten-year study of immunogenicity and safety of the AS04-HPV-16/18 vaccine in adolescent girls aged 10–14 years. *Hum. Vaccin. Immunother.* **2019**, *15*, 1970–1979. [CrossRef]
245. Donken, R.; Dobson, S.R.M.; Marty, K.D.; Cook, D.; Sauvageau, C.; Gilca, V.; Dionne, M.; McNeil, S.; Krajden, M.; Money, D.; et al. Immunogenicity of 2 and 3 Doses of the Quadrivalent Human Papillomavirus Vaccine up to 120 Months Postvaccination: Follow-up of a Randomized Clinical Trial. *Clin. Infect. Dis.* **2020**, *71*, 1022–1029. [CrossRef]
246. Arbyn, M.; Ronco, G.; Anttila, A.; Meijer, C.J.; Poljak, M.; Ogilvie, G.; Koliopoulos, G.; Naucler, P.; Sankaranarayanan, R.; Peto, J. Evidence regarding human papillomavirus testing in secondary prevention of cervical cancer. *Vaccine* **2012**, *30* (Suppl. 5), F88–F99. [CrossRef]
247. International Agency for Research on Cancer. *European Guidelines for Quality Assurance in Cervical Cancer Screening*; International Agency for Research on Cancer: Lyon, France, 2008.
248. Martinez, M.E.; Schmeler, K.M.; Lajous, M.; Newman, L.A. Cancer Screening in Low- and Middle-Income Countries. *Am. Soc. Clin. Oncol. Educ. Book.* **2024**, *44*, e431272. [CrossRef] [PubMed]
249. Ramírez, A.T.; Valls, J.; Baena, A.; Rojas, F.D.; Ramírez, K.; Álvarez, R.; Cristaldo, C.; Henríquez, O.; Moreno, A.; Reynaga, D.C.; et al. Performance of cervical cytology and HPV testing for primary cervical cancer screening in Latin America: An analysis within the ESTAMPA study. *Lancet Reg. Health Am.* **2023**, *26*, 100593. [CrossRef] [PubMed]
250. Lemp, J.M.; De Neve, J.W.; Bussmann, H.; Chen, S.; Manne-Goehler, J.; Theilmann, M.; Marcus, M.E.; Ebert, C.; Probst, C.; Tsabedze-Sibanyoni, L.; et al. Lifetime Prevalence of Cervical Cancer Screening in 55 Low- and Middle-Income Countries. *JAMA* **2020**, *324*, 1532–1542. [CrossRef] [PubMed]
251. Alfaro, K.; Maza, M.; Cremer, M.; Masch, R.; Soler, M. Removing global barriers to cervical cancer prevention and moving towards elimination. *Nat. Rev. Cancer* **2021**, *21*, 607–608. [CrossRef]

252. Lazcano-Ponce, E.; Lorincz, A.T.; Cruz-Valdez, A.; Salmerón, J.; Uribe, P.; Velasco-Mondragón, E.; Nevarez, P.H.; Acosta, R.D.; Hernández-Avila, M. Self-collection of vaginal specimens for human papillomavirus testing in cervical cancer prevention (MARCH): A community-based randomised controlled trial. *Lancet* **2011**, *378*, 1868–1873. [CrossRef]
253. Suba, E.J.; Donnelly, A.D.; Duong, D.V.; Gonzalez Mena, L.E.; Neethling, G.S.; Thai, N.V. WHO should adjust its global strategy for cervical cancer prevention. *BMJ Glob. Health* **2023**, *8*, e012031. [CrossRef] [PubMed]
254. Suba, E.J.; Zarka, M.A.; Raab, S.S. Human papillomavirus screening for low and middle-income countries. *Prev. Med.* **2017**, *100*, 296. [CrossRef]
255. Suba, E.J. Researchers should no longer delay implementation of Pap screening in low and middle income countries pending research into novel screening approaches. *Infect. Agent. Cancer* **2024**, *19*, 18. [CrossRef] [PubMed]
256. World Health Organization. *WHO Guideline for Screening and Treatment of Cervical Pre-Cancer Lesions for Cervical Cancer Prevention*; WHO: Geneva, Switzerland, 2021.
257. Hall, M.T.; Simms, K.T.; Murray, J.M.; Keane, A.; Nguyen, D.T.N.; Caruana, M.; Lui, G.; Kelly, H.; Eckert, L.O.; Santesso, N.; et al. Benefits and harms of cervical screening, triage and treatment strategies in women living with HIV. *Nat. Med.* **2023**, *29*, 3059–3066. [CrossRef]
258. Simms, K.T.; Keane, A.; Nguyen, D.T.N.; Caruana, M.; Hall, M.T.; Lui, G.; Gauvreau, C.; Demke, O.; Arbyn, M.; Basu, P.; et al. Benefits, harms and cost-effectiveness of cervical screening, triage and treatment strategies for women in the general population. *Nat. Med.* **2023**, *29*, 3050–3058. [CrossRef]
259. Bruni, L.; Serrano, B.; Roura, E.; Alemany, L.; Cowan, M.; Herrero, R.; Poljak, M.; Murillo, R.; Broutet, N.; Riley, L.M.; et al. Cervical cancer screening programmes and age-specific coverage estimates for 202 countries and territories worldwide: A review and synthetic analysis. *Lancet Glob. Health* **2022**, *10*, e1115–e1127. [CrossRef]
260. Kundrod, K.A.; Jeronimo, J.; Vetter, B.; Maza, M.; Murenzi, G.; Phoolcharoen, N.; Castle, P.E. Toward 70% cervical cancer screening coverage: Technical challenges and opportunities to increase access to human papillomavirus (HPV) testing. *PLOS Glob. Public Health* **2023**, *3*, e0001982. [CrossRef] [PubMed]
261. World Health Organization. Existing HIV and TB Laboratory Systems Facilitating COVID-19 Testing in Africa. Available online: https://www.who.int/news/item/26-11-2020-existing-hiv-and-tb-laboratory-systems-facilitating-covid-19-testing-in-africa (accessed on 22 April 2024).
262. Adesina, A.; Chumba, D.; Nelson, A.M.; Orem, J.; Roberts, D.J.; Wabinga, H.; Wilson, M.; Rebbeck, T.R. Improvement of pathology in sub-Saharan Africa. *Lancet Oncol.* **2013**, *14*, e152–e157. [CrossRef] [PubMed]
263. Adeyi, O.A. Pathology services in developing countries-the West African experience. *Arch. Pathol. Lab. Med.* **2011**, *135*, 183–186. [CrossRef]
264. The Pathologist. Constant Demand, Patchy Supply. Available online: https://thepathologist.com/outside-the-lab/constant-demand-patchy-supply (accessed on 24 April 2024).
265. Albayrak, A.; Akhan, A.U.; Calik, N.; Capar, A.; Bilgin, G.; Toreyin, B.U.; Muezzinoglu, B.; Turkmen, I.; Durak-Ata, L. A whole-slide image grading benchmark and tissue classification for cervical cancer precursor lesions with inter-observer variability. *Med. Biol. Eng. Comput.* **2021**, *59*, 1545–1561. [CrossRef]
266. Cho, B.J.; Kim, J.W.; Park, J.; Kwon, G.Y.; Hong, M.; Jang, S.H.; Bang, H.; Kim, G.; Park, S.T. Automated Diagnosis of Cervical Intraepithelial Neoplasia in Histology Images via Deep Learning. *Diagnostics* **2022**, *12*, 548. [CrossRef] [PubMed]
267. Sornapudi, S.; Addanki, R.; Stanley, R.J.; Stoecker, W.V.; Long, R.; Zuna, R.; Frazier, S.R.; Antani, S. Automated Cervical Digitized Histology Whole-Slide Image Analysis Toolbox. *J. Pathol. Inform.* **2021**, *12*, 26. [CrossRef] [PubMed]
268. Sornapudi, S.; Stanley, R.J.; Stoecker, W.V.; Long, R.; Xue, Z.; Zuna, R.; Frazier, S.R.; Antani, S. DeepCIN: Attention-Based Cervical histology Image Classification with Sequential Feature Modeling for Pathologist-Level Accuracy. *J. Pathol. Inform.* **2020**, *11*, 40. [CrossRef]
269. Kyrgiou, M.; Athanasiou, A.; Kalliala, I.E.J.; Paraskevaidi, M.; Mitra, A.; Martin-Hirsch, P.P.; Arbyn, M.; Bennett, P.; Paraskevaidis, E. Obstetric outcomes after conservative treatment for cervical intraepithelial lesions and early invasive disease. *Cochrane Database Syst. Rev.* **2017**, *11*, Cd012847. [CrossRef] [PubMed]
270. Brenes, D.; Salcedo, M.P.; Coole, J.B.; Maker, Y.; Kortum, A.; Schwarz, R.A.; Carns, J.; Vohra, I.S.; Possati-Resende, J.C.; Antoniazzi, M.; et al. Multiscale Optical Imaging Fusion for Cervical Precancer Diagnosis: Integrating Widefield Colposcopy and High-Resolution Endomicroscopy. *IEEE Trans. Biomed. Eng.* **2024**, *71*, 2547–2556. [CrossRef]
271. Hunt, B.; Fregnani, J.; Brenes, D.; Schwarz, R.A.; Salcedo, M.P.; Possati-Resende, J.C.; Antoniazzi, M.; de Oliveira Fonseca, B.; Santana, I.V.V.; de Macêdo Matsushita, G.; et al. Cervical lesion assessment using real-time microendoscopy image analysis in Brazil: The CLARA study. *Int. J. Cancer* **2021**, *149*, 431–441. [CrossRef] [PubMed]
272. Kundrod, K.A.; Barra, M.; Wilkinson, A.; Smith, C.A.; Natoli, M.E.; Chang, M.M.; Coole, J.B.; Santhanaraj, A.; Lorenzoni, C.; Mavume, C.; et al. An integrated isothermal nucleic acid amplification test to detect HPV16 and HPV18 DNA in resource-limited settings. *Sci. Transl. Med.* **2023**, *15*, eabn4768. [CrossRef]
273. Inturrisi, F.; de Sanjosé, S.; Desai, K.T.; Dagnall, C.; Egemen, D.; Befano, B.; Rodriguez, A.C.; Jeronimo, J.A.; Zuna, R.E.; Hoffman, A.; et al. A rapid HPV typing assay to support global cervical cancer screening and risk-based management: A cross-sectional study. *Int. J. Cancer* **2024**, *154*, 241–250. [CrossRef]
274. American Cancer Society. Treatment Options for Cervical Cancer, by Stage. Available online: https://www.cancer.org/cancer/types/cervical-cancer/treating/by-stage.html (accessed on 20 July 2024).

275. U.S. National Cancer Institute. Cervical Cancer Treatment. Available online: https://www.cancer.gov/types/cervical/treatment (accessed on 20 July 2024).
276. Shiels, M.S.; Lipkowitz, S.; Campos, N.G.; Schiffman, M.; Schiller, J.T.; Freedman, N.D.; Berrington de González, A. Opportunities for Achieving the Cancer Moonshot Goal of a 50% Reduction in Cancer Mortality by 2047. *Cancer Discov.* **2023**, *13*, 1084–1099. [CrossRef]
277. Holmer, H.; Shrime, M.G.; Riesel, J.N.; Meara, J.G.; Hagander, L. Towards closing the gap of the global surgeon, anaesthesiologist, and obstetrician workforce: Thresholds and projections towards 2030. *Lancet* **2015**, *385* (Suppl. S2), 40. [CrossRef] [PubMed]
278. Sullivan, R.; Alatise, O.I.; Anderson, B.O.; Audisio, R.; Autier, P.; Aggarwal, A.; Balch, C.; Brennan, M.F.; Dare, A.; D'Cruz, A.; et al. Global cancer surgery: Delivering safe, affordable, and timely cancer surgery. *Lancet Oncol.* **2015**, *16*, 1193–1224. [CrossRef]
279. Desai, K.T.; de Sanjosé, S.; Schiffman, M. Treatment of Cervical Precancers is the Major Remaining Challenge in Cervical Screening Research. *Cancer Prev. Res.* **2023**, *16*, 649–651. [CrossRef] [PubMed]
280. Shaffi, A.F.; Odongo, E.B.; Itsura, P.M.; Tonui, P.K.; Mburu, A.W.; Hassan, A.R.; Rosen, B.P.; Covens, A.L. Cervical cancer management in a low resource setting: A 10-year review in a tertiary care hospital in Kenya. *Gynecol. Oncol. Rep.* **2024**. [CrossRef] [PubMed]
281. Batman, S.; Rangeiro, R.; Monteiro, E.; Changule, D.; Daud, S.; Ribeiro, M.; Tsambe, E.; Bila, C.; Osman, N.; Carrilho, C.; et al. Expanding Cervical Cancer Screening in Mozambique: Challenges Associated With Diagnosing and Treating Cervical Cancer. *JCO Glob. Oncol.* **2023**, *9*, e2300139. [CrossRef]
282. Kassa, R.; Irene, Y.; Woldetsadik, E.; Kidane, E.; Higgins, M.; Dejene, T.; Wells, J. Survival of women with cervical cancer in East Africa: A systematic review and meta-analysis. *J. Obstet. Gynaecol.* **2023**, *43*, 2253308. [CrossRef]
283. Anakwenze, C.P.; Allanson, E.; Ewongwo, A.; Lumley, C.; Bazzett-Matabele, L.; Msadabwe, S.C.; Kamfwa, P.; Shouman, T.; Lombe, D.; Rubagumya, F.; et al. Mapping of Radiation Oncology and Gynecologic Oncology Services Available to Treat the Growing Burden of Cervical Cancer in Africa. *Int. J. Radiat. Oncol. Biol. Phys.* **2024**, *118*, 595–604. [CrossRef] [PubMed]
284. Definitive Healthcare. How many Oncologists Are in the U.S.? Available online: https://www.definitivehc.com/resources/healthcare-insights/how-many-oncologists-in-us#:~:text=As%20of%20August%202023,%20the,a%20total%20of%2026,241%20oncologists. (accessed on 20 July 2024).
285. Ige, T.A.; Jenkins, A.; Burt, G.; Angal-Kalinin, D.; McIntosh, P.; Coleman, C.N.; Pistenmaa, D.A.; O'Brien, D.; Dosanjh, M. Surveying the Challenges to Improve Linear Accelerator-based Radiation Therapy in Africa: A Unique Collaborative Platform of All 28 African Countries Offering Such Treatment. *Clin. Oncol.* **2021**, *33*, e521–e529. [CrossRef] [PubMed]
286. CERNCOURIER. Developing Medical Linacs for Challenging Regions. Available online: https://cerncourier.com/a/developing-medical-linacs-for-challenging-regions/ (accessed on 13 May 2024).
287. IAEA Directory of Radiotherapy Centers. Number of Radiotherapy Machines Per Million Population. Available online: https://dirac.iaea.org/Query/Map (accessed on 21 August 2024).
288. World Health Organization. The Global Health Observatory: Radiotherapy Units (Per Million Population), Total Density. Available online: https://www.who.int/data/gho/data/indicators/indicator-details/GHO/total-density-per-million-population-radiotherapy-units (accessed on 21 August 2024).
289. Maitre, P.; Krishnatry, R.; Chopra, S.; Gondhowiardjo, S.; Likonda, B.M.; Hussain, Q.M.; Zubizarreta, E.H.; Agarwal, J.P. Modern Radiotherapy Technology: Obstacles and Opportunities to Access in Low- and Middle-Income Countries. *JCO Glob. Oncol.* **2022**, *8*, e2100376. [CrossRef] [PubMed]
290. Chuang, L.T.; Temin, S.; Camacho, R.; Dueñas-Gonzalez, A.; Feldman, S.; Gultekin, M.; Gupta, V.; Horton, S.; Jacob, G.; Kidd, E.A.; et al. Management and Care of Women With Invasive Cervical Cancer: American Society of Clinical Oncology Resource-Stratified Clinical Practice Guideline. *J. Glob. Oncol.* **2016**, *2*, 311–340. [CrossRef]
291. Chuang, L.; Rainville, N.; Byrne, M.; Randall, T.; Schmeler, K. Cervical cancer screening and treatment capacity: A survey of members of the African Organisation for Research and Training in Cancer (AORTIC). *Gynecol. Oncol. Rep.* **2021**, *38*, 100874. [CrossRef]
292. Beltrán Ponce, S.E.; Abunike, S.A.; Bikomeye, J.C.; Sieracki, R.; Niyonzima, N.; Mulamira, P.; Kibudde, S.; Ortiz de Choudens, S.; Siker, M.; Small, C.; et al. Access to Radiation Therapy and Related Clinical Outcomes in Patients With Cervical and Breast Cancer Across Sub-Saharan Africa: A Systematic Review. *JCO Glob. Oncol.* **2023**, *9*, e2200218. [CrossRef]
293. Swanson, M.; Ueda, S.; Chen, L.M.; Huchko, M.J.; Nakisige, C.; Namugga, J. Evidence-based improvisation: Facing the challenges of cervical cancer care in Uganda. *Gynecol. Oncol. Rep.* **2018**, *24*, 30–35. [CrossRef]
294. International Atomic Energy Agency. From Emergency to Expansion: With IAEA Support, Uganda Recovers and Improves its Radiotherapy Services. Available online: https://www.iaea.org/newscenter/news/from-emergency-to-expansion-with-iaea-support-uganda-recovers-and-improves-its-radiotherapy-services (accessed on 21 August 2024).
295. International Gynecologic Cancer Society. Global Gynecologic Oncology Fellowship Program. Available online: https://igcs.org/mentorship-and-training/global-curriculum/ (accessed on 13 May 2024).
296. International Gynecologic Cancer Society. Radiation Oncology Consortium. Available online: https://igcs.org/radiation-oncology-consortium/ (accessed on 13 May 2024).
297. IAEA. Rays of Hope. Available online: https://www.iaea.org/raysofhope (accessed on 13 May 2024).
298. Chuang, L.; Kanis, M.J.; Miller, B.; Wright, J.; Small, W., Jr.; Creasman, W. Treating Locally Advanced Cervical Cancer With Concurrent Chemoradiation Without Brachytherapy in Low-resource Countries. *Am. J. Clin. Oncol.* **2016**, *39*, 92–97. [CrossRef]

299. Ngabonziza, E.; Ghebre, R.; DeBoer, R.J.; Ntasumbumuyange, D.; Magriples, U.; George, J.; Grover, S.; Bazzett-Matabele, L. Outcomes of neoadjuvant chemotherapy and radical hysterectomy for locally advanced cervical cancer at Kigali University Teaching Hospital, Rwanda: A retrospective descriptive study. *BMC Womens Health* **2024**, *24*, 204. [CrossRef]
300. Kokka, F.; Bryant, A.; Olaitan, A.; Brockbank, E.; Powell, M.; Oram, D. Hysterectomy with radiotherapy or chemotherapy or both for women with locally advanced cervical cancer. *Cochrane Database Syst. Rev.* **2022**, *8*, Cd010260. [CrossRef] [PubMed]
301. Miriyala, R.; Mahantshetty, U.; Maheshwari, A.; Gupta, S. Neoadjuvant chemotherapy followed by surgery in cervical cancer: Past, present and future. *Int. J. Gynecol. Cancer* **2022**, *32*, 260–265. [CrossRef] [PubMed]
302. Nguyen, V.T.; Winterman, S.; Playe, M.; Benbara, A.; Zelek, L.; Pamoukdjian, F.; Bousquet, G. Dose-Intense Cisplatin-Based Neoadjuvant Chemotherapy Increases Survival in Advanced Cervical Cancer: An Up-to-Date Meta-Analysis. *Cancers* **2022**, *14*, 842. [CrossRef]
303. Wang, D.; Fang, X. Meta-analysis of the efficacy of neoadjuvant chemotherapy for locally advanced cervical cancer. *Eur. J. Obstet. Gynecol. Reprod. Biol.* **2024**, *297*, 202–208. [CrossRef] [PubMed]
304. Desai, K.T.; Hansen, N.; Rodriguez, A.C.; Befano, B.; Egemen, D.; Gage, J.C.; Wentzensen, N.; Lopez, C.; Jeronimo, J.; de Sanjose, S.; et al. Squamocolumnar junction visibility, age, and implications for cervical cancer screening programs. *Prev. Med.* **2024**, *180*, 107881. [CrossRef] [PubMed]
305. Gonçalves, C.A.; Pereira-da-Silva, G.; Silveira, R.; Mayer, P.C.M.; Zilly, A.; Lopes-Júnior, L.C. Safety, Efficacy, and Immunogenicity of Therapeutic Vaccines for Patients with High-Grade Cervical Intraepithelial Neoplasia (CIN 2/3) Associated with Human Papillomavirus: A Systematic Review. *Cancers* **2024**, *16*, 672. [CrossRef]
306. Alouini, S.; Pichon, C. Therapeutic Vaccines for HPV-Associated Cervical Malignancies: A Systematic Review. *Vaccines* **2024**, *12*, 428. [CrossRef]
307. Trimble, C.L.; Levinson, K.; Maldonado, L.; Donovan, M.J.; Clark, K.T.; Fu, J.; Shay, M.E.; Sauter, M.E.; Sanders, S.A.; Frantz, P.S.; et al. A first-in-human proof-of-concept trial of intravaginal artesunate to treat cervical intraepithelial neoplasia 2/3 (CIN2/3). *Gynecol. Oncol.* **2020**, *157*, 188–194. [CrossRef]
308. Stoler, M.H.; Schiffman, M. Interobserver reproducibility of cervical cytologic and histologic interpretations: Realistic estimates from the ASCUS-LSIL Triage Study. *JAMA* **2001**, *285*, 1500–1505. [CrossRef]
309. Çuburu, N.; Khan, S.; Thompson, C.D.; Kim, R.; Vellinga, J.; Zahn, R.; Lowy, D.R.; Scheper, G.; Schiller, J.T. Adenovirus vector-based prime-boost vaccination via heterologous routes induces cervicovaginal CD8(+) T cell responses against HPV16 oncoproteins. *Int. J. Cancer* **2018**, *142*, 1467–1479. [CrossRef]
310. Stelzle, D.; Tanaka, L.F.; Lee, K.K.; Ibrahim Khalil, A.; Baussano, I.; Shah, A.S.V.; McAllister, D.A.; Gottlieb, S.L.; Klug, S.J.; Winkler, A.S.; et al. Estimates of the global burden of cervical cancer associated with HIV. *Lancet Glob. Health* **2021**, *9*, e161–e169. [CrossRef]
311. Athanasiou, A.; Veroniki, A.A.; Efthimiou, O.; Kalliala, I.; Naci, H.; Bowden, S.; Paraskevaidi, M.; Arbyn, M.; Lyons, D.; Martin-Hirsch, P.; et al. Comparative effectiveness and risk of preterm birth of local treatments for cervical intraepithelial neoplasia and stage IA1 cervical cancer: A systematic review and network meta-analysis. *Lancet Oncol.* **2022**, *23*, 1097–1108. [CrossRef]
312. Clark, D.; Baur, N.; Clelland, D.; Garralda, E.; López-Fidalgo, J.; Connor, S.; Centeno, C. Mapping Levels of Palliative Care Development in 198 Countries: The Situation in 2017. *J. Pain. Symptom Manage* **2020**, *59*, 794–807.e794. [CrossRef] [PubMed]
313. Clark, J.; Crowther, L.; Johnson, M.J.; Ramsenthaler, C.; Currow, D.C. Calculating worldwide needs for morphine for pain in advanced cancer and proportions feasibly met by country estimates of requirements and consumption. Retrospective, time-series analysis (1997–2017). *PLOS Glob. Public Health* **2022**, *2*, e0000533. [CrossRef]
314. World Health Organization. Palliative Care. Available online: https://www.who.int/news-room/fact-sheets/detail/palliative-care (accessed on 22 April 2024).
315. International Narcotics Control Board. Availability of Narcotic Drugs for Medical Use. Available online: https://www.incb.org/incb/en/narcotic-drugs/Availability/availability.html (accessed on 23 April 2024).
316. Reichenvater, H.; Matias, L.D. Is Africa a 'Graveyard' for Linear Accelerators? *Clin. Oncol.* **2016**, *28*, e179–e183. [CrossRef]
317. Marks, I.H.; Thomas, H.; Bakhet, M.; Fitzgerald, E. Medical equipment donation in low-resource settings: A review of the literature and guidelines for surgery and anaesthesia in low-income and middle-income countries. *BMJ Glob. Health* **2019**, *4*, e001785. [CrossRef] [PubMed]
318. Palefsky, J.M.; Lee, J.Y.; Jay, N.; Goldstone, S.E.; Darragh, T.M.; Dunlevy, H.A.; Rosa-Cunha, I.; Arons, A.; Pugliese, J.C.; Vena, D.; et al. Treatment of Anal High-Grade Squamous Intraepithelial Lesions to Prevent Anal Cancer. *N. Engl. J. Med.* **2022**, *386*, 2273–2282. [CrossRef] [PubMed]
319. Stier, E.A.; Clarke, M.A.; Deshmukh, A.A.; Wentzensen, N.; Liu, Y.; Poynten, I.M.; Cavallari, E.N.; Fink, V.; Barroso, L.F.; Clifford, G.M.; et al. International Anal Neoplasia Society's consensus guidelines for anal cancer screening. *Int. J. Cancer* **2024**, *154*, 1694–1702. [CrossRef]
320. Manne, V.; Ryan, J.; Wong, J.; Vengayil, G.; Basit, S.A.; Gish, R.G. Hepatitis C Vaccination: Where We Are and Where We Need to Be. *Pathogens* **2021**, *10*, 1619. [CrossRef]
321. Zhong, L.; Krummenacher, C.; Zhang, W.; Hong, J.; Feng, Q.; Chen, Y.; Zhao, Q.; Zeng, M.S.; Zeng, Y.X.; Xu, M.; et al. Urgency and necessity of Epstein-Barr virus prophylactic vaccines. *NPJ Vaccines* **2022**, *7*, 159. [CrossRef]
322. Cohen, J.I. Vaccine Development for Epstein-Barr Virus. *Adv. Exp. Med. Biol.* **2018**, *1045*, 477–493. [CrossRef]
323. Bjornevik, K.; Münz, C.; Cohen, J.I.; Ascherio, A. Epstein-Barr virus as a leading cause of multiple sclerosis: Mechanisms and implications. *Nat. Rev. Neurol.* **2023**, *19*, 160–171. [CrossRef] [PubMed]

324. Chen, W.-J.; Yu, X.; Lu, Y.-Q.; Pfeiffer, R.M.; Ling, W.; Xie, S.-H.; Wu, Z.-C.; Li, X.-Q.; Fan, Y.-Y.; Wu, B.-H.; et al. Impact of an EBV Serology-Based Screening Program on Nasopharyngeal Carcinoma Mortality: A Cluster Randomized Controlled Trial. *J. Clin. Oncol.* 2024; in press.
325. Morgan, E.; Arnold, M.; Camargo, M.C.; Gini, A.; Kunzmann, A.T.; Matsuda, T.; Meheus, F.; Verhoeven, R.H.A.; Vignat, J.; Laversanne, M.; et al. The current and future incidence and mortality of gastric cancer in 185 countries, 2020–2040: A population-based modelling study. *EClinicalMedicine* 2022, *47*, 101404. [CrossRef]
326. Huang, R.J.; Epplein, M.; Hamashima, C.; Choi, I.J.; Lee, E.; Deapen, D.; Woo, Y.; Tran, T.; Shah, S.C.; Inadomi, J.M.; et al. An Approach to the Primary and Secondary Prevention of Gastric Cancer in the United States. *Clin. Gastroenterol. Hepatol.* 2022, *20*, 2218–2228.e2212. [CrossRef]
327. Lee, E.; Tsai, K.Y.; Zhang, J.; Hwang, A.E.; Deapen, D.; Koh, J.J.; Kawaguchi, E.S.; Buxbaum, J.; Ahn, S.H.; Liu, L. Population-based evaluation of disparities in stomach cancer by nativity among Asian and Hispanic populations in California, 2011–2015. *Cancer* 2024, *130*, 1092–1100. [CrossRef]
328. In, H.; Solsky, I.; Castle, P.E.; Schechter, C.B.; Parides, M.; Friedmann, P.; Wylie-Rosett, J.; Kemeny, M.M.; Rapkin, B.D. Utilizing Cultural and Ethnic Variables in Screening Models to Identify Individuals at High Risk for Gastric Cancer: A Pilot Study. *Cancer Prev. Res.* 2020, *13*, 687–698. [CrossRef]
329. Greenberg, E.R.; Anderson, G.L.; Morgan, D.R.; Torres, J.; Chey, W.D.; Bravo, L.E.; Dominguez, R.L.; Ferreccio, C.; Herrero, R.; Lazcano-Ponce, E.C.; et al. 14-day triple, 5-day concomitant, and 10-day sequential therapies for Helicobacter pylori infection in seven Latin American sites: A randomised trial. *Lancet* 2011, *378*, 507–514. [CrossRef] [PubMed]
330. Morgan, D.R.; Torres, J.; Sexton, R.; Herrero, R.; Salazar-Martínez, E.; Greenberg, E.R.; Bravo, L.E.; Dominguez, R.L.; Ferreccio, C.; Lazcano-Ponce, E.C.; et al. Risk of recurrent Helicobacter pylori infection 1 year after initial eradication therapy in 7 Latin American communities. *JAMA* 2013, *309*, 578–586. [CrossRef]
331. Sarıkaya, B.; Çetinkaya, R.A.; Özyiğitoğlu, D.; Işık, S.A.; Kaplan, M.; Kırkık, D.; Görenek, L. High antibiotic resistance rates in Helicobacter pylori strains in Turkey over 20 years: Implications for gastric disease treatment. *Eur. J. Gastroenterol. Hepatol.* 2024, *36*, 545–553. [CrossRef]
332. Garvey, E.; Rhead, J.; Suffian, S.; Whiley, D.; Mahmood, F.; Bakshi, N.; Letley, D.; White, J.; Atherton, J.; Winter, J.A.; et al. High incidence of antibiotic resistance amongst isolates of Helicobacter pylori collected in Nottingham, UK, between 2001 and 2018. *J. Med. Microbiol.* 2023, *72*, 1. [CrossRef]
333. Dutta, S.; Jain, S.; Das, K.; Verma, P.; Som, A.; Das, R. Primary antibiotic resistance of Helicobacter pylori in India over the past two decades: A systematic review. *Helicobacter* 2024, *29*, e13057. [CrossRef]
334. Shrestha, A.B.; Pokharel, P.; Sapkota, U.H.; Shrestha, S.; Mohamed, S.A.; Khanal, S.; Jha, S.K.; Mohanty, A.; Padhi, B.K.; Asija, A.; et al. Drug Resistance Patterns of Commonly Used Antibiotics for the Treatment of Helicobacter pylori Infection among South Asian Countries: A Systematic Review and Meta-Analysis. *Trop. Med. Infect. Dis.* 2023, *8*, 172. [CrossRef] [PubMed]
335. National Cancer Institute Clinical Trials and Translational Researchadvisory Committee (CTAC) Gastric and Esophageal Cancers Working Group. Work Group Report. 2022. Available online: https://deainfo.nci.nih.gov/advisory/ctac/workgroup/gec/2022-11-09-GECWG-Report.pdf (accessed on 21 August 2024).
336. Huang, Y.K.; Yu, J.C.; Kang, W.M.; Ma, Z.Q.; Ye, X.; Tian, S.B.; Yan, C. Significance of Serum Pepsinogens as a Biomarker for Gastric Cancer and Atrophic Gastritis Screening: A Systematic Review and Meta-Analysis. *PLoS ONE* 2015, *10*, e0142080. [CrossRef]
337. Syrjänen, K. Accuracy of Serum Biomarker Panel (GastroPanel(®)) in the Diagnosis of Atrophic Gastritis of the Corpus. Systematic Review and Meta-analysis. *Anticancer. Res.* 2022, *42*, 1679–1696. [CrossRef]
338. Lee, S.Y.; Ahn, Y.S.; Moon, H.W. Comparison between the GastroPanel test and the serum pepsinogen assay interpreted with the ABC method-A prospective study. *Helicobacter* 2024, *29*, e13056. [CrossRef]
339. Dos Santos Viana, I.; Cordeiro Santos, M.L.; Santos Marques, H.; Lima de Souza Gonçalves, V.; Bittencourt de Brito, B.; França da Silva, F.A.; Oliveira, E.S.N.; Dantas Pinheiro, F.; Fernandes Teixeira, A.; Tanajura Costa, D.; et al. Vaccine development against Helicobacter pylori: From ideal antigens to the current landscape. *Expert. Rev. Vaccines* 2021, *20*, 989–999. [CrossRef]
340. Robinson, K.; Lehours, P. Review—Helicobacter, inflammation, immunology and vaccines. *Helicobacter* 2020, *25* (Suppl. 1), e12737. [CrossRef]
341. Sedarat, Z.; Taylor-Robinson, A.W. Helicobacter pylori Outer Membrane Proteins and Virulence Factors: Potential Targets for Novel Therapies and Vaccines. *Pathogens* 2024, *13*, 392. [CrossRef]
342. Best, L.M.; Takwoingi, Y.; Siddique, S.; Selladurai, A.; Gandhi, A.; Low, B.; Yaghoobi, M.; Gurusamy, K.S. Non-invasive diagnostic tests for Helicobacter pylori infection. *Cochrane Database Syst. Rev.* 2018, *3*, Cd012080. [CrossRef]
343. Khadangi, F.; Yassi, M.; Kerachian, M.A. Review: Diagnostic accuracy of PCR-based detection tests for Helicobacter Pylori in stool samples. *Helicobacter* 2017, *22*. [CrossRef]
344. Nieuwenburg, S.A.V.; Mommersteeg, M.C.; Wolters, L.M.M.; van Vuuren, A.J.; Erler, N.; Peppelenbosch, M.P.; Fuhler, G.M.; Bruno, M.J.; Kuipers, E.J.; Spaander, M.C.W. Accuracy of H. pylori fecal antigen test using fecal immunochemical test (FIT). *Gastric Cancer* 2022, *25*, 375–381. [CrossRef]
345. Lei, W.Y.; Lee, J.Y.; Chuang, S.L.; Bair, M.J.; Chen, C.L.; Wu, J.Y.; Wu, D.C.; Tien O'Donnell, F.; Tien, H.W.; Chen, Y.R.; et al. Eradicating Helicobacter pylori via (13)C-urea breath screening to prevent gastric cancer in indigenous communities: A population-based study and development of a family index-case method. *Gut* 2023, *72*, 2231–2240. [CrossRef] [PubMed]

346. Kaur, G.; Danovaro-Holliday, M.C.; Mwinnyaa, G.; Gacic-Dobo, M.; Francis, L.; Grevendonk, J.; Sodha, S.V.; Sugerman, C.; Wallace, A. Routine Vaccination Coverage—Worldwide, 2022. *MMWR Morb. Mortal. Wkly. Rep.* **2023**, *72*, 1155–1161. [CrossRef] [PubMed]
347. Global burden of 288 causes of death and life expectancy decomposition in 204 countries and territories and 811 subnational locations, 1990-2021: A systematic analysis for the Global Burden of Disease Study 2021. *Lancet* **2024**, *403*, 2100–2132. [CrossRef] [PubMed]
348. World Health Organization. The Top 10 Causes of Death. Available online: https://www.who.int/news-room/fact-sheets/detail/the-top-10-causes-of-death#:~:text=The%20top%20global%20causes%20of,birth%20asphyxia%20and%20birth%20trauma, (accessed on 23 April 2024).
349. Ritchie, H.; Spooner, F.; Roser, M. Clean water. Available online: https://ourworldindata.org/clean-water (accessed on 23 April 2024).
350. Guida, F.; Kidman, R.; Ferlay, J.; Schüz, J.; Soerjomataram, I.; Kithaka, B.; Ginsburg, O.; Mailhot Vega, R.B.; Galukande, M.; Parham, G.; et al. Global and regional estimates of orphans attributed to maternal cancer mortality in 2020. *Nat. Med.* **2022**, *28*, 2563–2572. [CrossRef] [PubMed]
351. Nguyen, D.T.N.; Hughes, S.; Egger, S.; LaMontagne, D.S.; Simms, K.; Castle, P.E.; Canfell, K. Risk of childhood mortality associated with death of a mother in low-and-middle-income countries: A systematic review and meta-analysis. *BMC Public Health* **2019**, *19*, 1281. [CrossRef] [PubMed]
352. Woldemariam, M.T.; Jimma, W. Adoption of electronic health record systems to enhance the quality of healthcare in low-income countries: A systematic review. *BMJ Health Care Inform.* **2023**, *30*, e100704. [CrossRef]

Disclaimer/Publisher's Note: The statements, opinions and data contained in all publications are solely those of the individual author(s) and contributor(s) and not of MDPI and/or the editor(s). MDPI and/or the editor(s) disclaim responsibility for any injury to people or property resulting from any ideas, methods, instructions or products referred to in the content.

Article

HPV16 *E6* Oncogene Contributes to Cancer Immune Evasion by Regulating PD-L1 Expression through a miR-143/HIF-1a Pathway

Georgios Konstantopoulos [1,†], Danai Leventakou [2,†], Despoina-Rozi Saltiel [1], Efthalia Zervoudi [3], Eirini Logotheti [1], Spyros Pettas [1], Korina Karagianni [1], Angeliki Daiou [1], Konstantinos E. Hatzistergos [1], Dimitra Dafou [1], Minas Arsenakis [1], Amanda Psyrri [4,*] and Christine Kottaridi [1,*]

1. Department of Genetics, Development and Molecular Biology, School of Biology, Aristotle University of Thessaloniki, 54124 Thessaloniki, Greece; konstanto@bio.auth.gr (G.K.); dessalton@bio.auth.gr (D.-R.S.); eirinilg@bio.auth.gr (E.L.); spyrospg@bio.auth.gr (S.P.); korinagk@bio.auth.gr (K.K.); angeldaiou@bio.auth.gr (A.D.); kchatzistergos@bio.auth.gr (K.E.H.); dafoud@bio.auth.gr (D.D.); arsenaki@bio.auth.gr (M.A.)
2. 2nd Department of Pathology, University General Hospital Attikon, School of Medicine, National and Kapodistrian University of Athens, 12462 Athens, Greece; dleventakou@med.uoa.gr
3. Research Unit—Oncology Unit, University General Hospital Attikon, School of Medicine, National and Kapodistrian University of Athens, 12462 Athens, Greece; t.zervoudi@hotmail.com
4. Section of Medical Oncology, Department of Internal Medicine, Attikon University Hospital, Faculty of Medicine, National and Kapodistrian University of Athens, 12462 Athens, Greece
* Correspondence: dpsyrri@med.uoa.gr or psyrri237@yahoo.com (A.P.); ckottaridi@bio.auth.gr (C.K.)
† These authors contributed equally to this work.

Abstract: Human Papillomaviruses have been associated with the occurrence of cervical cancer, the fourth most common cancer that affects women globally, while 70% of cases are caused by infection with the high-risk types HPV16 and HPV18. The integration of these viruses' oncogenes *E6* and *E7* into the host's genome affects a multitude of cellular functions and alters the expression of molecules. The aim of this study was to investigate how these oncogenes contribute to the expression of immune system control molecules, using cell lines with integrated HPV16 genome, before and after knocking out *E6* viral gene using the CRISPR/Cas9 system, delivered with a lentiviral vector. The molecules studied are the T-cell inactivating protein PD-L1, its transcription factor HIF-1a and the latter's negative regulator, miR-143. According to our results, in the E6 knock out (E6KO) cell lines an increased expression of miR-143 was recorded, while a decrease in the expression of HIF-1a and PD-L1 was exhibited. These findings indicate that E6 protein probably plays a significant role in enabling cervical cancer cells to evade the immune system, while we propose a molecular pathway in cervical cancer, where PD-L1's expression is regulated by E6 protein through a miR-143/HIF-1a axis.

Keywords: HPV16; cervical cancer; immune escape; hypoxia; microRNAs; E6; PD-L1; HIF-1a; miR-143

1. Introduction

Cervical cancer is the fourth most common type of cancer among women worldwide, while more than 95% of total cases are linked to infection with the Human Papillomavirus (HPV) [1,2]. In 2020, there were 604,000 cases of cervical cancer, 342,000 of which led to death [2]. The vast majority of these cases were limited to low- and middle-income countries, considering the lack of prophylactic vaccines and screening methods that are widely used in high-income countries and serve as means for the prevention and early diagnosis of the disease [1,3].

Human Papillomaviruses can be classified according to their ability to either cause benign lesions (low-risk, LR) or lead to several types of cancer (high-risk, HR) [4]. Two of these, HPV16 and HPV18, are responsible for most HPV-related cancers and are the causative agent for approximately 70% of all cervical cancer cases, while HPV16 by its own is responsible for 55% of all cases [4,5].

The HPV genome is a small circular double-stranded DNA of almost 8 kb and it is segmented into three regions: the early region (E) that encodes proteins E1, E2, E4, E5, E6 and E7, the late region (L) which encodes proteins—and L2, and the long control region (LCR) also known as non-coding region (NCR) or upstream regulatory region (URR) [6,7]. The early proteins are necessary for genome replication and transcription, with E5, E6, and E7 being responsible for oncogenesis [4,6]. *L1* and *L2* are important for the viral structure, given that they code the major and minor capsid proteins, respectively, whereas the LCR region does not code any proteins but contains various binding sites for transcription factors [6].

During HPV infection, the viral genome that naturally exists in a circular episomal form can break and integrate into the host's genome, an event that aids cancer progression. The most common site of integration has been reported to be the E2 ORF, resulting in the loss of the E2 protein, which normally negatively regulates the E6 and E7 oncoproteins [7,8]. Additionally, throughout persistent HPV infection, multiple HPV genes can be expressed by a single strand as a polycistronic pre-mRNA, while several transcripts are produced by alternative splicing, which generates different mRNA expression patterns. Alternative splicing within E6–E7 ORFs is a really common for HR-HPVs, in contrast to LR-HPVs where no splicing in this region has been noticed [9]. Apart from the full-length E6, which is produced from mRNAs with no splicing within E6 ORF, alternative splicing can generate several transcripts containing E6 truncated mRNAs, named E6*I, E6*II, and E6^E7, which are derived from a donor splicing site within the E6 ORF and one of the various acceptor sites located in the early mRNA [9,10]. Protein products generated from the HPV16 E6*I and E6*II transcripts are quite similar. However, it is suggested that they might play different cellular roles, enriching the ways HPV16 can dysregulate the host's molecular networks and pathways [10].

E6 and E7 activation plays a pivotal role in the development of cancer, considering these proteins' ability to interfere with many cellular pathways, but most importantly by dysregulating cell cycle, proliferation and apoptosis [6,11]. The way to achieve that is with the well-established process of ubiquitin-dependent proteasome degradation of p53—which regulates apoptosis—by E6 and the inhibition of the retinoblastoma protein (pRb) —which promotes cell cycle progression—by E7. However, E6 seems to participate in another crucial part of malignancy progression, the evasion of host's immune system [11,12].

HPV is considered a successful pathogen as it has the ability to evade host immune responses and establish long-term persistent infection. The immune checkpoints are critical to maintain tolerance against autoimmunity in physiologic conditions [13]. Programmed cell death protein 1 (PD-1) is a transmembrane protein that acts as a checkpoint molecule on T cells and is overexpressed in the tumor environment [13,14]. Its ligand, programmed death-ligand 1 (PD-L1), is a critical immune checkpoint molecule that has also been observed to be overexpressed on several types of tumors, and cervical cancer appears to be no exception [15,16]. PD-L1 (encoded by *CD274*) is a transmembrane protein synthesized in the endoplasmic reticulum of tumor cells and its interaction with the programmed cell death protein 1 on T-cells restrains antitumor immunity by T-cell activation inhibition or apoptosis, thus leading to cancer's immune evasion [15,17]. This information renders PD-L1 a possible candidate as a biomarker for cancer prognosis as well as a target for cancer treatment [14,16]. PD-L1 has also been reported to be upregulated under hypoxic conditions, a significant characteristic of tumor microenvironment [18,19].

HIF-1α is a transcription factor that plays a central role in the response to low oxygen levels, or hypoxia, within the tumor microenvironment [20]. HIF-1α's primary function is to enable cells to adapt to low oxygen, making it a critical player in the survival of both normal and cancer cells [19]. The interaction between PD-L1 and HIF-1α is complex. Under conditions of hypoxia, HIF-1α can upregulate the expression of PD-L1 in cancer cells. This means that in the hypoxic regions of tumors, where immune cells often struggle to function due to low oxygen levels, cancer cells can increase their expression of PD-L1 [18,21,22]. Consequently, this makes the tumor microenvironment even more inhospitable to immune cells, allowing the cancer to evade detection and destruction by the immune system [21,22].

MicroRNAs are small non-coding RNA molecules of 19–25 nucleotides that target and regulate a multitude of mRNAs [23]. The observation that these molecules' expression is differentiated in several diseases, including cancer, has put a magnifying lens on them as possible biomarkers or therapeutic targets [24,25]. As far as HPV-related cervical cancer is concerned, it has been reported that HPV's oncoproteins, E6 and E7, seem to target and modify the expression of a plethora of miRNAs, consequently intervening in cellular pathways [23]. HIF-1a appears to be targeted by various microRNAs, one of which is miR-143 that has been reported to negatively regulate the expression of HIF-1a [20,26,27]. Finally, studies on miR-143 have shown the molecule's aberrant expression in different types of cancer, with the example of cervical cancer, where miR-143 is down-regulated [24,27].

The aim of the present study is to investigate whether HPV16 E6 oncoprotein plays an interplay with a host's critical immune checkpoint molecule, as well as a known transcription factor that regulates its expression. Undertaking this endeavor, we are committed to understanding the mechanism behind this interaction, with the exploration of a network or a possible molecular pathway that includes HPV16 E6, a miRNA, HIF-1a and PD-L1 that probably promotes cervical cancer's immune evasion.

2. Materials and Methods

2.1. Cell Cultures

SiHa, CaSki and HEK293T cell lines were purchased from the American Type Culture Collection (ATCC) (Manassas, VA, USA) and grown in Dulbecco's Modified Eagle medium (DMEM, Biowest #L0103) supplemented with 10% fetal bovine serum (FBS, Biowest #S1810) (Gibco/Invitrogen; Thermo Fisher Scientific, Inc., Waltham, MA, USA), 1% L-Glutamine (Biowest #X0550) and 1% Penicillin-Streptomycin (Biowest #L0022). According to the ATCC, SiHa cells contain 1–2 copies of the HPV16 genome per cell, whereas CaSki cells contain approximately 600 copies per cell. HCK1T cervical keratinocytes were purchased from Dr Tohru Kiyono of the National Cancer Center Research Institute (Chuo-ku, Tokyo, Japan) [28] to be used as a control and were cultured in KSFM (Keratinocyte serum-free medium, Gibco, #17005042) supplemented with 25 mg Bovine Pituitary Extract (BPE), 2.5 μg EGF, 1% L-Glutamine and 1% Penicillin-Streptomycin as proposed [29]. All cell lines were cultured in a humidified incubator at 37 °C with 5% CO_2. Wild type cells were harvested after reaching approximately 80% confluence in 100 mm cell culture dishes.

2.2. Lentivirus Construction and Cell Transfection

The CRISPRdirect online tool (https://crispr.dbcls.jp/ accessed on 10 January 2023) was used to design HPV16 E6 specific sgRNAs that include the PAM sequence, necessary for the recognition from the CRISPR-Cas9 system. Several proposed sgRNAs were tested in order to opt for the sgRNA set that knocks E6 out sufficiently. The sgRNAs we ended up using were 16E6T2A (5′-CACCGTCCATAATATAAGGGGTCGG-3′) and 16E6T2B (5′-AAACCCGACCCCTTATATTATGGAC-3′) and they were used for ligation into the lentiCRISPRv2 plasmid (Addgene #52961) which was digested with the BsmBI-v2 digestion enzyme (New England Biolabs, #R0739). The ligated plasmid was cloned into TOP10 competent cells via heat shock and grown on LB agar plates supplemented with ampicillin (100 μg/mL). Colonies were subjected to colony PCR to ensure successful insertion of the sgRNAs, using the universal primer hU6-F (5′-GAGGGCCTATTTCCCATGATT-3′) as a forward primer and as a reverse primer, the reverse sgRNA of each pair. Positive colonies were grown overnight in LB broth supplemented with ampicillin (100 μg/mL). The plasmid was extracted using the MACHEREY-NAGEL Plasmid DNA purification NucleoBond Xtra Maxi (#740414) and was used for transfection of HEK293T cells, using the calcium phosphate method, with the packaging and envelope plasmids psPAX2 (Addgene

#12260) and pMD2.G (Addgene #12259). The produced lentivirus was isolated 3 days later by penetrating the media of the transfected cells through a 0.45 mm filter and was used for the transduction of SiHa and CaSki cells which have the HPV16 genome integrated, aiming to knock-out the *E6* oncogene. Optimal lentivirus concentration was determined by using various concentrations of a lentiviral system expressing the green fluorescent protein (GFP). Transfected cells were selected with puromycin (4 µg/mL). In order to have sufficient RNA and protein to extract from the KO cells and to avoid extensive cell-death, transfection was performed in ~80% confluent cells in 100 mm culture dishes and the cells were harvested 4 days post-transfection. Concurrently, we conducted an experiment in which we possessed 3 flasks of the same cell line: one control (untreated cells), one transfected flask (harvested 4 days after puromycin treatment which is the flask used for in vitro experiments) and one flask as apoptosis «observatory», in order to evaluate both changes to cell morphology and decrease in number of viable cells. Successful *E6* knock-out was confirmed by checking p53 protein levels.

2.3. Western Blot

Protein was extracted from harvested cells using an RIPA buffer (Cell Signaling, #9806) supplemented with PMSF (Cell Signaling, #8553) and protein concentration was calculated with Bradford assay. Total protein extracts were subjected to electrophoresis on 10% SDS-polyacrylamide gels and transferred on PVDF membranes. After blocking with 5% non-fat milk in TBS-T, the membranes were probed overnight at 4 °C with the following antibodies diluted in the same blocking buffer: anti-p53 (1:2000, mouse, Dako, #M7001), anti-HIF-1a (1:1000, rabbit, Cell Signaling Technology, #36169), anti-PD-L1 (1:500 mouse, Origene, #TA808771), and anti-β-actin (1:2000, mouse, Cell Signaling Technology, #3700). Then, the membranes were washed with TBS-T and incubated for 1 h at room temperature with the following species-specific HRP-linked secondary antibodies: anti-mouse (1:4000 Cell Signaling Technology, #7076) and anti-rabbit (1: 4000 Cell Signaling Technology, #7074). After brief washing with TBS-T, membranes were incubated with LumiGLO chemiluminescent substrate and hydrogen peroxide (Cell Signaling Technology, #7003) and pictures were captured using the Invitrogen iBright FL1500 Imaging System.

2.4. qPCR

Harvested cells were subjected to RNA extraction using the TRIzol™ Reagent. Then, the RNA was used for cDNA synthesis, using both SuperScript III Reverse Transcriptase (Invitrogen, #18080) and Mir-X™ miRNA First Strand Synthesis Kit (Takara, #638315). The cDNA was used as a template for qPCR, for which we selected the following primer sets: HIF-1aF (5′-TCTCCATCT-CCTACCCACATACA-3′) with HIF-1aR (5′-TGCTCTGTTTGGTG AGGCTGT-3′), PD-L1F (5′-TATGGTGGTGCCGACTACAA-3′) with PD-L1R (5′-TGGCTCC CAGAATTACCAAG-3′), and GUSBF (5′-CTCATTTGGAATTTTGCCGATT-3′) with GUSBR (5′-CCGAGTGAAGATCCCCTTTTTA-3′). GUSB was used as the internal control for comparative CT analysis. For miR-143 detection, a miR-143 forward primer was designed using the miRprimer2 software version 2.0 (5′-TGCAGTGCTGCATCTCT-3′) and a universal miRNA reverse primer was used that was supplied from the Mir-X™ miRNA First Strand Synthesis Kit. The same kit provided us with a U6 forward and reverse primer set to use as the internal control for comparative CT analysis. The mastermix used was Xpert Fast SYBR (GRiSP, #GE20). Samples were run in an Applied Biosystems StepOnePlus™ Real-Time PCR System and results were received through the StepOne Software v2.3.

2.5. Statistical Analysis

Western blot images were quantified using ImageJ (v1.54g) and protein expression was normalized to β-actin expression levels. qPCR results were analyzed using the ΔΔCt method on Microsoft Excel for Microsoft 365 MSO (Version 2309). All experiments were conducted in triplicates. The graphs were created in GraphPad Prism 8 and presented as

3. Results

3.1. p53 Protein Levels as a Marker for Successful E6 Knock-Out

To confirm the successful knock-out of the *E6* oncogene in the transfected cell lines that carry the HPV16 genome, we determined p53 protein levels via Western blot, taking into consideration the fact that *E6* integration and activation into the host's genome leads to p53 degradation and contributes to the establishment of the proliferative profile of cancer. As it is presented in Figure 1, the E6KO SiHa and CaSki cell lines exhibit a statistically significant rise in the p53 protein levels when compared to the wild type (WT) control cells. To be precise, in the E6 knock-out cell lines, a second band appears in the blots which can be attributed to the presence of the Δ40p53 isoform of the p53 protein that is mainly targeted and degraded by the E6*II splice variant of E6 [10]. These results show that p53 degradation is reduced in the E6KO cell lines, meaning that *E6* is sufficiently silenced.

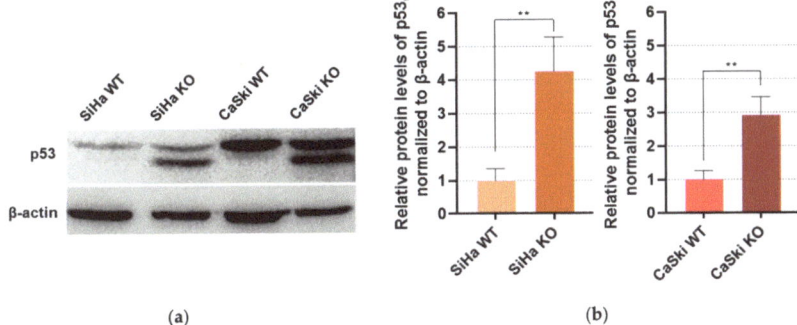

Figure 1. (a) Western blot for p53 in SiHa and CaSki cell lines, before and after E6 knock-out. β-actin served as the internal control; (b) Bar graphs depicting p53 levels in the cell protein extracts. ** $p \leq 0.01$.

3.2. E6KO in Cervical Cancer Cell Lines Downregulates PD-L1 Expression

Firstly, the mRNA levels of PD-L1 were calculated via qPCR to determine whether PD-L1's gene expression levels are upregulated in SiHa and CaSki wild type cell lines in comparison with the normal cervical keratinocytes HCK1T. As shown in Figure 2a, we indeed noticed a more than threefold increase in PD-L1's transcript levels in the cancer cell lines. However, PD-L1 is significantly downregulated in the E6KO cell lines. This was further confirmed with Western blot targeting PD-L1 in protein extracts derived from SiHa and CaSki cells before and after E6KO, shown in Figure 2b,c. Additionally, PD-L1 levels of E6KO cells were compared to HCK1T cells and displayed non-significant differences (Figure S1). These results suggest that PD-L1 overexpression in HPV16 positive cervical cancer is related to the activation of E6 in the tumor microenvironment.

3.3. HIF-1a Expression Is Controlled by E6 in Cervical Cancer

In order to assess HIF-1a expression, we conducted qPCR on the cDNAs created by the cell lines' RNA extracts. As it can be observed in Figure 3a, hypoxia-inducible factor-1a is upregulated in cervical cancer cells in comparison to the normal cervical cells. Conversely, the knock-out of *E6* appears to result in a decrease in the transcript levels of HIF-1a, proposing that the aforementioned upregulation is an aftereffect of the E6 activation in HPV16 derived cancer. Moreover, after knocking *E6* out, HIF-1a levels seem to be similar to the normal cervical keratinocytes (Figure S2). Additionally, as shown in Figure 3b,c, HIF-1a protein levels seem to significantly drop in the KO cell lines, further supporting this hypothesis.

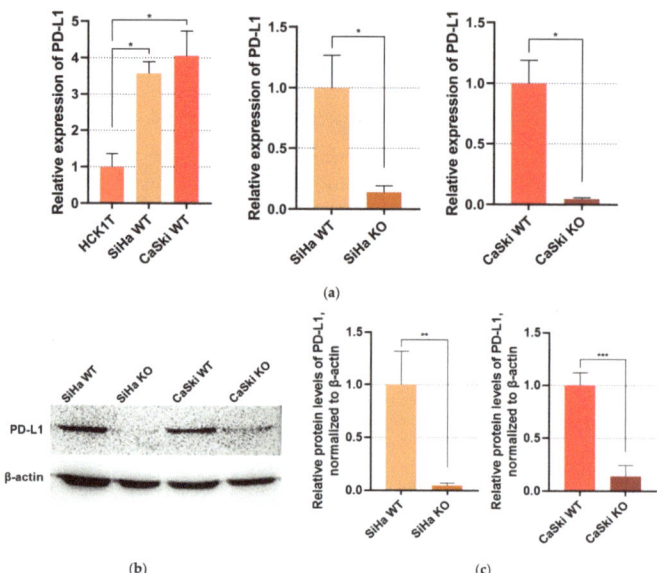

Figure 2. (**a**) Bar graphs representing qPCR results. WT cervical cancer cell lines SiHa and CaSki were compared to normal cervical keratinocytes HCK1T, while E6KO SiHa and CaSki were compared to the WT strains. PD-L1 expression was normalized with GUSB; (**b**) Western blot for PD-L1 in SiHa and CaSki cell lines, before and after *E6* knock-out. β-actin served as the internal control; (**c**) Bar graphs depicting PD-L1 levels in the cell protein extracts. * $p \leq 0.05$, ** $p \leq 0.01$, *** $p \leq 0.001$.

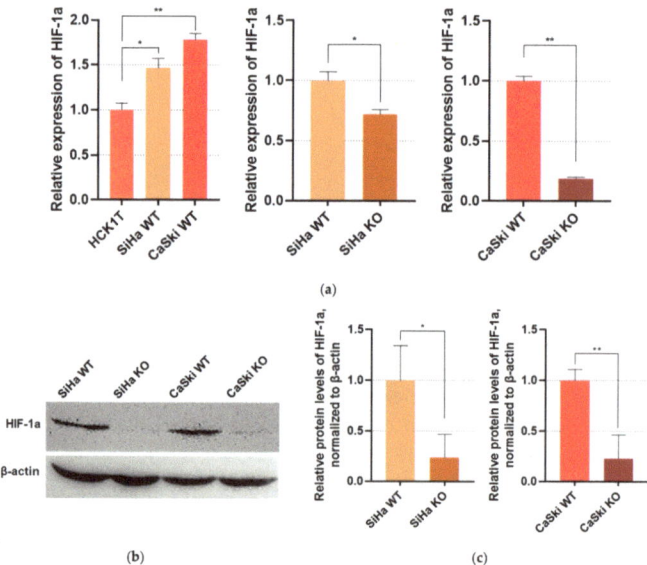

Figure 3. (**a**) Bar graphs representing qPCR results. WT cervical cancer cell lines SiHa and CaSki were compared to normal cervical keratinocytes HCK1T, while E6KO SiHa and CaSki were compared to the WT strains. HIF-1a expression was normalized with GUSB; (**b**) Western blot for HIF-1a in SiHa and CaSki cell lines, before and after *E6* knock-out. β-actin served as the internal control; (**c**) Bar graphs depicting HIF-1a levels in the cell protein extracts. * $p \leq 0.05$, ** $p \leq 0.01$.

3.4. E6 Inactivation Increases miR-143 Levels

Lastly, we needed to evaluate microRNA-143 expression levels in the cell extracts. To this end, we conducted qPCR using microRNA-specific cDNA libraries of the cell lines and the results we received are presented in Figure 4. miR-143 seems to be downregulated in WT SiHa and CaSki cells when compared to the HCK1T keratinocytes. Nonetheless, miR-143 is considerably upregulated in the cancer cell lines subjected to *E6* knock-out and does not show significant difference in expression when compared to the HCK1T cells (Figure S3).

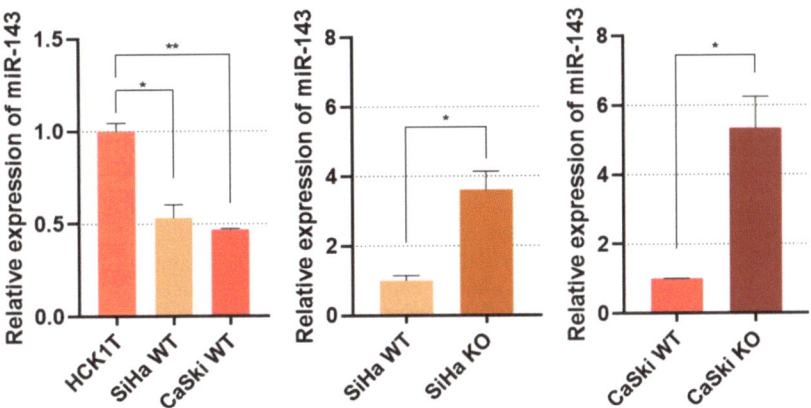

Figure 4. Bar graphs representing qPCR results. WT cervical cancer cell lines SiHa and CaSki were compared to normal cervical keratinocytes HCK1T, while E6KO SiHa and CaSki were compared to the WT strains. miR-143 expression was normalized with U6. * $p \leq 0.05$, ** $p \leq 0.01$.

4. Discussion

Cervical cancer is the most common HPV-related disease with an overall 5-year relative survival rate of 67% [2,30]. Patients diagnosed with cervical cancer may be subjected to a variety of treatment schemes consisting of radiation therapy, chemotherapy and immunotherapy, to name but a few [30]. An immunotherapy drug that has shown potential in increasing survival rate to patients with different types of cervical cancer is Pembrolizumab, a monoclonal antibody that targets and binds on the PD-1 protein on the surface of T-cells, thus denying PD-1/PD-L1 interaction and allowing T-cell mediated destruction of cancer cells [31,32]. Several studies have reported that a great number of cervical carcinomas overexpress PD-L1 [15,16,31,32], findings that go in line with the results of our study, where we showed upregulated expression of the specific molecule in cervical cancer cell lines that carry the HPV16 genome. So, our initial scientific question was the possible role of viral oncogenes and specifically of *E6*, in pathways that take part in PD-L1 regulation, to answer this question regarding the knocking-out of *E6* oncogene constituted our strategy. Definitely, we strongly kept in mind that *E6* knockouts lead to apoptosis and cell death of HPV containing cell lines [33]. Provided that for the apoptotic response 4–6 days are needed in order to notice any difference in cell viability [34], cells in our experimental model were harvested 4 days post-transfection while an additional flask with *E6* KO cells evaluated in parallel both for changes to cell morphology and decrease in number of viable cells.

As far as HPV16-related cervical cancer is concerned, our results indicate that the E6 oncoprotein seems to contribute to the PD-L1 overexpression, considering that PD-L1 levels drop significantly in the cell lines that have gone through E6 knock-out. This implies that *E6* integration in the host's genome triggers a number of alterations that ultimately lead to cancer cells escaping immunosurveillance. In order to unravel the mystery of which molecules take part in this event, it was important to examine PD-L1's transcription factors.

Hypoxia-inducible factor-1a is an important transcription factor that has been proven to act as a master regulator of quite a few genes, especially in the hypoxic tumor microenvironment where HIF-1a thrives. In a normal aerobic environment, HIF-1a is regulated by the ubiquitin-protease system, so its expression in normal cells is not stable. On the contrary, in the tumor microenvironment, hypoxia leads to the continuous accumulation of HIF-1α, making cancer cells continuously adapt to hypoxia [35]. HIF-1a is in an interplay with all hallmarks of cancer, like genomic instability, inflammation, vascularization, tumor invasion and survival, amongst others [36,37]. Furthermore, there is strong evidence that HIF-1a reinforces cancer's immune evasion by dysregulating various characteristic mechanisms of immune response, like the production of cytokines, assisting the activity of immunosuppressive M2 macrophages in addition to inducing the expression of immune checkpoint inhibitors [38,39]. PD-L1 is one of these immune checkpoint molecules that fall under the regulatory control of HIF-1a.

Studies in the past have showcased HIF-1a's ability to positively regulate PD-L1 under hypoxic conditions, as well as HPV16 E6's upregulation of HIF-1a in the tumor microenvironment [40,41]. However, the molecular mechanism of the interaction between HIF-1a and PD-L1 in the presence of HPV16 in cervical cancer has not been studied. Our research strongly supports the existing data, given that HIF-1a mRNA levels appear significantly increased in the cervical cancer cell lines when compared to the normal cervical keratinocytes, and correlates E6's presence in the cancer cells with HIF-1a's expression increase. To elaborate, knocking *E6* out considerably decreases HIF-1a's levels, a change that, in combination with PD-L1's decrease in the E6KO cell lines, implicates that PD-L1's upregulation in HPV16-caused cervical cancer happens in a HIF-1a related manner.

An additional effect of the presence and accumulation of HIF-1a in tumors is presumed to be the contribution to tumor chemoresistance by obstructing drug transport and uptake, whereas its overexpression is linked to worse prognosis for patients with cervical cancer [39,42]. On the other hand, a molecule that has given signs of decreasing cancer cell resistance to chemotherapeutics in addition to inhibiting several of the hallmarks of cancer, like proliferation, tumor invasion and metastasis, is microRNA-143 [43–46].

MicroRNAs regulate a wide range of biological processes in the host-pathogen interactions and are commonly encoded by viruses that undergo long-term persistent infection, including HPV, acting either as oncogenes or as tumor suppressors by targeting different mRNAs. Dysregulation of miRNA expression causes abnormal cell growth and differentiation, assisting to the development of cancer or other diseases [24]. The expression of several miRNAs in cervical cancer has been studied in order to further understand the way the Human Papillomaviruses interact with the host's cellular pathways, and this research still has a lot to unravel. MicroRNAs' expression profiles seem to differ depending on the tissue studied and the cancer differentiation state, making the classification of each biomolecule difficult. MicroRNA-143 has been reported to be up- or downregulated in the tumor microenvironment of different tissues [47]. However, when it comes to cervical cancer, many studies agree on miR-143's down-regulation throughout all the stages of cancer progression when compared to healthy tissue [23,24,27,47]. Our study's findings are consistent with this data, given that miR-143 levels are decreased in SiHa and CaSki cell lines in comparison with the HCK1T normal cervical keratinocytes.

Induced expression of miR-143 in cervical cancer cells resulted into increased apoptosis as well as improved reaction to Cisplatin treatment, data that renders miR-143 a possible tumor-suppressing microRNA, as well as a candidate biomarker for prognosis or the optimization of cervical cancer treatment [27,44] Zhao et al. demonstrated, using dual-luciferase reporter gene assay, that miR-143 directly targets and silences HIF-1a by binding on its 3′UTR, thus, negating the transcription factor's effects in the cervical tumor microenvironment and ameliorating the cancerous phenotype. As mentioned above, in our experiments, miR-143 expression drops in the cells that carry the HPV16 genome, however, this downregulation seems to reverse after the knock-out of *E6* in the same cell lines, where a significant increase in the specific microRNA's levels is exhibited. These results suggest that the expression of miR-143 is regulated by the activation of E6 after its integration into the host's genome.

miR-143 is definitely not the first case of a microRNA being regulated by E6 to promote immune escape of cervical cancer by targeting PD-L1. As Ling et al. have already shown, another miRNA—the miR-142-5p, seems to follow the same expression pattern of miR-143 in cervical cancer, whereas when overexpressed it appears to directly interact with PD-L1 and negatively regulate its expression [48]. Likewise, our results indicate that miR-143 is in an interplay with the expression of PD-L1 in cervical cancer cells, yet this interaction possibly happens in an indirect way, via the HIF-1a inhibition. However, regardless of the way these miRNAs act on the immune checkpoint molecule, they both seem to be targets of the HPV16's E6 oncoprotein.

The way E6 acts on miR-143 is yet to be investigated. A hypothetical way in which E6 affects miR-143's expression could be via the p53 degradation, for there is evidence that supports that p53 post-transcriptionally upregulates miR-143's expression [49,50]. This interaction could explain how *E6* integration into the host's genome results in miR-143's negative regulation, since p53 gets degraded by E6 and can no longer enhance miR-143's expression. Nonetheless, the scenario that E6 directly targets miR-143 in either stage of the microRNA's biogenesis and maturation cannot be ruled out, but more research needs to be conducted. Future experiments, including transfections with synthetic circRNA sponges, represent a strategy for achieving targeted loss of miR143 function where the link between E6–p53–miR143–HIF-1a–PD-L1 would be further enlightened.

5. Conclusions

In order to enhance PD-L1 targeting in cervical cancer treatment and improve response rate, it is crucial to further investigate the molecules and the pathways that take part in PD-L1 regulation. Towards this direction, our endeavor shows our preliminary data regarding a mechanistic pathway were HPV16 viral oncogenes have a possible role. Our data could propose a molecular network that leads to PD-L1's upregulation in HPV16 related cervical cancer through a mir-143/HIF-1a mediated axis and, consequently, to cervical cancer's ability to escape immunosurveillance.

Supplementary Materials: The following supporting information can be downloaded at: https://www.mdpi.com/article/10.3390/v16010113/s1, Figure S1: Bar graphs representing qPCR results. KO cervical cancer cell lines SiHa and CaSki were compared to normal cervical keratinocytes HCK1T. PD-L1 expression was normalized with GUSB. ns = non-significant; Figure S2: Bar graphs representing qPCR results. KO cervical cancer cell lines SiHa and CaSki were compared to normal cervical keratinocytes HCK1T. HIF-1a expression was normalized with GUSB. ns = non-significant; Figure S3: Bar graphs representing qPCR results. KO cervical cancer cell lines SiHa and CaSki were compared to normal cervical keratinocytes HCK1T. miR-143 expression was normalized with U6. ns = non-significant.

Author Contributions: Conceptualization, study design, and supervision, C.K., K.E.H. and D.D.; conducted the experimental work, G.K., D.L., D.-R.S. and E.L.; contributed to the interpretation of the data, E.Z., S.P., K.K. and A.D.; writing—original draft preparation, G.K. and C.K.; conceptualization and supervision, A.P.; review and editing, C.K., K.E.H., D.D. and M.A. All authors have read and agreed to the published version of the manuscript.

Funding: This research was partly funded by the postgraduate program "Applications in Biology", specialization "Applied Genetics and Biodiagnosis".

Institutional Review Board Statement: Not applicable.

Informed Consent Statement: Not applicable.

Data Availability Statement: Data are contained within the article and Supplementary Materials.

Conflicts of Interest: The authors declare no conflicts of interest. The funders had no role in the design of the study; in the collection, analyses, or interpretation of data; in the writing of the manuscript; or in the decision to publish the results.

References

1. Sung, H.; Ferlay, J.; Siegel, R.L.; Laversanne, M.; Soerjomataram, I.; Jemal, A.; Bray, F. Global Cancer Statistics 2020: GLOBOCAN Estimates of Incidence and Mortality Worldwide for 36 Cancers in 185 Countries. *CA Cancer J. Clin.* **2021**, *71*, 209–249. [CrossRef]
2. Cervical Cancer. Available online: https://www.who.int/news-room/fact-sheets/detail/cervical-cancer (accessed on 22 June 2023).
3. Zhu, Y.; Wang, Y.; Hirschhorn, J.; Welsh, K.J.; Zhao, Z.; Davis, M.R.; Feldman, S. Human Papillomavirus and Its Testing Assays, Cervical Cancer Screening, and Vaccination. In *Advances in Clinical Chemistry*; Elsevier: Amsterdam, The Netherlands, 2017; Volume 81, pp. 135–192.
4. Graham, S.V. Human Papillomavirus: Gene Expression, Regulation and Prospects for Novel Diagnostic Methods and Antiviral Therapies. *Future Microbiol.* **2010**, *5*, 1493–1506. [CrossRef] [PubMed]
5. Human Papillomavirus (HPV). Available online: https://www.who.int/teams/health-product-policy-and-standards/standards-and-specifications/vaccine-standardization/human-papillomavirus (accessed on 22 June 2023).
6. Pal, A.; Kundu, R. Human Papillomavirus E6 and E7: The Cervical Cancer Hallmarks and Targets for Therapy. *Front. Microbiol.* **2020**, *10*, 3116. [CrossRef] [PubMed]
7. Zygouras, I.; Leventakou, D.; Pouliakis, A.; Panagiotou, S.; Tsakogiannis, D.; Konstantopoulos, G.; Logotheti, E.; Samaras, M.; Kyriakopoulou, Z.; Beloukas, A.; et al. Human Papillomavirus 16 DNA Methylation Patterns and Investigation of Integration Status in Head and Neck Cancer Cases. *Int. J. Mol. Sci.* **2023**, *24*, 14593. [CrossRef] [PubMed]
8. Williams, V.M.; Filippova, M.; Soto, U.; Duerksen-Hughes, P.J. HPV-DNA Integration and Carcinogenesis: Putative Roles for Inflammation and Oxidative Stress. *Future Virol.* **2011**, *6*, 45–57. [CrossRef] [PubMed]
9. Olmedo-Nieva, L.; Muñoz-Bello, J.O.; Contreras-Paredes, A.; Lizano, M. The Role of E6 Spliced Isoforms (E6*) in Human Papillomavirus-Induced Carcinogenesis. *Viruses* **2018**, *10*, 45. [CrossRef]
10. Antonio-Véjar, V.; Ortiz-Sánchez, E.; Rosendo-Chalma, P.; Patiño-Morales, C.C.; Guido-Jiménez, M.C.; Alvarado-Ortiz, E.; Hernández, G.; García-Carrancá, A. New Insights into the Interactions of HPV-16 E6*I and E6*II with P53 Isoforms and Induction of Apoptosis in Cancer-Derived Cell Lines. *Pathol. Res. Pract.* **2022**, *234*, 153890. [CrossRef]
11. Bhattacharjee, R.; Das, S.S.; Biswal, S.S.; Nath, A.; Das, D.; Basu, A.; Malik, S.; Kumar, L.; Kar, S.; Singh, S.K.; et al. Mechanistic Role of HPV-Associated Early Proteins in Cervical Cancer: Molecular Pathways and Targeted Therapeutic Strategies. *Crit. Rev. Oncol. Hematol.* **2022**, *174*, 103675. [CrossRef]
12. Balasubramaniam, S.D.; Balakrishnan, V.; Oon, C.E.; Kaur, G. Key Molecular Events in Cervical Cancer Development. *Medicina* **2019**, *55*, 384. [CrossRef]
13. Sharpe, A.H.; Wherry, E.J.; Ahmed, R.; Freeman, G.J. The Function of Programmed Cell Death 1 and Its Ligands in Regulating Autoimmunity and Infection. *Nat. Immunol.* **2007**, *8*, 239–245. [CrossRef]
14. Dermani, F.K.; Samadi, P.; Rahmani, G.; Kohlan, A.K.; Najafi, R. PD-1/PD-L1 Immune Checkpoint: Potential Target for Cancer Therapy. *J. Cell. Physiol.* **2019**, *234*, 1313–1325. [CrossRef] [PubMed]
15. Reddy, O.L.; Shintaku, P.I.; Moatamed, N.A. Programmed Death-Ligand 1 (PD-L1) Is Expressed in a Significant Number of the Uterine Cervical Carcinomas. *Diagn. Pathol.* **2017**, *12*, 45. [CrossRef] [PubMed]
16. Nicol, A.F.; de Andrade, C.V.; Gomes, S.C.; Brusadelli, M.G.; Lodin, H.M.; Wells, S.I.; Nuovo, G.J. The Distribution of Novel Biomarkers in Carcinoma-in-Situ, Microinvasive, and Squamous Cell Carcinoma of the Uterine Cervix. *Ann. Diagn. Pathol.* **2019**, *38*, 115–122. [CrossRef] [PubMed]
17. Yi, M.; Niu, M.; Xu, L.; Luo, S.; Wu, K. Regulation of PD-L1 Expression in the Tumor Microenvironment. *J. Hematol. Oncol.* **2021**, *14*, 10. [CrossRef] [PubMed]
18. Wen, Q.; Han, T.; Wang, Z.; Jiang, S. Role and Mechanism of Programmed Death-Ligand 1 in Hypoxia-Induced Liver Cancer Immune Escape. *Oncol. Lett.* **2020**, *19*, 2595–2601. [CrossRef]
19. Rashid, M.; Zadeh, L.R.; Baradaran, B.; Molavi, O.; Ghesmati, Z.; Sabzichi, M.; Ramezani, F. Up-down Regulation of HIF-1α in Cancer Progression. *Gene* **2021**, *798*, 145796. [CrossRef]
20. Movafagh, S.; Crook, S.; Vo, K. Regulation of Hypoxia-Inducible Factor-1a by Reactive Oxygen Species: New Developments in an Old Debate. *J. Cell. Biochem.* **2015**, *116*, 696–703. [CrossRef]
21. Barsoum, I.B.; Smallwood, C.A.; Siemens, D.R.; Graham, C.H. A Mechanism of Hypoxia-Mediated Escape from Adaptive Immunity in Cancer Cells. *Cancer Res.* **2014**, *74*, 665–674. [CrossRef]
22. Chen, Z.Q.; Zuo, X.L.; Cai, J.; Zhang, Y.; Han, G.Y.; Zhang, L.; Ding, W.Z.; Wu, J.D.; Wang, X.H. Hypoxia-Associated CircPRDM4 Promotes Immune Escape via HIF-1α Regulation of PD-L1 in Hepatocellular Carcinoma. *Exp. Hematol. Oncol.* **2023**, *12*, 17. [CrossRef]
23. Nahand, J.S.; Taghizadeh-boroujeni, S.; Karimzadeh, M.; Borran, S.; Pourhanifeh, M.H.; Moghoofei, M.; Bokharaei-Salim, F.; Karampoor, S.; Jafari, A.; Asemi, Z.; et al. MicroRNAs: New Prognostic, Diagnostic, and Therapeutic Biomarkers in Cervical Cancer. *J. Cell. Physiol.* **2019**, *234*, 17064–17099. [CrossRef]
24. Sammarco, M.L.; Tamburro, M.; Pulliero, A.; Izzotti, A.; Ripabelli, G. Human Papillomavirus Infections, Cervical Cancer and MicroRNAs: An Overview and Implications for Public Health. *MicroRNA* **2020**, *9*, 174. [CrossRef] [PubMed]
25. Menon, A.; Abd-Aziz, N.; Khalid, K.; Poh, C.L.; Naidu, R. MiRNA: A Promising Therapeutic Target in Cancer. *Int. J. Mol. Sci.* **2022**, *23*, 11502. [CrossRef]

26. Sun, Z.; Zhang, Q.; Yuan, W.; Li, X.; Chen, C.; Guo, Y.; Shao, B.; Dang, Q.; Zhou, Q.; Wang, Q.; et al. MiR-103a-3p Promotes Tumour Glycolysis in Colorectal Cancer via Hippo/YAP1/HIF1A Axis. *J. Exp. Clin. Cancer Res.* **2020**, *39*, 250. [CrossRef]
27. Zhao, Y.; Liu, X.; Lu, Y.X. MicroRNA-143 Regulates the Proliferation and Apoptosis of Cervical Cancer Cells by Targeting HIF-1α. *Eur. Rev. Med. Pharmacol. Sci.* **2021**, *21*, 5580–5586. [CrossRef]
28. Narisawa-Saito, M.; Handa, K.; Yugawa, T.; Ohno, S.; Fujita, M.; Kiyono, T. HPV16 E6-Mediated Stabilization of ErbB2 in Neoplastic Transformation of Human Cervical Keratinocytes. *Oncogene* **2007**, *26*, 2988–2996. [CrossRef] [PubMed]
29. Yugawa, T.; Handa, K.; Narisawa-Saito, M.; Ohno, S.; Fujita, M.; Kiyono, T. Regulation of Notch1 Gene Expression by P53 in Epithelial Cells. *Mol. Cell. Biol.* **2007**, *27*, 3732. [CrossRef]
30. NCI. What Is Cervical Cancer? Available online: https://www.cancer.gov/types/cervical (accessed on 31 October 2023).
31. Colombo, N.; Dubot, C.; Lorusso, D.; Caceres, M.V.; Hasegawa, K.; Shapira-Frommer, R.; Tewari, K.S.; Salman, P.; Hoyos Usta, E.; Yañez, E.; et al. Pembrolizumab for Persistent, Recurrent, or Metastatic Cervical Cancer. *N. Engl. J. Med.* **2021**, *385*, 1856–1867. [CrossRef]
32. Mauricio, D.; Zeybek, B.; Tymon-Rosario, J.; Harold, J.; Santin, A. Immunotherapy in Cervical Cancer. *Curr. Oncol. Rep.* **2021**, *23*, 61. [CrossRef]
33. Bonetta, A.C.; Mailly, L.; Robinet, E.; Trave, G.; Masson, M.; Deryckere, F. Artificial microRNAs against the viral E6 protein provoke apoptosis in HPV positive cancer cells. *Biochem. Biophys. Res. Commun.* **2015**, *465*, 658–664. [CrossRef]
34. Kennedy, E.M.; Kornepati, A.V.R.; Goldstein, M.; Bogerd, H.P.; Poling, B.C.; Whisnant, A.W.; Kastan, M.B.; Cullen, B.R. Inactivation of the Human Papillomavirus E6 or E7 Gene in Cervical Carcinoma Cells by Using a Bacterial CRISPR/Cas RNA-Guided Endonuclease. *J. Virol.* **2014**, *88*, 11965–11972. [CrossRef]
35. Semenza, G.L. Oxygen Sensing, Homeostasis, and Disease. *N. Engl. J. Med.* **2011**, *365*, 537–547. [CrossRef]
36. Wigerup, C.; Påhlman, S.; Bexell, D. Therapeutic Targeting of Hypoxia and Hypoxia-Inducible Factors in Cancer. *Pharmacol. Ther.* **2016**, *164*, 152–169. [CrossRef] [PubMed]
37. Metin, C.U.; Ozcan, G. The HIF-1α as a Potent Inducer of the Hallmarks in Gastric Cancer. *Cancers* **2022**, *14*, 2711. [CrossRef]
38. Wu, Q.; You, L.; Nepomiova, E.; Heger, Z.; Wu, W.; Kuca, K.; Adam, V. Hypoxia-Inducible Factors: Master Regulators of Hypoxic Tumor Immune Escape. *J. Hematol. Oncol.* **2022**, *15*, 77. [CrossRef] [PubMed]
39. Multhoff, G.; Vaupel, P. Hypoxia Compromises Anti-Cancer Immune Responses. *Adv. Exp. Med. Biol.* **2020**, *1232*, 131–143. [CrossRef] [PubMed]
40. Fan, R.; Hou, W.J.; Zhao, Y.J.; Liu, S.L.; Qiu, X.S.; Wang, E.H.; Wu, G.P. Overexpression of HPV16 E6/E7 Mediated HIF-1α Upregulation of GLUT1 Expression in Lung Cancer Cells. *Tumor Biol.* **2016**, *37*, 4655–4663. [CrossRef]
41. Liu, F.; Lin, B.; Liu, X.; Zhang, W.; Zhang, E.; Hu, L.; Ma, Y.; Li, X.; Tang, X. ERK Signaling Pathway Is Involved in HPV-16 E6 but Not E7 Oncoprotein-Induced HIF-1α Protein Accumulation in NSCLC Cells. *Oncol. Res.* **2016**, *23*, 109–118. [CrossRef]
42. Priego-Hernández, V.D.; Arizmendi-Izagaza, A.; Soto-Flores, D.G.; Santiago-Ramón, N.; Feria-Valadez, M.D.; Navarro-Tito, N.; Jiménez-Wences, H.; Martínez-Carrillo, D.N.; Salmerón-Bárcenas, E.G.; Leyva-Vázquez, M.A.; et al. Expression of HIF-1α and Genes Involved in Glucose Metabolism Is Increased in Cervical Cancer and HPV-16-Positive Cell Lines. *Pathogens* **2023**, *12*, 33. [CrossRef]
43. Bajhan, E.; Mansoori, B.; Mohammadi, A.; Shanehbandi, D.; Khaze Shahgoli, V.; Baghbani, E.; Hajiasgharzadeh, K.; Baradaran, B. MicroRNA-143 Inhibits Proliferation and Migration of Prostate Cancer Cells. *Arch. Physiol. Biochem.* **2022**, *128*, 1323–1329. [CrossRef]
44. Esfandyari, Y.B.; Doustvandi, M.A.; Amini, M.; Baradaran, B.; Zaer, S.J.; Mozammel, N.; Mohammadzadeh, M.; Mokhtarzadeh, A. MicroRNA-143 Sensitizes Cervical Cancer Cells to Cisplatin: A Promising Anticancer Combination Therapy. *Reprod. Sci.* **2021**, *28*, 2036–2049. [CrossRef]
45. Zhang, P.; Zhang, J.; Quan, H.; Wang, J.; Liang, Y. MicroRNA-143 Expression Inhibits the Growth and the Invasion of Osteosarcoma. *J. Orthop. Surg. Res.* **2022**, *17*, 236. [CrossRef] [PubMed]
46. Liu, Y.F.; Luo, D.; Li, X.; Li, Z.Q.; Yu, X.; Zhu, H.W. PVT1 Knockdown Inhibits Autophagy and Improves Gemcitabine Sensitivity by Regulating the MiR-143/HIF-1α/VMP1 Axis in Pancreatic Cancer. *Pancreas* **2021**, *50*, 227–234. [CrossRef]
47. Asghariazar, V.; Kadkhodayi, M.; Sarailoo, M.; Jolfayi, A.G.; Baradaran, B. MicroRNA-143 as a Potential Tumor Suppressor in Cancer: An Insight into Molecular Targets and Signaling Pathways. *Pathol. Res. Pract.* **2023**, *250*, 154792. [CrossRef] [PubMed]
48. Ling, J.; Sun, Q.; Tian, Q.; Shi, H.; Yang, H.; Ren, J. Human Papillomavirus 16 E6/E7 Contributes to Immune Escape and Progression of Cervical Cancer by Regulating MiR-142-5p/PD-L1 Axis. *Arch. Biochem. Biophys.* **2022**, *731*, 109449. [CrossRef] [PubMed]
49. Karimi, L.; Mansoori, B.; Shanebandi, D.; Mohammadi, A.; Aghapour, M.; Baradaran, B. Function of MicroRNA-143 in Different Signal Pathways in Cancer: New Insights into Cancer Therapy. *Biomed. Pharmacother.* **2017**, *91*, 121–131. [CrossRef]
50. Zhang, J.; Sun, Q.; Zhang, Z.; Ge, S.; Han, Z.G.; Chen, W.T. Loss of MicroRNA-143/145 Disturbs Cellular Growth and Apoptosis of Human Epithelial Cancers by Impairing the MDM2-P53 Feedback Loop. *Oncogene* **2013**, *32*, 61–69. [CrossRef]

Disclaimer/Publisher's Note: The statements, opinions and data contained in all publications are solely those of the individual author(s) and contributor(s) and not of MDPI and/or the editor(s). MDPI and/or the editor(s) disclaim responsibility for any injury to people or property resulting from any ideas, methods, instructions or products referred to in the content.

Article

A Single-Cell Transcriptome Atlas of Epithelial Subpopulations in HPV-Positive and HPV-Negative Head and Neck Cancers

Mary C. Bedard [1,2,*], Cosette M. Rivera-Cruz [1], Tafadzwa Chihanga [1], Andrew VonHandorf [3,4], Alice L. Tang [5], Chad Zender [5], Matthew T. Weirauch [3,4,6], Robert Ferris [7], Trisha M. Wise-Draper [8], Mike Adam [1,*] and Susanne I. Wells [1,9,*]

[1] Division of Oncology, Cincinnati Children's Hospital Medical Center, Cincinnati, OH 45229, USA
[2] Medical Scientist Training Program, University of Cincinnati College of Medicine, Cincinnati, OH 45267, USA
[3] Division of Allergy and Immunology, Cincinnati Children's Hospital Medical Center, Cincinnati, OH 45229, USA
[4] Center for Autoimmune Genomics and Etiology, Cincinnati Children's Hospital Medical Center, Cincinnati, OH 45229, USA
[5] Department of Otolaryngology, University of Cincinnati College of Medicine, Cincinnati, OH 45267, USA; zendercd@ucmail.uc.edu (C.Z.)
[6] Divisions of Human Genetics, Biomedical Informatics, and Developmental Biology, Cincinnati Children's Hospital Medical Center, Cincinnati, OH 45229, USA
[7] UNC Lineberger Comprehensive Cancer Center, UNC Health Care System, Chapel Hill, NC 27599, USA; robert_ferris@med.unc.edu
[8] Division of Hematology/Oncology, Department of Internal Medicine, University of Cincinnati College of Medicine, Cincinnati, OH 45267, USA
[9] Department of Pediatrics, University of Cincinnati College of Medicine, Cincinnati, OH 45267, USA
* Correspondence: mary.bedard@cchmc.org (M.C.B.); mike.adam@cchmc.org (M.A.); susanne.wells@cchmc.org (S.I.W.)

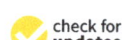

Academic Editors: Hossein H. Ashrafi and Mustafa Ozdogan

Received: 11 February 2025
Revised: 13 March 2025
Accepted: 14 March 2025
Published: 24 March 2025

Citation: Bedard, M.C.; Rivera-Cruz, C.M.; Chihanga, T.; VonHandorf, A.; Tang, A.L.; Zender, C.; Weirauch, M.T.; Ferris, R.; Wise-Draper, T.M.; Adam, M.; et al. A Single-Cell Transcriptome Atlas of Epithelial Subpopulations in HPV-Positive and HPV-Negative Head and Neck Cancers. *Viruses* 2025, 17, 461. https://doi.org/10.3390/v17040461

Copyright: © 2025 by the authors. Licensee MDPI, Basel, Switzerland. This article is an open access article distributed under the terms and conditions of the Creative Commons Attribution (CC BY) license (https://creativecommons.org/licenses/by/4.0/).

Abstract: Persistent infection with HPV causes nearly 5% of all cancers worldwide, including cervical and oropharyngeal cancers. Compared to HPV-negative (HPV−) head and neck squamous cell carcinomas (HNSCCs), HPV-positive (HPV+) HNSCCs exhibit a significantly improved treatment response; however, established treatment regimens were largely developed for HPV− disease. Effectively de-escalating therapy and optimizing treatment protocols to minimize toxicity for both HPV+ and HPV− tumors has been variably successful, in part due to the heterogeneity of cellular subpopulations. Single-cell RNA sequencing (scRNAseq) has primarily been used to define immune cell populations rather than the cell type of origin, epithelial cells. To address this, we analyzed published scRNAseq data of HPV+ and HPV− HNSCCs to distinguish epithelial tumor cell populations as a function of HPV status. We identified the transcriptome signatures, ontologies, and candidate biomarkers of newly identified epithelial subpopulations with attention to those that are shared or enriched in HPV+ or HPV− HNSCCs. We hypothesize that distinct epithelial cell populations and reprogramming in HPV− versus HPV+ HNSCC represent important components of the pro-tumor environment. These are described here as a foundation for the identification of new epithelial-cell-specific biomarkers, effectors, and candidate targets for optimizing the treatment of HNSCC.

Keywords: human papillomavirus; HPV; head and neck cancer; HNSCC; single-cell transcriptomics; scRNAseq; epithelial cells; cancer therapy

1. Introduction

Although a causal relationship between HPV infection and head and neck squamous cell carcinoma (HNSCC) development was first reported over two decades ago [1] and a preventive vaccine is available, the incidence of HPV+ HNSCCs has continued to increase and is predicted to represent the majority of HNSCCs in the future [2,3]. This trend reflects the continued prevalence of oral HPV infection (i.e., ~7% of the US population, higher amongst men) [4] that is associated with a 50-fold increased risk for developing HPV+ HNSCC [5]. It is well established that HPV+ and HPV− HNSCCs differ in anatomical distribution, molecular drivers, patient demographics, treatment response, and clinical course, and as such, can be considered distinct cancer types that warrant distinct treatment algorithms [6]. For example, HPV-positive and HPV-negative HNSCCs tend to arise in different anatomical locations: HPV-negative HNSCCs primarily occur in the oral cavity, larynx, and hypopharynx, whereas HPV-positive HNSCCs commonly occur in the oropharynx (e.g., tonsils, base of tongue, soft palate). This distinction aligns with epidemiological data showing that approximately 90% of oral cavity HNSCCs are HPV-negative [7], while around 70% of oropharyngeal HNSCCs are HPV-positive [8]. Altogether, these differences support ongoing efforts to tailor HNSCC treatments based on patient and/or tumor characteristics. For example, window-of-opportunity studies in HPV− HNSCCs utilizing PD1 or PDL1-targeting immune therapy have shown improved outcomes in intermediate-risk HNSCC patients [9] and in locally advanced resectable HNSCC (KEYNOTE-689). However, additional studies are needed to understand why some patients will respond favorably to de-escalation and how to optimize treatment paradigms based on tumor characteristics, for example, by HPV status.

With regards to HPV+ HNSCCs, various deintensification strategies have been tested in clinical trials to maximize response while minimizing toxicity. These approaches have included (1) replacement [10,11], reduction [12–14], or omission of cytotoxic chemotherapy [15], (2) de-escalated adjuvant (chemo)radiotherapy following ablative surgery [16,17], (3) reduction in dose of radiation following induction chemotherapy [18–22], and (4) reduction in dose of radiation during definitive (chemo)radiotherapy [23]. Unfortunately, recent phase III clinical trials aimed at de-escalation approaches in HPV+ tumors (De-ESCALate HPV [10], RTOG 1016 [11]) resulted in inferior outcomes and have demonstrated the need for caution in deviation from standard of care [24]. In the wake of these studies, there is a renewed interest in predictive and prognostic biomarkers that may help guide patient selection for treatment tailoring [24,25]. For example, ongoing research on the utility of serum HPV circulating tumor DNA assays [26–29] has led to promising initial results. Other studies have correlated genomic biomarkers representative of tumor biology subtypes with patient outcomes. These have included p53 status [30], PIK3CA mutation [31], MATH score/ER-alpha expression [32], and TRAF/CYLD loss [33]. Thus, there is a clear need to better understand the biology of HPV-driven carcinogenesis and the profiles and/or reprogramming of key cell subpopulations specific to HPV+ disease.

Given that HPV exclusively infects the mucosal epithelium, and that squamous epithelial cells are the cells of origin for HNSCCs, defining the effects of infection on epithelial subpopulations is essential to advance new insights into HPV-reprogrammed host biology, candidate biomarkers, and targeted therapeutic strategies. Recent advances in single-cell technologies such as single-cell RNA sequencing (scRNAseq) have enabled the bioinformatic identification of distinct subpopulations within heterogenous tissues. With scRNAseq, the transcriptomic signature of distinct epithelial subpopulations can be identified and analyzed to identify their respective gene and pathway signatures. A previous publication [34] described scRNAseq data on HPV+ and HPV− HNSCCs to define distinct cell types, and explored immune-cell-related processes and interactions that shape the tumor immune microenvironment. Herein, we systematically analyzed the corresponding epithelial compartment to identify cellular subpopulations and ontologies enriched in

HPV+ vs. HPV− HNSCCs as a foundation for the discovery of novel biomarkers and subtype-specific therapeutic targets.

2. Materials and Methods

2.1. scRNAseq Data Processing

Publicly available preprocessed single-cell RNA sequencing (scRNAseq) data were downloaded from the Gene Expression Omnibus database: accession ID GSE164690 [34] (Table S1). The R v4.1.1 library Seurat v4.4 was used for cell-type clustering and marker gene identification [35]. Each sample was normalized by SCTransform, using the glmGamPoi method and the number of RNA molecules per cell was regressed out. Samples were integrated with common anchor genes using the rPCA method to minimize sample-to-sample variation. Cell clusters were determined by the Louvain algorithm. UMAP dimension reduction was performed using the first 30 principal components. Marker genes for each cell type were calculated using the Wilcoxon rank-sum test returning only genes that are present in a minimum of 25% of the analyzed cluster. Epithelial cells were subset by isolating the CD45- cells, reintegrating the data and curating the epithelial cells of interest by using gene expression markers. Original annotations of HPV status, defined based on clinical p16 IHC testing and confirmed by detection of viral genes, were retained for all samples. Global expression of all epithelial cells originating from HPV− versus HPV+ tumors was compared to define globally differentially expressed genes (DEGs). Each scRNAseq cluster was considered a distinct epithelial subpopulation.

2.2. Ontology Analysis and Cytoscape Visualization

The transcriptomes and DEGs of select clusters were analyzed using the gProfiler web server [36] for Gene Ontology (GO) terms, which includes Gene Ontology (GO) terms, curated by the Ensembl database [37], and pathways from KEGG (https://www.genome.jp/kegg/, accessed on 1 January 2025), WikiPathways (https://www.wikipathways.org/index.php/WikiPathways, accessed on 3 January 2025), and Reactome (https://reactome.org/, accessed on 4 January 2025). Complex enriched gene sets were visualized using the Enrichment Map App [38] within Cytoscape 3 using parameters previously defined [39]. In brief, enrichment files and gene sets outputs from g:Profiler were processed using Enrichment Map and terms with a false discovery rate less than 0.01 were considered significantly enriched. Nodes represent pathways, and they are connected by edges (lines) between nodes with genes in common. Node size is dependent on the enrichment score associated with that pathway, while edges thickness is relative to the number of genes shared between nodes.

3. Results

3.1. Identification of Epithelial Cells by Joint scRNAseq Analysis of HPV+ and HPV− HNSCCs

We sought to define the epithelial subpopulations present in HNSCC tumors and their gene signatures, which have not been previously reported. To this end, published scRNAseq data for six HPV+ and nine HPV− HNSCC tumors were processed with batch correction (Figure 1A). UMAPs of all cells split by the HPV status of the parent tumor confirmed a high level of overlap (Figure 1B). Unbiased clustering revealed 20 distinct populations whose ontologies (Figure 1C) were assigned based on the corresponding distinct transcriptomic signatures visualized by heatmap (Figure 1D). The identified cellular populations included immune, epithelial, and stromal cells, demonstrating the heterogeneous cell types present in the tumors.

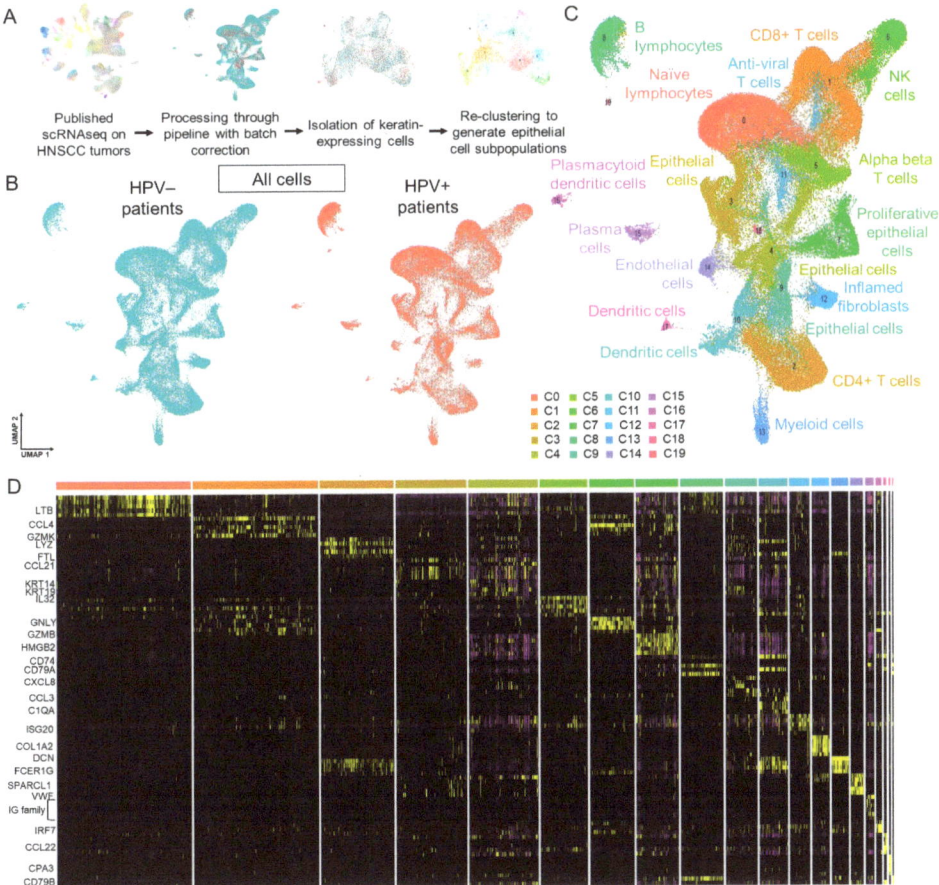

Figure 1. Joint analysis of HPV+ and HPV− HNSCC tumors with batch correction. (**A**) Overview of the bioinformatic pipeline to identify transcriptomically distinct epithelial subpopulations in scRNAseq data of HPV+ ($n = 6$) and HPV− ($n = 9$) HNSCCs. (**B**) Resulting UMAP of all cells separated by patient HPV status. (**C**) Cell clustering demonstrates a mix of immune, epithelial, and stromal cell types. (**D**) Heatmap of transcriptomically distinct clusters with select genes labeled.

3.2. Identification of Global Transcriptomes and Pathways Distinguished by HPV Status

Keratin-expressing clusters were jointly re-clustered to isolate epithelial cells from other cell types (UMAP Figure 2A). The global signature of epithelial cells in HPV+ vs. HPV− HNSCCs was first analyzed (heatmap, Figure S1). The cytoscape visualization of GO biological processes upregulated in HPV− vs. HPV+ HNSCCs revealed pathways related to immune activation, peptidase activity, and processes such as adhesion, angiogenesis, and apoptosis (Figure 2B). Conversely, a similar analysis for processes upregulated in HPV+ vs. HPV− HNSCCs included pathways related to metabolism, migration, and differentiation (Figure 2C). Additionally, KEGG pathway (Figure 2D) and reactome pathway (Figure 2E) enrichment was assessed. Relative to HPV− HNSCCs, there was an upregulation in HPV+ HNSCCs in processes related to metabolism, tissue development, migration, and signal transduction. In HPV− HNSCCs, there was an upregulation of immune response, cell motility, and peptidase activity, which notably indicated a relative downregulation in immune response activation, cytokine signaling, and T-cell proliferation.

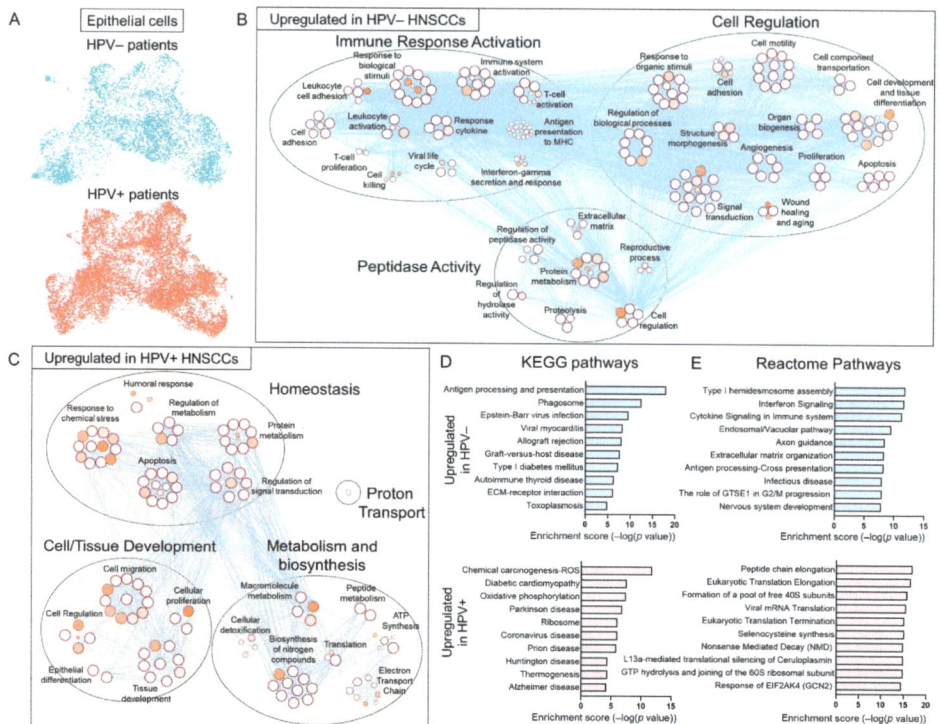

Figure 2. Signatures upregulated in epithelial cells from HPV+ and HPV− HNSCCs. (**A**) UMAP of keratinocytes isolated from the published scRNAseq data and re-clustered, separated by HPV status to show extensive overlap. (**B–D**) Global differential expression analysis by HPV status. (**B**) Cytoscape visualization of GO biological processes upregulated in HPV− vs. HPV+ HNSCCs reveals pathways related to immune activation, peptidase activity, and processes such as adhesion, angiogenesis, and apoptosis. (**C**) Cytoscape visualization of GO biological processes upregulated in HPV+ HNSCCs includes pathways related to metabolism, migration, and differentiation. Top 10 KEGG pathways (**D**) and reactome pathways (**E**) upregulated in HPV− and HPV+ HNSCCs.

3.3. Distinct Epithelial Cell Subpopulations Are Present in HPV− vs. HPV+ HNSCC Tumors

Epithelial subpopulations were identified by unbiased clustering (UMAP Figure 3A, heatmap Figure 3B, dot plot Figure 3C. Cells from both HPV+ and HPV− HNSCCs were represented in all subpopulations. Enrichment (defined as ≥30% difference by cell number) of subpopulations in HPV+ versus HPV− HNSCCs was determined by analyzing the distribution of tumor cells across clusters (Figure 3D, arrows indicating enrichment). C1, C4, C5, C7 were found to be enriched in HPV+ HNSCCs, C2 and C3 in HPV− HNSCCs, and C0 and C6 were roughly equally represented in HPV+ and HPV− HNSCCs. C8 had too few cells to be confidently assessed. Each cluster/subpopulation was defined by a distinct transcriptomic profile, although in some subpopulations, there were differences in the signature between HPV+ and HPV− specimens (heatmap, Figure S2).

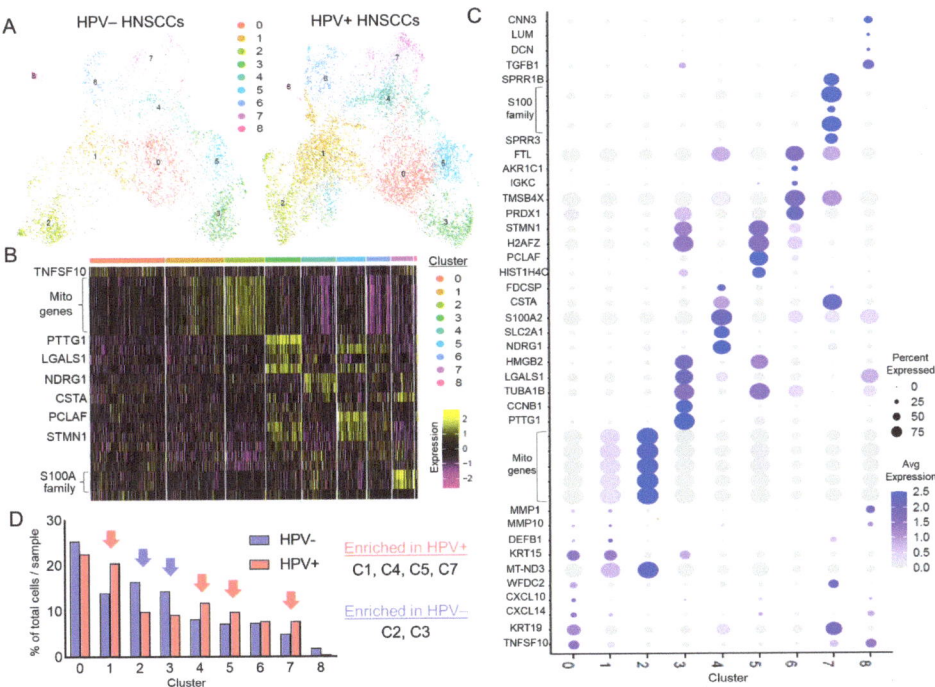

Figure 3. Enrichment of distinct epithelial subpopulations in HPV+ and HPV− HNSCC. (**A**) UMAP showing transcriptomically distinct clusters representing distinct epithelial subpopulations, separated by HPV status of HNSCC tumor. (**B**) Heatmap corresponding to clusters with select genes labeled. (**C**) Dot plot of top genes expressed per cluster. (**D**) Distribution of cells from HPV+ and HPV− HNSCCs across scRNAseq clusters, with those enriched ≥30% by cell counts highlighted by arrows.

3.4. HPV+ and HPV− Epithelial Subpopulations Are Defined by Differentiation Status and Cell-Cycle Phase

We determined the differentiation status and cell-cycle phase of epithelial subpopulations as previously described [39]. To this end, we probed for markers of embryonic/basal (COL17A+/KRT5+) (Figure 4A) versus differentiated (KRT13+/DMKN+) (Figure 4B) character, and markers of S (PCNA) (Figure 4C) and G2/M (MKI67) (Figure 4D) phase based on a well-defined set of markers for each [40,41]. This allowed the predominant differentiation state and cell-cycle phase(s) of each epithelial subpopulation to be defined and provide context into major biological processes that may appear in pathway analyses. We find that cells in S phase were predominately in C5, cells in G2/M phase in C3, and cells in C6 were in a mix of S and G2/M phases (Figure 4E). When broken down by HPV status, an increase in cells in S phase was observed for HPV+ vs. HPV− HNSCCs (Figure 4F).

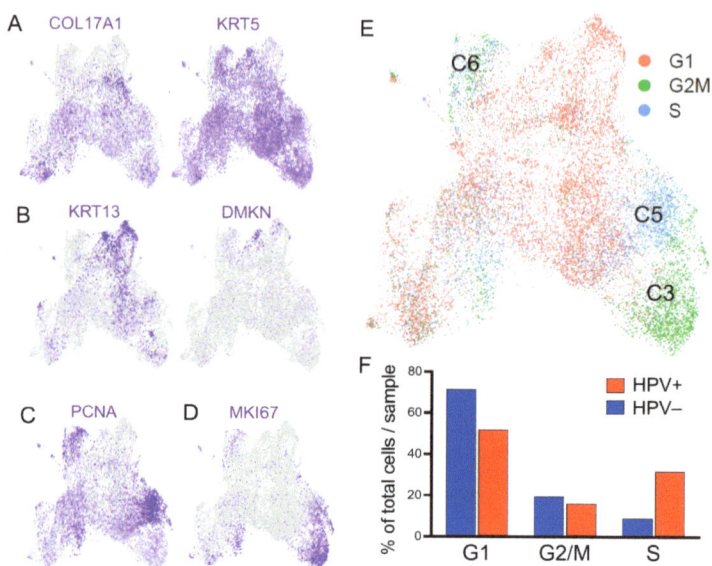

Figure 4. Analysis of differentiation status and cell-cycle phase in epithelial subpopulations. Feature plots demonstrating distribution of select basal (**A**), differentiated (**B**), S phase (**C**), and G2/M phase (**D**) markers. (**E**) Distribution of G1, G2/M, and S-phase cells. C5 harbors predominately cells in S, C3 cells in G2/M, and C6 a mix of S and G2/M cells. (**F**) Distribution of epithelial cells across cell-cycle phases by HPV status.

3.5. Genes Ontologies of Epithelial Subpopulations Enriched in HPV+ HNSCCs

The C1, C4, C5, and C7 subpopulations were proportionately increased in HPV+ HNSCCs. We have previously discussed C7, which most closely matches the previously reported HIDDEN cell signature, as being upregulated in HPV+ HNSCCs [39]. For each of these subpopulations, we sought to determine the defining processes and gene ontologies to elucidate the identity of these epithelial cell subtypes. We analyzed each of these subpopulations using Cytoscape visualization (Figures 5A, 6A, 7A and 8A) and defined the top hits for GO biological processes (Figures 5B, 6B, 7B and 8B), KEGG pathways (Figures 5C, 6C, 7C and 8D), and reactome pathways (Figures 5D, 6D, 7D and 8C). To identify candidate drivers of each subpopulation, transcription factor binding site enrichment analysis was performed through Transfac analysis (Figures 5E, 6E, 7E and 8E). Altogether, we found that C1 was predominated by mitochondrial-related processes, e.g., cellular respiration and oxidative phosphorylation, C4 by cell migration, p53 signaling, and cancer cell metabolism, C5 by processes related to the S phase of the cell cycle such as DNA replication, and C7 by migration and tissue differentiation.

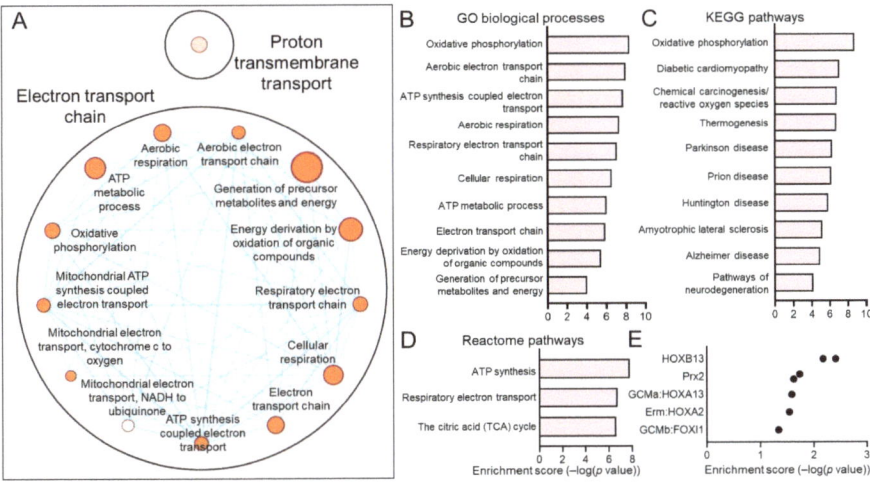

Figure 5. Gene ontologies of the HPV+ enriched C1 HNSCC epithelial subpopulation. (**A**) Cytoscape visualization of GO biological processes highlight genes related to the electron transport chain and aerobic respiration. Summary of top GO biological processes (**B**), KEGG pathways (**C**), and reactome pathways (**D**) demonstrates that the transcriptome of C1 centers on mitochondrial processes and ATP generation. (**E**) Transfac analysis for transcription factor drivers of the C1 subpopulation.

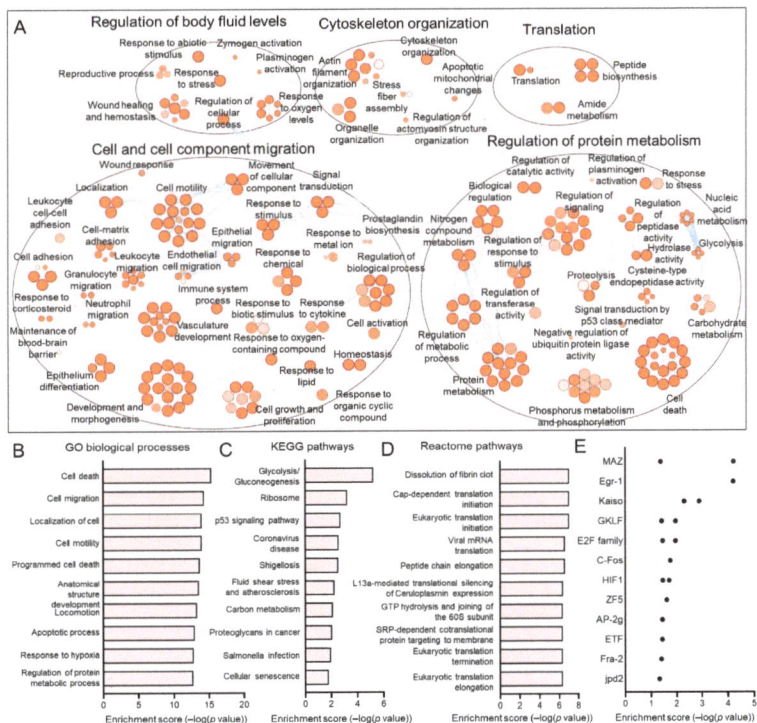

Figure 6. Gene ontologies of the HPV+ enriched C4 HNSCC epithelial subpopulation. (**A**) Cytoscape visualization of GO biological processes highlights pathways related to migration, cytoskeleton organization, and metabolic processes. Summary of top GO biological processes (**B**), KEGG pathways (**C**), and reactome pathways (**D**). (**E**) Transfac analysis for transcription factor drivers of the C4 subpopulation.

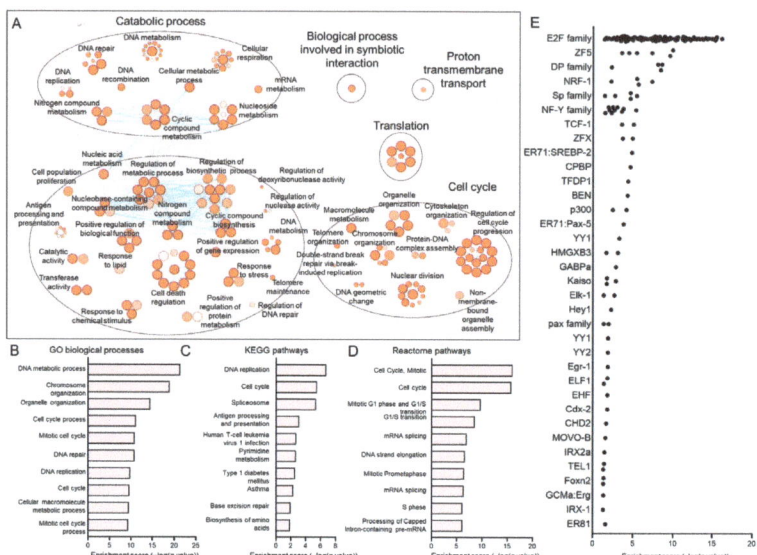

Figure 7. Gene ontologies of the HPV+ enriched C5 HNSCC epithelial subpopulation. (**A**) Cytoscape visualization of GO biological processes highlights pathways related to proliferation. Summary of top GO biological processes (**B**), KEGG pathways (**C**), and reactome pathways (**D**) centers on cell-cycle processes, particularly S phase. (**E**) Transfac analysis for candidate transcription factor drivers of the C5 subpopulation.

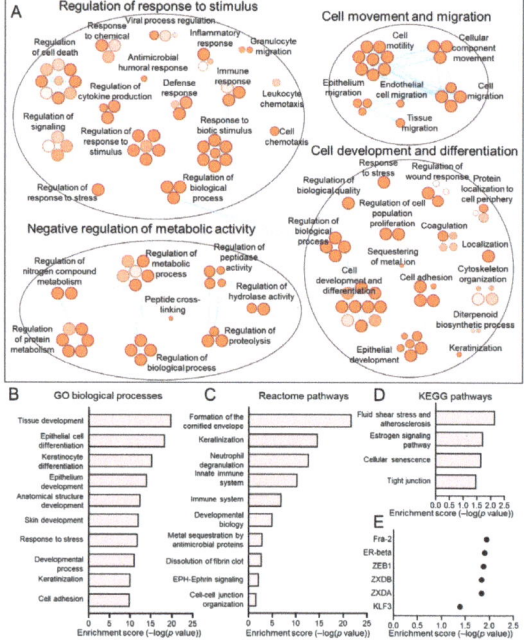

Figure 8. Gene ontologies of the HPV+ enriched C7 HNSCC epithelial subpopulation. (**A**) Cytoscape visualization of GO biological processes highlights pathways related to migration, development, and metabolism. Summary of top GO biological processes (**B**), reactome pathways (**C**), and KEGG pathways (**D**) include keratinocyte differentiation related processes. (**E**) Transfac analysis discover candidate transcription factor drivers of the C7 subpopulation.

3.6. Ontologies of Epithelial Subpopulations Enriched in HPV− HNSCCs

Similarly, we examined the subpopulations proportionately increased in HPV− HNSCCs, namely, C2 and C3, using Cytoscape (Figures 9A and 10A) and by defining top hits for GO biological processes (Figures 9B and 10B), KEGG pathways (Figures 9C and 10C), and reactome pathways (Figures 9D and 10D). We also determined transcription factor binding site enrichment by Transfac analysis (Figures 9E and 10E). C2 was dominated by mitochondrial-related pathways such as biosynthesis and cellular respiration, signatures shared with HPV+ enriched C1 cells. Lastly, C3 was defined by genes involved in the G2/M cell-cycle regulation, including processes of organelle and chromosome organization, nuclear division, cytokinesis, and nucleic acid metabolism.

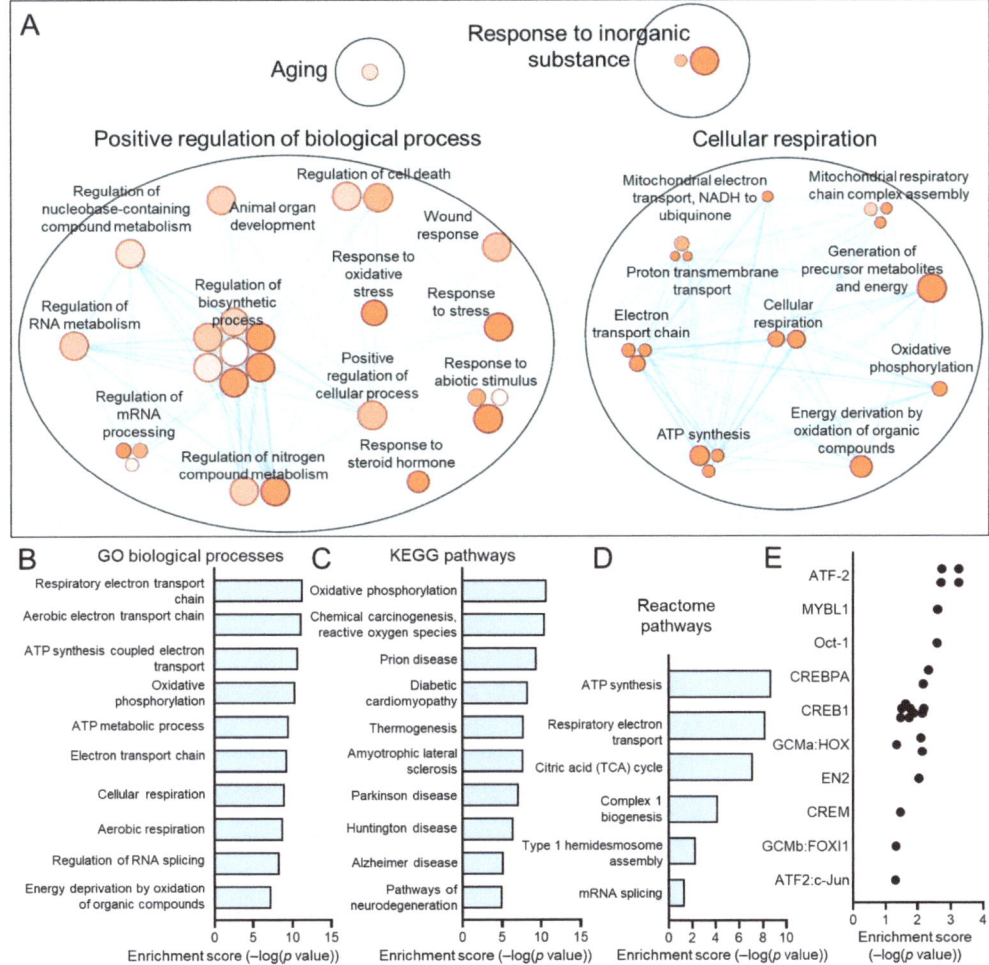

Figure 9. Gene ontologies of the HPV− enriched C2 HNSCC epithelial subpopulation. (**A**) Cytoscape visualization of GO biological processes highlights pathways related to biosynthesis and cellular respiration. Summary of top GO biological processes (**B**), KEGG pathways (**C**), and reactome pathways (**D**) centers on mitochondrial and ATP metabolic processes. (**E**) Transfac analysis for transcription factor drivers of the C2 subpopulation.

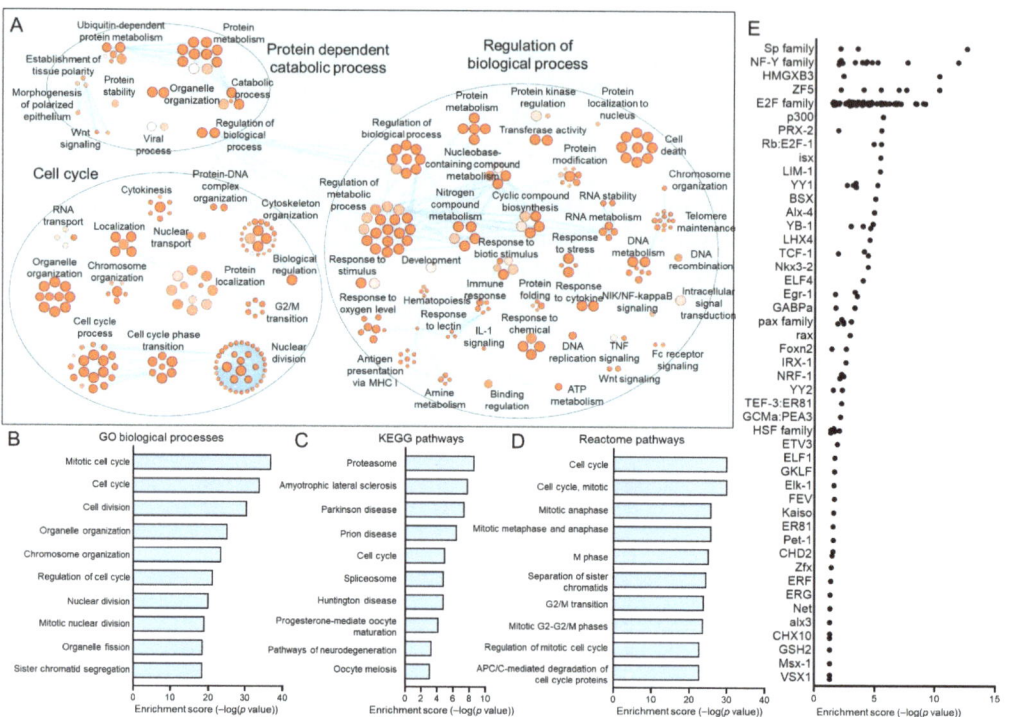

Figure 10. Gene ontologies of the HPV− enriched C3 HNSCC epithelial subpopulation. (**A**) Cytoscape visualization of GO biological processes highlights pathways related to cell cycle and proliferation. Summary of top GO biological processes (**B**), KEGG pathways (**C**), and reactome pathways (**D**) centers on the G2/M phase of the cell cycle. (**E**) Transfac analysis for transcription factor drivers of the C3 subpopulation.

3.7. Ontologies of Epithelial Subpopulations Equally Represented in HPV− and HPV+ HNSCCs

Two epithelial subpopulations (C0 and C6) were found to be present in HNSCC tumors regardless of HPV status. The same analysis for these subpopulations was performed to define ontologies: Cytoscape (Figures 11A and 12A), GO biological processes (Figures 11B and 12B), KEGG pathways (Figures 11C and 12C), reactome pathways (Figures 11D and 12D), and transcription factor binding site enrichment by Transfac (Figures 11E and 12E). C0 processes predominantly related to immune responses, biosynthesis, and cell differentiation, while C6 featured a range of pathways related to the S and G2/M phases of the cell cycle, including ATP synthesis, translation, biosynthesis, and p53 class mediator signaling.

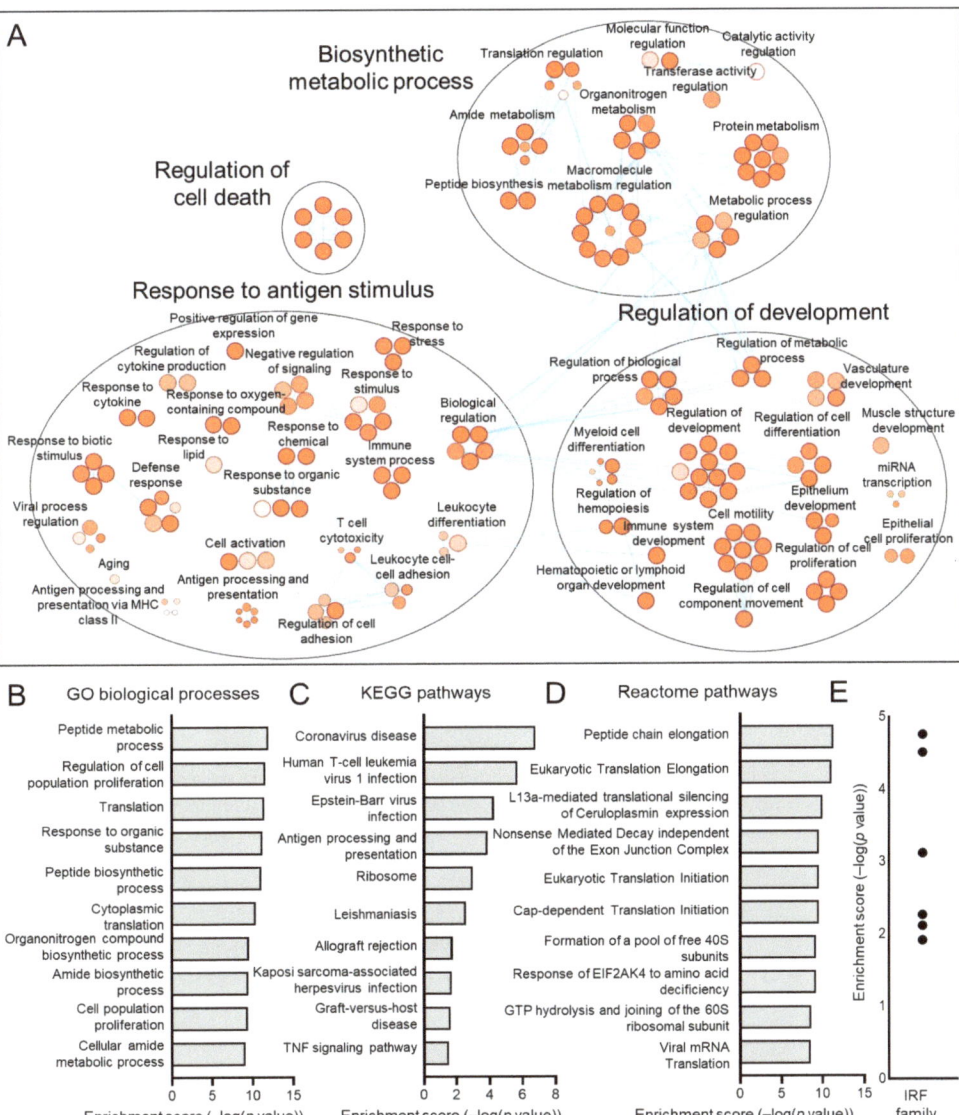

Figure 11. Gene ontologies of the shared C0 HNSCC epithelial subpopulation. (**A**) Cytoscape visualization of GO biological processes highlights pathways related to immune response and proliferation. Summary of top GO biological processes (**B**), KEGG pathways (**C**), and reactome pathways (**D**) centers on antigen processing and translation. (**E**) Transfac analysis for transcription factor drivers of the C0 subpopulation.

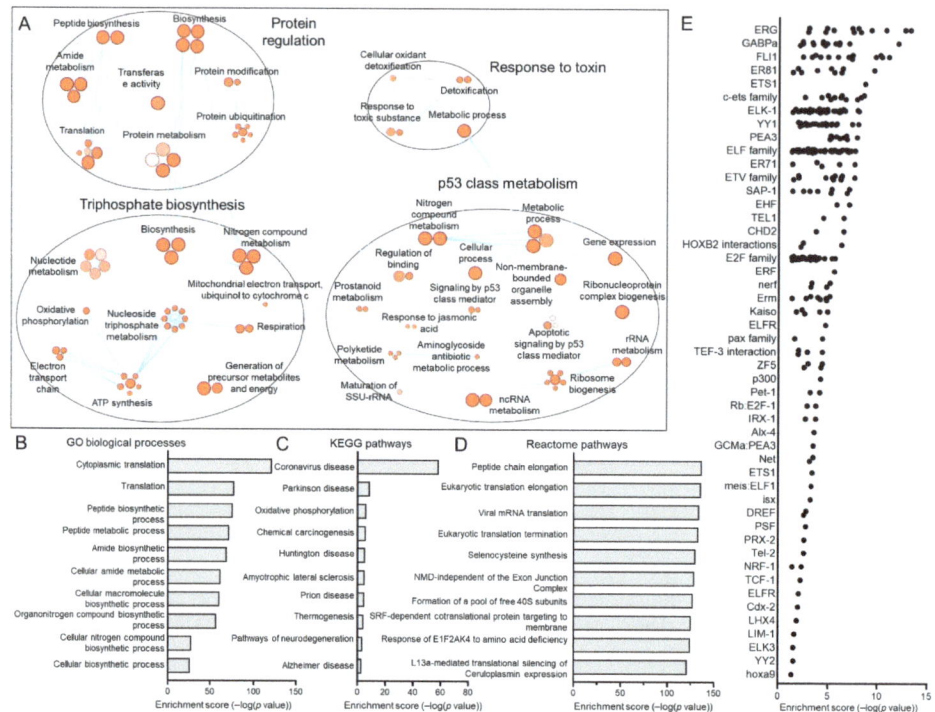

Figure 12. Gene ontologies of the shared C6 HNSCC epithelial subpopulation. (**A**) Cytoscape visualization of GO biological processes highlights pathways related to biosynthesis and p53. Summary of top GO biological processes (**B**), KEGG pathways (**C**), and reactome pathways (**D**) centers on translation and biosynthesis. (**E**) Transfac analysis for transcription factor drivers of the C6 subpopulation.

3.8. Summary of Newly Identified Transcriptome Signatures

Signatures discovered by Cytoscape visualization, GO biological processes, KEGG pathways, and reactome pathways for each epithelial subpopulation and global expression comparison are summarized in Table 1. Potential avenues for targeting cellular subpopulations based on defining signatures were added.

Table 1. Summary of select signatures and potentially targetable phenotypes of cellular subpopulations identified by scRNAseq analysis.

	Enrichment	Select Signatures	Candidate Targetable Phenotypes
Global	HPV−	- Immune response - Cell motility - Peptidase activity	- Peptidases
Global	HPV+	- Biosynthesis - Epithelial differentiation - Migration - Signal transduction	- Metabolic pathways - Immune reactivation - Plasticity
C0	Shared	- Biosynthesis - Antigen processing and presentation - Cell differentiation	- Metabolic pathways - Immune reactivation

Table 1. Cont.

	Enrichment	Select Signatures	Candidate Targetable Phenotypes
C6	Shared	- S and G2/M phase of cell cycle - Biosynthesis - Oxidative phosphorylation - Signaling by p53 class mediators	- Cell-cycle checkpoints - Mitochondrial processes - p53 signaling
C2	HPV−	- Cellular respiration - Electron transport chain	- Mitochondrial processes
C3	HPV−	- G2/M phase of cell cycle - Organelle and chromosome organization - Nuclear division and cytokinesis - RNA/DNA metabolism	- Cell division - Mitotic machinery - Nucleotide metabolism
C1	HPV+	- Oxidative phosphorylation - Electron transport chain	- Mitochondrial processes
C4	HPV+	- Cell migration - Protein metabolism - p53 signaling - Glycolysis/gluconeogenesis	- Invasion - p53 signaling - Cancer cell metabolism
C5	HPV+	- S phase of cell cycle - DNA replication - Chromosome and cytoskeletal organization - Translation	- DNA replication machinery - Translation machinery
C7	HPV+	- Cell migration - Epithelial differentiation	- Aberrant HPV-driven differentiation (HIDDEN cells)

4. Discussion

Ongoing deintensification efforts and the study of new therapies in the treatment of HPV+ and HPV− HNSCCs will benefit from the definition of differences within specific cellular populations and signatures. These offer opportunities for targeted treatment and/or prognostic biomarkers towards improved treatment stratification, especially with the increasing interest in neoadjuvant immunotherapy. Single-cell technologies enable such studies by discovering cellular subpopulations and their respective transcriptomes for greater granularity in our understanding of tumor- and microenvironment-specific HNSCC heterogeneity. Recent studies using scRNAseq have largely focused on differences in immune cell and stromal subpopulations and transcriptomic profiles, which may impact immunotherapy development [34,42]. For example, transcriptome profiles of tumor-infiltrating leukocytes isolated from immunotherapy naïve HPV− vs. HPV+ HNSCC tumors revealed that certain cell types, such as B cells, myeloid cells, and conventional CD4$^+$ T cells, have divergent signatures by HPV status [43]. Thus, immunotherapeutic strategies targeting CD8$^+$ T cells or CD4$^+$ regulatory cells may be equally efficacious between HPV+ and HPV− HNSCCs since these cell types have similar signatures independent of HPV status; however, strategies targeting B cells, myeloid cells, and conventional CD4$^+$ T cells could require tailored designs to match the divergent signatures between HPV+ vs. HPV− HNSCCs. These findings highlight the clinical importance of understanding divergent cell subpopulations and signatures of HNSCCs by HPV status.

Because HNSCCs originate in epithelial tissues, we, therefore, reasoned that elucidating the signatures of epithelial subpopulations enriched in HPV+ vs. HPV− tumors may identify biomarkers, as well as drivers of malignancy that might be therapeutic targets. First, the global signature of epithelial cells was defined in HPV+ and HPV− tumors. HPV+

HNSCCs harbored relatively decreased immune response activation signatures, including decreased antigen presentation and interferon signaling. This signature is consistent with numerous reported immunosuppressive activities of the high-risk HPV E5, E6, and E7 oncoproteins [44,45], including the modulation of antigen presentation [46], MHC surface expression [47], and interferon signaling [48]. Additionally, this finding in epithelial cells complements recent scRNAseq data in tumor-infiltrating immune cells, wherein conventional CD4$^+$ T cells were found to differ in their differentiation trajectory by HPV status, having downregulated interferon responses and effector memory phenotypes [43]. There was also an upregulation in processes related to epithelial differentiation, consistent with the published disruption of the epithelial differentiation program by HPV towards the formation of an HPV-induced differentiation-dissonant epithelial nonconventional (HIDDEN) surface compartment [39]. Distinct differential signatures related to motility (HPV− HNSCCs) and migration (HPV+ HNSCCs) may reflect the HPV-dependent epithelial-to-mesenchymal transition (EMT) phenotypes. For example, EMT signature genes predicted worse five-year overall survival in HPV−, but not HPV+, HNSCCs [49,50], highlighting underlying mechanisms dependent on HPV. These differences may relate to distinct mechanisms whereby HPV reprograms epithelial cells and drives carcinogenesis, as the E6 and E7 oncogenes have been shown to downregulate E-Cadherin [51] and induce EMT-like processes [52,53]. Lastly, peptidase activity implicated in cancer progression was globally upregulated in epithelial HPV− but not HPV+ cells, indicating therapeutic potential for peptidase inhibitors tailored to HPV− tumors.

The particular advantage of scRNAseq technologies was next leveraged to delineate transcriptomically distinct epithelial subpopulations. Eight subpopulations were subsequently subjected to in-depth analysis. Two of these (C0 and C6) were roughly equally represented; two were enriched in HPV− HNSCCs (C2, C3), and four in HPV+ HNSCCs (C1, C4, C5, C7). First, we examined shared, and, therefore, likely HPV-independent, subpopulations. The C0 subpopulation was defined by metabolic biosynthetic processes while C6 contained cells expressing markers of the G2/M and S phases of the cell cycle, indicative of the HPV-independent presence of cells defined by metabolic and proliferative signatures. Studies of cancer cell metabolism have long highlighted the Warburg effect, unique metabolic rewiring that allows persistent aerobic glycolysis and fuels rapid biosynthesis, growth, and proliferation [54,55]. This signature was indeed observed in the shared C0 subpopulations, and also in the HPV+ enriched C4 subpopulation. In the C6 subpopulation harboring proliferative cells, signaling by p53 class mediators was observed, perhaps representing signaling downstream of the p53 pathway that permits cellular survival and uncontrolled growth. Given that the p53 tumor suppressor is the most commonly mutated gene in HPV− HNSCCs [56] and that high-risk HPV E6 causes the degradation of p53 [57–59], this ontology may reflect a shared functional loss of wild-type p53 followed by unrestricted cellular growth, despite the difference in p53 mutational status between HPV− and HPV+ tumors. This ontology was also shared with that of the HPV+ enriched C4 subpopulation. Altogether, standard therapeutic techniques such as chemo/radiation targeting shared proliferation and cancer cell metabolism signatures would be expected to demonstrate efficacy against these HNSCC subpopulations regardless of HPV status.

Next, we examined epithelial subpopulations relatively enriched in HPV− HNSCCs (C2 and C3). The C2 subpopulation was dominated by mitochondrial processes, such as cellular respiration and electron transport chain functions, while C3 consisted of cells in the G2/M phase of the cell cycle, featuring processes involved in organelle and chromosomal organization, nuclear division, and cytokinesis. Future functional analysis of C3 might yield therapeutic approaches targeting mitotic machineries in HNSCC specifically. This is particularly relevant in light of the recent literature elucidating mechanisms and agents to target cancer cell mitochondria as a novel therapeutic [60,61] and/or to improve the response to existing radiotherapy protocols [62]. Interestingly, a potentially analogous subpopulation for C2 was identified in the HPV+ enriched C1 population, which was also defined by mitochondrial and respiration processes. Several mechanisms of mitochondrial reprogramming by HPV have been reported [63], such as the induction of proapoptotic proteins, reactive oxygen species (ROS), and oxidative stress [64]. A comparative analysis of these subpopulations may further define mechanisms whereby HPV reprograms and dysregulates mitochondrial biology and/or ATP production. Differences and similarities between C3 and C1 may then guide similar and/or distinct mitochondrial targeting strategies for both HPV− and HPV+ HNSCCs.

Lastly, the remaining subpopulations enriched in HPV+ HNSCCs were considered. The defining ontologies of C1 (mitochondrial processes), C4 (cancer cell metabolism), and C7 (aberrant differentiation) were previously discussed, leaving the C5 subpopulation consisting of cells in the S phase of the cell cycle. This enrichment reflected a global shift in the distribution of cells defined by cell-cycle markers between HPV+ and HPV− tumors, wherein we observed a notable increase in cells in the S phase (C5) in HPV+ tumors. This finding was expected given that reprogramming of the cell cycle in high-risk HPV-infected SE by the E6 and E7 oncogenes is classically defined by dysplasia, hyperplasia, and hyperproliferation, and infected cells remain dependent on E6/E7 expression upon transformation into SCC. Thus, the enrichment of cells in the S phase of the cell cycle is anticipated for HPV+ tumors and underscores the validity of novel cell populations and their possible functions identified here based on gene expression patterns.

Altogether, this work represents the first step towards a detailed understanding of distinct epithelial subpopulations in HNSCCs, and their defining transcriptomes and associated biological processes as a function of HPV status. In-depth analysis and functional testing of differentially expressed genes, e.g., those regulating mitochondrial processes, may advance the translational goal of developing novel biomarkers and approaches for the tailored or joint suppression of HPV-driven and -independent effectors. Future analysis may permit the discovery of novel biomarkers and therapeutic targets to eliminate epithelial cells that are crucial for sustaining and promoting the development of each tumor subtype, and new treatment approaches that are shared or uniquely dependent on HPV status. A larger sample size of HPV+ tumors will be needed in the future to address the high clinical variability amongst HPV+ HNSCCs and to identify sub-classes of HPV+ tumors that can be used for stratification in de-escalation attempts.

5. Conclusions

We identify differentially expressed genes and pathways that define and distinguish HPV+ and HPV− epithelial subpopulations in HNSCC. These can now be used as a foundation for the discovery of biomarkers and, through functional laboratory testing, of effectors of HNSCC progression and therapy resistance. New treatment strategies shared by or tailored to HPV tumor status, both HPV+ and HPV−, may emerge from these data.

Supplementary Materials: The following supporting information can be downloaded at: https://www.mdpi.com/article/10.3390/v17040461/s1, Figure S1: Heatmap of genes differentially expressed in epithelial cells in HPV− vs HPV+ HNSCC tumors; Figure S2: Heatmap of genes differentially expressed in epithelial cells in HPV− vs HPV+ HNSCC tumors organized by clusters, with select clusters with distinct differences in gene profiles highlighted with arrows; Table S1: Data—scRNAseq gene lists.

Author Contributions: Conceptualization, M.C.B., R.F., M.A. and S.I.W.; Data curation, M.C.B., C.M.R.-C., R.F. and M.A.; Formal analysis, M.C.B., C.M.R.-C., T.C., A.V., M.T.W. and M.A.; Funding acquisition, M.C.B., M.T.W. and S.I.W.; Investigation, M.C.B., M.A. and S.I.W.; Methodology, M.C.B., T.C. and M.A.; Resources, S.I.W.; Software, M.A.; Supervision, S.I.W.; Writing—original draft, M.C.B.; Writing—review and editing, M.C.B., A.L.T., C.Z., M.T.W., R.F., T.M.W.-D. and S.I.W. All authors have read and agreed to the published version of the manuscript.

Funding: This research was funded by the NIH grants T32ES007250 (M.C.B.), F30AI157229 (M.C.B.), CA228113 (S.I.W.), R01HG010730 (M.T.W) and P30AR070549 (M.T.W.), as well as support from CancerFreeKids (M.C.B.) and the CCHMC ARC Award #53632 (M.T.W.).

Institutional Review Board Statement: Not applicable.

Informed Consent Statement: Not applicable.

Data Availability Statement: Data are contained within the article and Supplementary Materials.

Acknowledgments: We thank all members of the Wells laboratory for reagents and insightful discussions.

Conflicts of Interest: The authors declare no conflicts of interest.

References

1. Gillison, M.L.; Koch, W.M.; Capone, R.B.; Spafford, M.; Westra, W.H.; Wu, L.; Zahurak, M.L.; Daniel, R.W.; Viglione, M.; Symer, D.E.; et al. Evidence for a Causal Association Between Human Papillomavirus and a Subset of Head and Neck Cancers. *JNCI J. Natl. Cancer Inst.* **2000**, *92*, 709–720. [CrossRef] [PubMed]
2. Chaturvedi, A.K.; Engels, E.A.; Pfeiffer, R.M.; Hernandez, B.Y.; Xiao, W.; Kim, E.; Jiang, B.; Goodman, M.T.; Sibug-Saber, M.; Cozen, W.; et al. Human papillomavirus and rising oropharyngeal cancer incidence in the United States. *J. Clin. Oncol.* **2011**, *29*, 4294–4301. [CrossRef] [PubMed]
3. Sung, H.; Ferlay, J.; Siegel, R.L.; Laversanne, M.; Soerjomataram, I.; Jemal, A.; Bray, F. Global Cancer Statistics 2020: GLOBOCAN Estimates of Incidence and Mortality Worldwide for 36 Cancers in 185 Countries. *CA A Cancer J. Clin.* **2021**, *71*, 209–249. [CrossRef] [PubMed]
4. Gillison, M.L.; Broutian, T.; Pickard, R.K.L.; Tong, Z.-Y.; Xiao, W.; Kahle, L.; Graubard, B.I.; Chaturvedi, A.K. Prevalence of Oral HPV Infection in the United States, 2009–2010. *JAMA* **2012**, *307*, 693–703. [CrossRef] [PubMed]
5. Gillison, M.L.; D'Souza, G.; Westra, W.; Sugar, E.; Xiao, W.; Begum, S.; Viscidi, R. Distinct Risk Factor Profiles for Human Papillomavirus Type 16–Positive and Human Papillomavirus Type 16–Negative Head and Neck Cancers. *JNCI J. Natl. Cancer Inst.* **2008**, *100*, 407–420. [CrossRef] [PubMed]
6. Sabatini, M.E.; Chiocca, S. Human papillomavirus as a driver of head and neck cancers. *Br. J. Cancer* **2020**, *122*, 306–314. [CrossRef] [PubMed]
7. Katirachi, S.K.; Grønlund, M.P.; Jakobsen, K.K.; Grønhøj, C.; von Buchwald, C. The Prevalence of HPV in Oral Cavity Squamous Cell Carcinoma. *Viruses* **2023**, *15*, 451. [CrossRef] [PubMed]
8. Gooi, Z.; Chan, J.Y.K.; Fakhry, C. The epidemiology of the human papillomavirus related to oropharyngeal head and neck cancer. *Laryngoscope* **2016**, *126*, 894–900. [CrossRef]
9. Wise-Draper, T.M.; Gulati, S.; Palackdharry, S.; Hinrichs, B.H.; Worden, F.P.; Old, M.O.; Dunlap, N.E.; Kaczmar, J.M.; Patil, Y.; Riaz, M.K.; et al. Phase II Clinical Trial of Neoadjuvant and Adjuvant Pembrolizumab in Resectable Local-Regionally Advanced Head and Neck Squamous Cell Carcinoma. *Clin. Cancer Res.* **2022**, *28*, 1345–1352. [CrossRef]
10. Mehanna, H.; Robinson, M.; Hartley, A.; Kong, A.; Foran, B.; Fulton-Lieuw, T.; Dalby, M.; Mistry, P.; Sen, M.; O'Toole, L.; et al. Radiotherapy plus cisplatin or cetuximab in low-risk human papillomavirus-positive oropharyngeal cancer (De-ESCALaTE HPV): An open-label randomised controlled phase 3 trial. *Lancet* **2019**, *393*, 51–60. [CrossRef]
11. Gillison, M.L.; Trotti, A.M.; Harris, J.; Eisbruch, A.; Harari, P.M.; Adelstein, D.J.; Jordan, R.C.K.; Zhao, W.; Sturgis, E.M.; Burtness, B.; et al. Radiotherapy plus cetuximab or cisplatin in human papillomavirus-positive oropharyngeal cancer (NRG Oncology RTOG 1016): A randomised, multicentre, non-inferiority trial. *Lancet* **2019**, *393*, 40–50. [CrossRef] [PubMed]
12. Nguyen-Tan, P.F.; Zhang, Q.; Ang, K.K.; Weber, R.S.; Rosenthal, D.I.; Soulieres, D.; Kim, H.; Silverman, C.; Raben, A.; Galloway, T.J.; et al. Randomized Phase III Trial to Test Accelerated Versus Standard Fractionation in Combination With Concurrent Cisplatin for Head and Neck Carcinomas in the Radiation Therapy Oncology Group 0129 Trial: Long-Term Report of Efficacy and Toxicity. *J. Clin. Oncol.* **2014**, *32*, 3858–3867. [CrossRef] [PubMed]

13. Chera, B.S.; Amdur, R.J.; Green, R.; Shen, C.; Gupta, G.; Tan, X.; Knowles, M.; Fried, D.; Hayes, N.; Weiss, J.; et al. Phase II Trial of De-Intensified Chemoradiotherapy for Human Papillomavirus–Associated Oropharyngeal Squamous Cell Carcinoma. *J. Clin. Oncol.* **2019**, *37*, 2661–2669. [CrossRef] [PubMed]
14. Chera, B.S.; Amdur, R.J.; Tepper, J.E.; Tan, X.; Weiss, J.; Grilley-Olson, J.E.; Hayes, D.N.; Zanation, A.; Hackman, T.G.; Patel, S.; et al. Mature results of a prospective study of deintensified chemoradiotherapy for low-risk human papillomavirus-associated oropharyngeal squamous cell carcinoma. *Cancer* **2018**, *124*, 2347–2354. [PubMed]
15. Yom, S.S.; Torres-Saavedra, P.; Caudell, J.J.; Waldron, J.N.; Gillison, M.L.; Truong, M.T.; Jordan, R.; Subramaniam, R.; Yao, M.; Chung, C.; et al. NRG-HN002: A Randomized Phase II Trial for Patients With p16-Positive, Non-Smoking-Associated, Locoregionally Advanced Oropharyngeal Cancer. *Int. J. Radiat. Oncol. Biol. Phys.* **2019**, *105*, 684–685. [CrossRef]
16. Ferris, R.L.; Flamand, Y.; Weinstein, G.S.; Li, S.; Quon, H.; Mehra, R.; Garcia, J.J.; Chung, C.H.; Gillison, M.L.; Duvvuri, U.; et al. Phase II Randomized Trial of Transoral Surgery and Low-Dose Intensity Modulated Radiation Therapy in Resectable p16+ Locally Advanced Oropharynx Cancer: An ECOG-ACRIN Cancer Research Group Trial (E3311). *J. Clin. Oncol.* **2021**, *40*, 138–149. [PubMed]
17. Ma, D.J.; Price, K.A.; Moore, E.J.; Patel, S.H.; Hinni, M.L.; Garcia, J.J.; Graner, D.E.; Foster, N.R.; Ginos, B.; Neben-Wittich, M.; et al. Phase II Evaluation of Aggressive Dose De-Escalation for Adjuvant Chemoradiotherapy in Human Papillomavirus–Associated Oropharynx Squamous Cell Carcinoma. *J. Clin. Oncol.* **2019**, *37*, 1909–1918. [PubMed]
18. Fakhry, C.; Westra, W.H.; Li, S.; Cmelak, A.; Ridge, J.A.; Pinto, H.; Forastiere, A.; Gillison, M.L. Improved Survival of Patients With Human Papillomavirus–Positive Head and Neck Squamous Cell Carcinoma in a Prospective Clinical Trial. *JNCI J. Natl. Cancer Inst.* **2008**, *100*, 261–269.
19. Marur, S.; Li, S.; Cmelak, A.J.; Gillison, M.L.; Zhao, W.J.; Ferris, R.L.; Westra, W.H.; Gilbert, J.; Bauman, J.E.; Wagner, L.I.; et al. E1308: Phase II Trial of Induction Chemotherapy Followed by Reduced-Dose Radiation and Weekly Cetuximab in Patients With HPV-Associated Resectable Squamous Cell Carcinoma of the Oropharynx—ECOG-ACRIN Cancer Research Group. *J. Clin. Oncol.* **2016**, *35*, 490–497. [CrossRef]
20. Villaflor, V.M.; Melotek, J.M.; Karrison, T.G.; Brisson, R.J.; Blair, E.A.; Portugal, L.; De Souza, J.A.; Ginat, D.T.; Stenson, K.M.; Langerman, A.; et al. Response-adapted volume de-escalation (RAVD) in locally advanced head and neck cancer. *Ann. Oncol.* **2016**, *27*, 908–913. [CrossRef]
21. Seiwert, T.Y.; Foster, C.C.; Blair, E.A.; Karrison, T.G.; Agrawal, N.; Melotek, J.M.; Portugal, L.; Brisson, R.J.; Dekker, A.; Kochanny, S.; et al. OPTIMA: A phase II dose and volume de-escalation trial for human papillomavirus-positive oropharyngeal cancer. *Ann. Oncol.* **2019**, *30*, 297–302. [CrossRef] [PubMed]
22. Chen, A.M.; Felix, C.; Wang, P.-C.; Hsu, S.; Basehart, V.; Garst, J.; Beron, P.; Wong, D.; Rosove, M.H.; Rao, S.; et al. Reduced-dose radiotherapy for human papillomavirus-associated squamous-cell carcinoma of the oropharynx: A single-arm, phase 2 study. *Lancet Oncol.* **2017**, *18*, 803–811. [CrossRef] [PubMed]
23. Yom, S.S.; Harris, J.; Caudell, J.J.; Geiger, J.L.; Waldron, J.; Gillison, M.; Subramaniam, R.M.; Yao, M.; Xiao, C.; Kovalchuk, N.; et al. nterim Futility Results of NRG-HN005, A Randomized, Phase II/III Non-Inferiority Trial for Non-Smoking p16+ Oropharyngeal Cancer Patients. *Int. J. Radiat. Oncol. Biol. Phys.* **2024**, *120*, S2–S3. [CrossRef]
24. Rosenberg, A.J.; Vokes, E.E. Optimizing Treatment De-Escalation in Head and Neck Cancer: Current and Future Perspectives. *Oncologist* **2021**, *26*, 40–48. [CrossRef]
25. Farah, C.S. Molecular landscape of head and neck cancer and implications for therapy. *Ann. Transl. Med.* **2021**, *9*, 915. [CrossRef] [PubMed]
26. Routman, D.M.; Chera, B.S.; Jethwa, K.R.; Van Abel, K.; Kumar, S.; DeWees, T.A.; Garcia, J.J.; Price, D.L.; Kasperbauer, J.L.; Laack, N.N., II; et al. Detectable HPV ctDNA in Post-Operative Oropharyngeal Squamous Cell Carcinoma Patients is Associated With Progression. *Int. J. Radiat. Oncol. Biol. Phys.* **2019**, *105*, 682–683. [CrossRef]
27. Chera, B.S.; Kumar, S.; Shen, C.; Amdur, R.; Dagan, R.; Green, R.; Goldman, E.; Weiss, J.; Grilley-Olson, J.; Patel, S.; et al. Plasma Circulating Tumor HPV DNA for the Surveillance of Cancer Recurrence in HPV-Associated Oropharyngeal Cancer. *J. Clin. Oncol.* **2020**, *38*, 1050–1058. [CrossRef] [PubMed]
28. Naegele, S.; Efthymiou, V.; Das, D.; Sadow, P.M.; Richmon, J.D.; Iafrate, A.J.; Faden, D.L. Detection and Monitoring of Circulating Tumor HPV DNA in HPV-Associated Sinonasal and Nasopharyngeal Cancers. *JAMA Otolaryngol.–Head Neck Surg.* **2023**, *149*, 179–181. [CrossRef] [PubMed]
29. Yang, R.; Li, T.; Zhang, S.; Shui, C.; Ma, H.; Li, C. The effect of circulating tumor DNA on the prognosis of patients with head and neck squamous cell carcinoma: A systematic review and meta-analysis. *BMC Cancer* **2024**, *24*, 1434. [CrossRef]
30. Carlos de Vicente, J.; Junquera Gutiérrez, L.M.; Zapatero, A.H.; Fresno Forcelledo, M.F.; Hernández-Vallejo, G.; López Arranz, J.S. Prognostic significance of p53 expression in oral squamous cell carcinoma without neck node metastases. *Head Neck* **2004**, *26*, 22–30. [CrossRef]

31. Beaty, B.T.; Moon, D.H.; Shen, C.J.; Amdur, R.J.; Weiss, J.; Grilley-Olson, J.; Patel, S.; Zanation, A.; Hackman, T.G.; Thorp, B.; et al. PIK3CA Mutation in HPV-Associated OPSCC Patients Receiving Deintensified Chemoradiation. *JNCI J. Natl. Cancer Inst.* **2020**, *112*, 855–858. [CrossRef] [PubMed]
32. Patel, K.B.; Mroz, E.A.; Faquin, W.C.; Rocco, J.W. A combination of intra-tumor genetic heterogeneity, estrogen receptor alpha and human papillomavirus status predicts outcomes in head and neck squamous cell carcinoma following chemoradiotherapy. *Oral Oncol.* **2021**, *120*, 105421. [PubMed]
33. Hajek, M.; Sewell, A.; Kaech, S.; Burtness, B.; Yarbrough, W.G.; Issaeva, N. TRAF3/CYLD mutations identify a distinct subset of human papillomavirus-associated head and neck squamous cell carcinoma. *Cancer* **2017**, *123*, 1778–1790. [CrossRef] [PubMed]
34. Kürten, C.H.L.; Kulkarni, A.; Cillo, A.R.; Santos, P.M.; Roble, A.K.; Onkar, S.; Reeder, C.; Lang, S.; Chen, X.; Duvvuri, U.; et al. Investigating immune and non-immune cell interactions in head and neck tumors by single-cell RNA sequencing. *Nat. Commun.* **2021**, *12*, 7338. [PubMed]
35. Hao, Y.; Hao, S.; Andersen-Nissen, E.; Mauck, W.M., 3rd; Zheng, S.; Butler, A.; Lee, M.J.; Wilk, A.J.; Darby, C.; Zager, M.; et al. Integrated analysis of multimodal single-cell data. *Cell* **2021**, *184*, 3573–3587.e29. [CrossRef] [PubMed]
36. Raudvere, U.; Kolberg, L.; Kuzmin, I.; Arak, T.; Adler, P.; Peterson, H.; Vilo, J. g:Profiler: A web server for functional enrichment analysis and conversions of gene lists (2019 update). *Nucleic Acids Res.* **2019**, *47*, W191–W198. [PubMed]
37. Cunningham, F.; Achuthan, P.; Akanni, W.; Allen, J.; Amode, M.R.; Armean, I.M.; Bennett, R.; Bhai, J.; Billis, K.; Boddu, S.; et al. Ensembl 2019. *Nucleic Acids Res.* **2019**, *47*, D745–D751. [PubMed]
38. Merico, D.; Isserlin, R.; Stueker, O.; Emili, A.; Bader, G.D. Enrichment Map: A Network-Based Method for Gene-Set Enrichment Visualization and Interpretation. *PLoS ONE* **2010**, *5*, e13984.
39. Bedard, M.C.; Chihanga, T.; Carlile, A.; Jackson, R.; Brusadelli, M.G.; Lee, D.; VonHandorf, A.; Rochman, M.; Dexheimer, P.J.; Chalmers, J.; et al. Single cell transcriptomic analysis of HPV16-infected epithelium identifies a keratinocyte subpopulation implicated in cancer. *Nat. Commun.* **2023**, *14*, 1975.
40. Kowalczyk, M.S.; Tirosh, I.; Heckl, D.; Nageswara Rao, T.; Dixit, A.; Haas, B.J.; Schneider, R.; Wagers, A.J.; Ebert, B.L.; Regev, A. Single cell RNA-seq reveals changes in cell cycle and differentiation programs upon aging of hematopoietic stem cells. *Genome Res.* **2015**, *25*, 1860–1872.
41. Tirosh, I.; Izar, B.; Prakadan, S.M.; Wadsworth, M.H.; Treacy, D.; Trombetta, J.J.; Rotem, A.; Rodman, C.; Lian, C.; Murphy, G.; et al. Dissecting the multicellular ecosystem of metastatic melanoma by single-cell RNA-seq. *Science* **2016**, *352*, 189–196. [CrossRef] [PubMed]
42. Li, H.; Zandberg, D.P.; Kulkarni, A.; Chiosea, S.I.; Santos, P.M.; Isett, B.R.; Joy, M.; Sica, G.L.; Contrera, K.J.; Tatsuoka, C.M.; et al. Ferris, Distinct CD8+ T cell dynamics associate with response to neoadjuvant cancer immunotherapies. *Cancer Cell* **2025**. ahead of print. [CrossRef]
43. Cillo, A.R.; Kürten, C.H.L.; Tabib, T.; Qi, Z.; Onkar, S.; Wang, T.; Liu, A.; Duvvuri, U.; Kim, S.; Soose, R.J.; et al. Immune Landscape of Viral- and Carcinogen-Driven Head and Neck Cancer. *Immunity* **2020**, *52*, 183–199.e9. [CrossRef] [PubMed]
44. Kondoh, N.; Mizuno-Kamiya, M. The Role of Immune Modulatory Cytokines in the Tumor Microenvironments of Head and Neck Squamous Cell Carcinomas. *Cancers* **2022**, *14*, 2884. [CrossRef]
45. Conarty, J.P.; Wieland, A. The Tumor-Specific Immune Landscape in HPV+ Head and Neck Cancer. *Viruses* **2023**, *15*, 1296. [CrossRef] [PubMed]
46. de Freitas, A.C.; de Oliveira, T.H.A.; Barros, M.R.; Venuti, A. hrHPV E5 oncoprotein: Immune evasion and related immunotherapies. *J. Exp. Clin. Cancer Res.* **2017**, *36*, 71. [CrossRef] [PubMed]
47. Westrich, J.A.; Warren, C.J.; Pyeon, D. Evasion of host immune defenses by human papillomavirus. *Virus Res.* **2017**, *231*, 21–33. [CrossRef] [PubMed]
48. Miyauchi, S.; Kim, S.S.; Jones, R.N.; Zhang, L.; Guram, K.; Sharma, S.; Schoenberger, S.P.; Cohen, E.E.W.; Califano, J.A.; Sharabi, A.B. Human papillomavirus E5 suppresses immunity via inhibition of the immunoproteasome and STING pathway. *Cell Rep.* **2023**, *42*, 112508. [CrossRef] [PubMed]
49. Jung, A.R.; Jung, C.-H.; Noh, J.K.; Lee, Y.C.; Eun, Y.-G. Epithelial-mesenchymal transition gene signature is associated with prognosis and tumor microenvironment in head and neck squamous cell carcinoma. *Sci. Rep.* **2020**, *10*, 3652. [CrossRef]
50. van der Heijden, M.; Essers, P.B.M.; Verhagen, C.V.M.; Willems, S.M.; Sanders, J.; de Roest, R.H.; Vossen, D.M.; Leemans, C.R.; Verheij, M.; Brakenhoff, R.H.; et al. Epithelial-to-mesenchymal transition is a prognostic marker for patient outcome in advanced stage HNSCC patients treated with chemoradiotherapy. *Radiother. Oncol.* **2020**, *147*, 186–194. [CrossRef]
51. Matthews, K.; Leong Cheng, M.; Baxter, L.; Inglis, E.; Yun, K.; Bäckström, B.T.; Doorbar, J.; Hibma, M. Depletion of Langerhans Cells in Human Papillomavirus Type 16-Infected Skin Is Associated with E6-Mediated Down Regulation of E-Cadherin. *J. Virol.* **2003**, *77*, 8378–8385. [PubMed]
52. Jung, Y.-S.; Kato, I.; Kim, H.-R.C. A novel function of HPV16-E6/E7 in epithelial–mesenchymal transition. *Biochem. Biophys. Res. Commun.* **2013**, *435*, 339–344. [CrossRef] [PubMed]

53. Rezaei, M.; Mostafaei, S.; Aghaei, A.; Hosseini, N.; Darabi, H.; Nouri, M.; Etemadi, A.; Neill, A.O.; Nahand, J.S.; Mirzaei, H.; et al. The association between HPV gene expression, inflammatory agents and cellular genes involved in EMT in lung cancer tissue. *BMC Cancer* **2020**, *20*, 916. [CrossRef] [PubMed]
54. Hsu, P.P.; Sabatini, D.M. Cancer Cell Metabolism: Warburg and Beyond. *Cell* **2008**, *134*, 703–707.
55. Liberti, M.V.; Locasale, J.W. The Warburg Effect: How Does it Benefit Cancer Cells? *Trends Biochem Sci* **2016**, *41*, 211–218. [CrossRef] [PubMed]
56. Nathan, C.-A.; Khandelwal, A.R.; Wolf, G.T.; Rodrigo, J.P.; Mäkitie, A.A.; Saba, N.F.; Forastiere, A.A.; Bradford, C.R.; Ferlito, A. TP53 mutations in head and neck cancer. *Mol. Carcinog.* **2022**, *61*, 385–391.
57. Thomas, M.; Pim, D.; Banks, L. The role of the E6-p53 interaction in the molecular pathogenesis of HPV. *Oncogene* **1999**, *18*, 7690–7700. [PubMed]
58. Werness, B.A.; Levine, A.J.; Howley, P.M. Association of human papillomavirus types 16 and 18 E6 proteins with p53. *Science* **1990**, *248*, 76–79.
59. Scheffner, M.; Werness, B.A.; Huibregtse, J.M.; Levine, A.J.; Howley, P.M. The E6 oncoprotein encoded by human papillomavirus types 16 and 18 promotes the degradation of p53. *Cell* **1990**, *63*, 1129–1136. [CrossRef]
60. Wen, S.; Zhu, D.; Huang, P. Targeting Cancer Cell Mitochondria as a Therapeutic Approach. *Future Med. Chem.* **2013**, *5*, 53–67. [CrossRef]
61. Guo, X.; Yang, N.; Ji, W.; Zhang, H.; Dong, X.; Zhou, Z.; Li, L.; Shen, H.-M.; Yao, S.Q.; Huang, W. Mito-Bomb: Targeting Mitochondria for Cancer Therapy. *Adv. Mater.* **2021**, *33*, 2007778. [CrossRef] [PubMed]
62. McCann, E.; O'Sullivan, J.; Marcone, S. Targeting cancer-cell mitochondria and metabolism to improve radiotherapy response. *Transl. Oncol.* **2021**, *14*, 100905. [CrossRef] [PubMed]
63. Cruz-Gregorio, A.; Aranda-Rivera, A.K.; Roviello, G.N.; Pedraza-Chaverri, J. Targeting Mitochondrial Therapy in the Regulation of HPV Infection and HPV-Related Cancers. *Pathogens* **2023**, *12*, 402. [CrossRef] [PubMed]
64. Cruz-Gregorio, A.; Aranda-Rivera, A.K.; Pedraza-Chaverri, J. Human Papillomavirus-related Cancers and Mitochondria. *Virus Res.* **2020**, *286*, 198016. [CrossRef] [PubMed]

Disclaimer/Publisher's Note: The statements, opinions and data contained in all publications are solely those of the individual author(s) and contributor(s) and not of MDPI and/or the editor(s). MDPI and/or the editor(s) disclaim responsibility for any injury to people or property resulting from any ideas, methods, instructions or products referred to in the content.

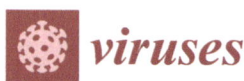

Article

Detection of High-Risk Human Papillomavirus (HPV), p16 and EGFR in Lung Cancer: Insights from the Mediterranean Region of Turkey

Arsenal Sezgin Alikanoğlu [1,*] and İrem Atalay Karaçay [2]

[1] Pathology Department, Antalya Education and Research Hospital, Health Sciences University, Antalya 07100, Turkey
[2] Pathology Department, Alanya Alaaddin Keykubat University, Antalya 07400, Turkey; irematalay@hotmail.com
* Correspondence: arsi75@hotmail.com; Tel.: +90-532-5829609

Abstract: Human papillomavirus (HPV) is an oncogenic DNA virus that plays a role in different cancer types. The aim of this study was to detect the prevalence and types of HPV and its relation with p16, EGFR and clinical findings in lung cancer. HPV and EGFR detection and genotyping of HPV were performed by polymerase chain reaction (PCR) and p16 by immunohistochemistry. Fifty lung cancer patients and seven patients with non-neoplastic lung disease were enrolled in this study. HPV was positive in 78% (39/50) of lung cancer cases. HPV 51 was the most frequent type, followed by HPV 16. Moreover, p16 was positive in 24% (12/50) of the cancer patients, and all of these patients were HPV-positive, while 27 HPV-positive patients showed no p16 expression. There was no relationship between HPV infection and p16 (p = 0.05), gender (p = 0.42), age (p = 0.38), or smoking history (p = 0.68). Although not statistically significant, the HPV prevalence was found to be higher in cancer patients compared to non-neoplastic patients. The prevalence of HPV in lung cancer varies across different studies, which may be due to differences in the detection methods, number of patients, geographic regions, and vaccination status. Further studies are necessary to understand the role of HPV in lung cancer pathogenesis.

Keywords: lung cancer; human papillomavirus (HPV); polymerase chain reaction (PCR); viral oncology; p16 protein

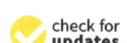

Citation: Alikanoğlu, A.S.; Karaçay, İ.A. Detection of High-Risk Human Papillomavirus (HPV), p16 and EGFR in Lung Cancer: Insights from the Mediterranean Region of Turkey. *Viruses* 2024, *16*, 1201. https://doi.org/10.3390/v16081201

Academic Editors: Daniel DiMaio, Hossein H. Ashrafi and Mustafa Ozdogan

Received: 12 June 2024
Revised: 15 July 2024
Accepted: 23 July 2024
Published: 26 July 2024

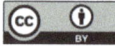

Copyright: © 2024 by the authors. Licensee MDPI, Basel, Switzerland. This article is an open access article distributed under the terms and conditions of the Creative Commons Attribution (CC BY) license (https:// creativecommons.org/licenses/by/ 4.0/).

1. Introduction

Lung cancer is the leading cause of cancer death in both men and women worldwide. Smoking ranks first among the etiological factors that cause the development of lung cancer [1–3]. The cases of lung cancer detected in non-smokers are more often seen in females and in Asian countries. Furthermore, these cases have different molecular characteristics compared to the cases of lung cancer in smokers. Genetic susceptibility, radiation, environmental pollution, occupational exposure, and infectious agents, especially those of viral origin, can be counted among the other factors that play a role in lung carcinogenesis, apart from smoking [4–6].

It is known that about 10–15% of cancers seen in humans all over the world are caused by Epstein–Barr virus, hepatitis B or C virus, human T-lymphotropic virus-1, human papillomavirus (HPV) and Merkel cell polyomavirus. The viruses can promote cancer as carcinogens or promoters.

HPV is a non-enveloped, small, double-stranded circular DNA virus and has "low-risk" or "high-risk" types, which are defined according to their relation with cancer development. HPV is known to dysregulate the cell cycle at the transition from the G1 to S phase and to promote DNA synthesis for viral replication. The expression of the most important viral oncoproteins, E6 and E7, is considered a first step in carcinogenesis since these oncoproteins inactivate the two important products of tumor suppressor genes p53 and retinoblastoma protein (pRb), respectively [7]. P16 is also a tumor suppressor protein that functions as an inhibitor of cyclin-dependent kinase 4 (CDK4) and regulates the cell cycle. Loss of p16, as reported in a variety of tumors, including lung cancer, causes phosphorylation of Rb, which ends up with uncontrolled cell proliferation [8–10].

The link between HPV and bronchial lesions was first established in the 1970s by Rubel and Reynold, who found that there is cytological and histological similarity between condyloma acuminatum and squamous cell papilloma of the respiratory tract. They detected koilocytes, which are characteristic of HPV infections in the sputum samples of patients with benign bronchial lesions [11]. There are also other studies presenting condylomatous histological changes in bronchial epithelium and bronchial squamous cell carcinoma, similar to the changes seen in the genital tract [4,12,13].

After these detections, the relationship between HPV infection and lung cancer has been investigated in several studies until today. These studies revealed a great difference in the HPV infection rate in lung cancer (0–78.3%) in different regions of the world. It is suggested that this wide range may be due to the difference in sensitivity and specificity of the methods used for HPV genotyping, the number of types of HPV analyzed, the diagnostic criteria, the number and characteristics of patients and the ethnicity of patients [1,3,14–19].

Epidermal growth factor receptor (EGFR) is a receptor tyrosine kinase that affects some signaling pathways in cell proliferation. Mutations in EGFR may cause uncontrolled growth and proliferation of cells, especially in non-small-cell lung cancer (NSCLC). EGFR mutations are detected more frequently in women, non-smokers, adenocarcinoma, and Asian populations [20–23]. The most commonly detected mutations in EGFR in NSCLC are exon 19 deletion (small in-frame deletions in exon 19) and L858R point mutation (amino acid substitution (leucine to arginine) at codon 858 in exon 21) [20,21]. EGFR tyrosine-kinase inhibitors (gefitinib, erlotinib) are considered the standard first-line treatment for patients with EGFR mutations and therefore it is recommended that screening for EGFR mutations should be a part of the routine clinical practice for NSCLC patients [20,23]. Previous studies demonstrated that HPV infection was found more frequently in lung adenocarcinoma patients with EGFR gene mutations than in patients without mutations, suggesting that the viral protein E6 regulates the inhibitors of apoptosis of the EGFR/PI3K/AKT signaling pathway [22,23].

In this study, we aimed to investigate the prevalence of HPV and its genotypes and the relation with EGFR mutations, p16 protein expression and clinicopathological findings in lung cancer.

2. Materials and Methods

2.1. Patient Selection and Data Collection

This study included 50 patients who had a histopathologic diagnosis of primary lung carcinoma in lobectomy specimens and 7 patients who had surgery for a non-tumoral lung pathology (bullous disease, infection) at a tertiary-level hospital between 1 January 2013 and 1 January 2019. None of the patients received HPV vaccination. This study was performed in accordance with the ethical standards of the Declaration of Helsinki, 2013. The study was approved by the Ethics Committee of Health Sciences University, Antalya Education and Research Hospital (date and register number: 2019-242, 19/9). Hematoxylin and eosin sections of the cases were obtained from the archive and examined histologically by the authors (A.S.A. and İ.A.K.). The demographic and clinical characteristics of the patients, including age, gender, smoking history (the patients who self-reported as a current or former smoker and had smoked ≥100 cigarettes in their lifetime were accepted as "smoker", based on the criteria proposed by the Centers for Disease Control and Prevention), and pathological data were obtained through patient records and pathology reports from the hospital database. The non-metastatic patients (42/50) received adjuvant chemotherapy, while the patients without EGFR and anaplastic lymphoma kinase (ALK) mutation received palliative platinum-based systemic chemotherapy at a metastatic setting. Eight of the patients had distant metastasis. According to the frequency of occurrence, metastases were detected in the brain, costa and liver.

2.2. DNA Extraction

DNA was extracted from the formalin-fixed paraffin-embedded blocks of 57 patients for HPV analysis and 50 patients for EGFR analysis. Eight tissue sections of 10 μm thickness were used per patient for DNA extraction. DNA was extracted and deparaffinized from the sections using the QIAamp DNA FFPE Tissue kit (Qiagen, Hilden, Germany) according to the manufacturer's instruction for real-time PCR analysis of HPV and EGFR. In order to avoid contamination, precautions were taken, including extensive cleaning of the work area, changing the microtome blades and cleaning of the microtome after cutting each sample, performing extraction of DNA in tumoral and non-tumoral samples separately and using appropriate protection equipment.

2.3. HPV DNA Detection and Genotyping

Detection and genotyping of human papillomavirus (16, 18, 31, 33, 35, 39, 45, 51, 52, 56, 58, 59, 66, 68) were performed using the HPV Genotypes 14 Real-TM Quant kit (Nuclear Laser Medicine, Milan, Italy), which was based on two major processes: isolation of DNA from specimens and multiplex real-time amplification of 4 PCR tubes for each sample, each tube amplifying "16-18-31-IC", "39-45-59-IC", "33-35-56-68" and "51-52-58-66". For each sample, negative and positive clinical samples were used as controls. The HPV Genotypes 14 Real-TM Quant kit contains the internal control (human beta-globin gene), which allows control of the presence of cellular material in the sample in order to avoid false-negative results.

HPV DNA amplification was carried out in the real-time PCR cycler (Rotor-Gene™ 3000/6000/Q (Qiagen, Hilden, Germany), and for the quantitative analysis, Microsoft® Excel HPV Genotype 14 Real-TM.xls, ver. 09.09.21 (Sacace Biotechnologies®, Como, Italy) was used according to the enclosed instructions.

2.4. EGFR Mutation Detection

The extracted DNA samples were assessed using real-time PCR (Rotor-Gene™ 3000/6000/Q, Qiagen, Hilden, Germany) with the Easy EGFR Real Time PCR kit (Diatech Pharmacogenetics, Jesi, Italy) following the manufacturer's protocol. Each DNA sample was analyzed for mutations on exon 18 (G719X), exon 19 (ex19del), exon 20 (T790M, S768I, ex20ins), and exon 21 (L858R, L861Q). A positive control was included with the kit, and distilled water was used as the negative control.

2.5. p16 Immunohistochemical Staining

For the detection of p16, monoclonal mouse anti-human antibody (clone INK4A, Clone IHC116, 1:200 dilution, GeneAb, Richmond, BC, Canada) was used according to the manufacturer's suggested protocol, using the automated staining system Bench-mark XT (Roche/Ventana Medical Systems, Tucson, AZ, USA). Deparaffinization at 75 °C was followed by antigen retrieval by CC1 buffer for 64 min. Incubation lasted for 44 min at 36 °C. Diaminobenzidine was used as a chromogen. After washing, the slides were placed in differently graded alcohol solution and xylene and finally mounted with entellan. Cervical cancer and parathyroid tissue were used as positive and negative controls, respectively. The slides were evaluated by the authors (A.S.A., İ.A.K.). Nuclear and cytoplasmic staining in $\geq$10% of the tumor cells was accepted as positive, while <10% was considered as negative for p16 [8].

2.6. Statistical Analysis

Statistical analyses were carried out using IBM SPSS Statistics for Windows, version 23.0 (IBM Corp., Armonk, NY, USA). The descriptive findings were presented as the mean $\pm$ standard deviation (SD) for the continuous data, and as the frequency and percentage for the categorical data. The normality assumptions were controlled by the

Shapiro–Wilk test. Categorical data were analyzed by the Pearson chi-square test and Fisher's exact test. Student's *t*-test was used for analysis of the normally distributed numerical data. Two-sided *p* values < 0.05 were considered statistically significant.

3. Results
3.1. Clinicopathological Characteristics of Patients

This study included 57 patients with a mean age of 63.2 ± 2.8 (range 27–83 years). In this study, the male gender prevailed (84.2%) and almost 60% of patients had a history of smoking. Thirty of the male patients and four of the female patients were smokers. All the patients with non-neoplastic disease were non-smokers. The two most common histological tumor types were squamous cell carcinoma (54.4%) and adenocarcinoma (22.8%).

The clinicopathologic characteristics of the patients are summarized in Table 1.

Table 1. The clinicopathological characteristics of the patients and their HPV status.

Characteristic		HPV Positive (n)	HPV Negative (n)	HPV and p16 Positive (n)
Age (years)	≤62	20	1	3
	>62	23	13	9
Gender	Female	8	7	3
	Male	35	7	9
Smoking history	Smoker	25	9	6
	Non-smoker	18	5	6
Histopathological diagnosis	Squamous cell carcinoma	20	11	7
	Adenocarcinoma	13	0	1
	Other tumors	6	0	4
	Non-neoplastic	4	3	-*
EGFR status	Wild type	36	11	11
	Mutated	3	0	1
	Not applied	4	3	0

n: number of patients, * p16 immunohistochemistry was not applied in non-neoplastic patients.

3.2. HPV Infection, Prevalence of HPV Types, and Their Relationship with Clinicopathologic Parameters

In total, 75.4% (43/57) of the patients were HPV-positive. The HPV positivity rate was 57.1% (4/7) in the non-neoplastic samples and 78% (39/50) in the neoplastic samples. All the adenocarcinomas (13/13, 100%) and 64.5% (20/31) of the squamous cell carcinomas showed positivity for high-risk HPV DNA. HPV 51 was the most frequent HPV type (49.1%, n = 27), followed by HPV 16 (43.9%), HPV 31 (15.8%), and HPV 18 (12.3%). Among the smokers, the HPV positivity rate was found to be 73.5% (25/34), and 28% (14/50) of the cancer patients were non-smokers and HPV-positive. In terms of the histopathological diagnosis and HPV status, the frequency of adenocarcinoma was higher in the HPV-positive cases.

The prevalence of the HPV types by gender and tumor type are represented in Figures 1 and 2. Higher rates of HPV 51 and 56 positivity were detected in women; however, there was no statistically significant relationship between HPV infection and gender ($p = 0.42$), age ($p = 0.38$), or smoking history ($p = 0.68$). HPV 16 positivity was more common in adenocarcinomas ($p = 0.006$). Furthermore, HPV 51 was more frequent in adenocarcinomas and other histological types of carcinomas, including large- and small-cell carcinoma and large-cell neuroendocrine carcinoma ($p < 0.001$), and it was the only type detected in the histological types of carcinomas other than adenocarcinoma and squamous cell carcinoma.

When the HPV and p16 positive tumors were analyzed as one category, HPV 51 was the most frequent type, followed by HPV 16, as shown in Figure 3.

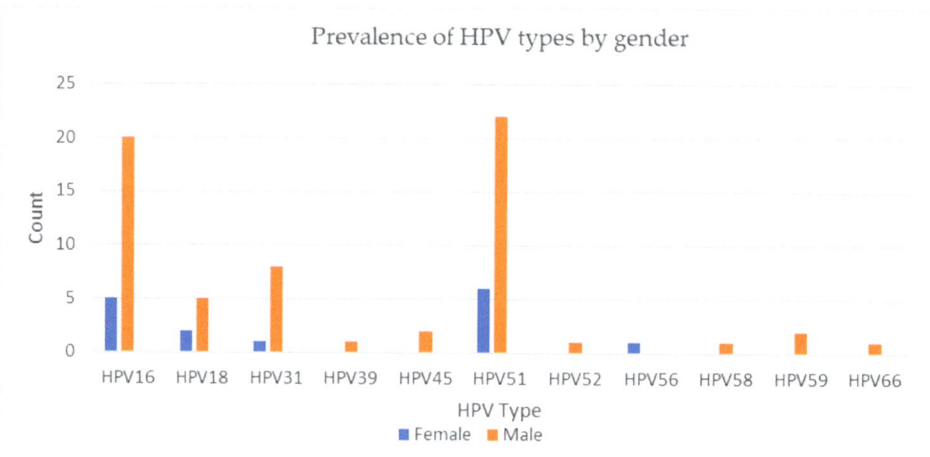

Figure 1. Prevalence of HPV types by gender.

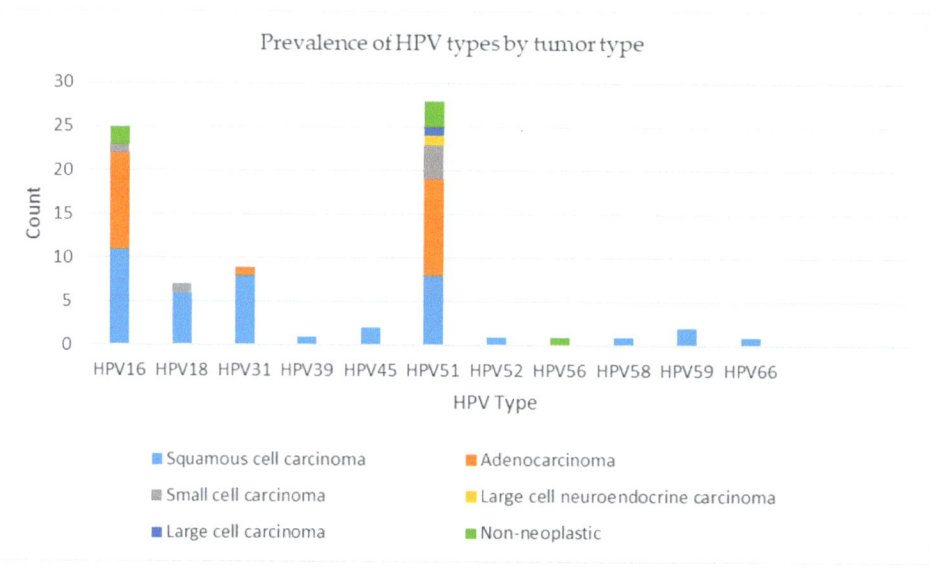

Figure 2. Prevalence of HPV types by tumor type.

Most samples (58.1%, 25/43) contained multiple HPV types, with HPV16 and HPV51 being the most prevalent. Figure 4 displays the occurrence of multiple HPV genotypes among the different types of tumors and non-neoplastic lung tissue.

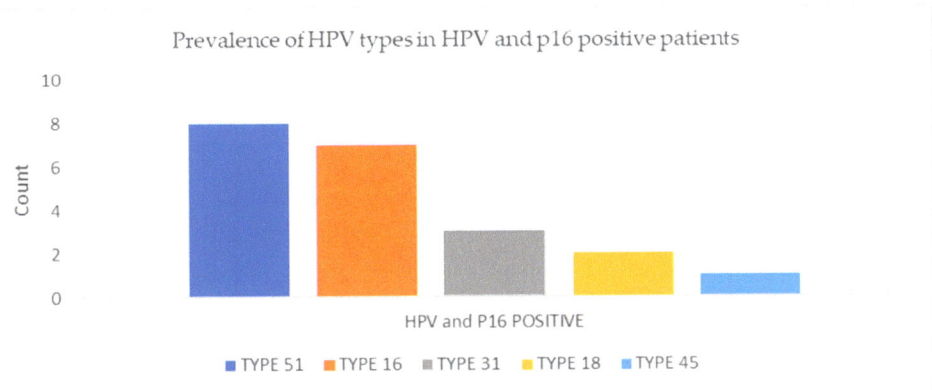

Figure 3. Prevalence of HPV types in HPV- and p16-positive patients.

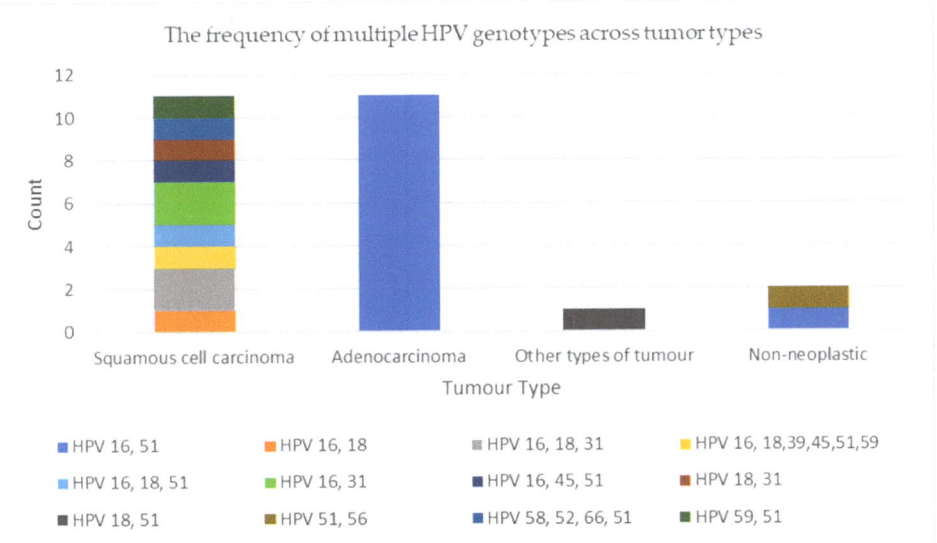

Figure 4. The frequency of multiple HPV genotypes across tumor types.

3.3. Presence of EGFR Mutation and Its Relation with HPV

EGFR mutation was detected in 3/50 (6%) of lung cancer cases, and all the cases with EGFR mutation revealed exon 19 deletion. All the EGFR-mutated patients had a histopathological diagnosis of adenocarcinoma and revealed multiple infection of HPV types 16 and 51, and two of them were smokers. There was no significant relationship between HPV positivity and the presence of EGFR mutation in the lung cancer cases ($p > 0.999$).

3.4. Detection of p16 by Immunohistochemistry

The expression of the p16 protein was detected in 12 of the 50 (24%) cancer patients. HPV was positive in 100% of the p16-positive cases. A total of 11 cases were both p16-negative and HPV-negative. The number of HPV-positive and p16-negative cases was found to be 27. There was no significant relationship between HPV status and p16 protein expression ($p = 0.05$), as shown in Table 2. The p16 expression showed variation in the different histological types of tumors. The highest expression was found in squamous cell carcinoma (7/12), followed by small-cell carcinoma (3/12), large-cell adenocarcinoma (1/12) and adenocarcinoma (1/12), as shown in Table 1.

Table 2. HPV rates in the p16-positive and -negative groups.

		HPV-Positive (n = 39)	HPV-Negative (n = 11)	p *
P16	Positive	12 (30.8)	0 (0)	0.05
	Negative	27 (69.2)	11 (100)	

* Fisher's exact test, n (%).

Figure 5 shows the immunohistochemical expression of p16 in the positive control and cancer tissue samples.

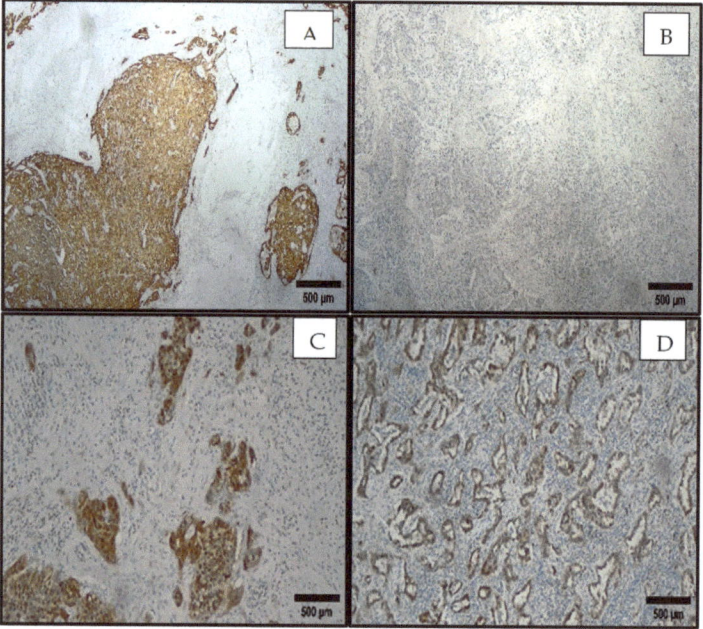

Figure 5. p16 staining, immunohistochemistry, Nikon Ci-L light microscope. (Nikon Corporation, Yokohama, Japan) (**A**) Positive in cervix cancer as a positive control, ×40. (**B**) Negative in lung adenocarcinoma, ×40. (**C**) Positive in lung squamous cell carcinoma, ×100. (**D**) Positive in lung adenocarcinoma, ×100.

4. Discussion

Since lung cancer is the leading cause of cancer death worldwide, studies on the etiological factors and carcinogenesis are important, especially for guiding prophylactic therapy with vaccines and targeted therapy. Although there is some supporting evidence concerning the relation between HPV infection and lung carcinogenesis, the subject is still controversial, and because of this, studies on this issue are ongoing.

The rate of HPV positivity in lung cancer reported in several studies is between 0 and 78.3%. Some of the studies report that there is a close relationship between HPV and lung cancer [3,14,24–26], while some of them report the very low prevalence of HPV in lung cancer [1,2,27–29]. HPV seems to be more associated with lung cancer in certain geographical regions of the world [6]. In many studies, it is evidenced that the prevalence of HPV in lung cancer is higher in Asian countries than on the other continents [15,30–35]. Furthermore, the HPV prevalence rate ranging from 0% to 61% in different studies conducted in Greece indicates that the results can be discrepant even within the same country [14,27].

In previous studies, the HPV positivity rate was found to be higher in cancer patients than in non-neoplastic controls [15,26,36]. The most recent meta-analysis study reported the prevalence difference of HPV to be 22% in lung cancer compared to control cases [24]. In our study, HPV positivity was detected in 78% of the cancer group and 57% in the non-neoplastic group. The prevalence difference was found to be 21%, similar to the meta-analysis study mentioned above.

To date, few studies have investigated the prevalence of HPV in lung cancer in Turkey. The rate of HPV positivity reported in these studies is between 1.54 and 11.5% and the most commonly detected HPV type is HPV 16/18 [37–39]. The differences in the sample types and sizes, as well as the HPV detection/genotyping methods used, may be the reason for the different results.

The high rate of HPV prevalence detected in our study in both cancer and non-neoplastic tissue may be due to factors including the vaccination status and the number of the patients selected from a single region. The FDA-approved HPV vaccine has been on the Turkish market since April 2007. But, in Turkey, the HPV vaccine is not included in the national vaccination program, and people who want to be vaccinated are vaccinated at their own expense. None of the patients included in our study were vaccinated.

In previous studies, there are conflicting results regarding the association between smoking and HPV infection. Some studies have shown that the interaction of smoking and HPV induces viral oncoproteins [40] and that the majority of HPV-positive lung cancers are smokers [36], whereas others concluded that smoking is an independent factor in lung cancer [41]. It is suggested that some other factors, such as the number of lifetime sexual partners, other lifestyle habits and additional molecular alterations may play a role in HPV-related carcinogenesis in smokers [42]. In our study, the rate of HPV positivity was higher in females and close between smokers and non-smokers with a little difference (73.5% and 78.2%), and no statistically significant difference was found between HPV infection, age, gender, and smoking history, similar to the results of some other studies [1,27].

The relation between the presence of HPV and the histopathological type of lung cancer is discrepant between studies. Some studies have observed the higher prevalence of HPV in squamous cell carcinoma [3,10,14,15,24], while others have found a greater presence in adenocarcinomas [9,32,43,44]. Our findings support the latter. The most frequently detected HPV types worldwide are types 16 and 18 [3,24,26,29], while the other commonly detected high-risk types are known to be types 31 and 33 [31]. In our study, the two most commonly detected types were type 51 (49.1%) and type 16 (43.9%), followed by type 31 (15.8%) and type 18 (12.3%).

Although some studies found that HPV 16/18 is significantly associated with squamous cell carcinoma, some reported that there is no statistically significant relation between HPV 16/18 and the histopathological subtypes of cancer [3,26]. In a study by Baba et al., HPV type 16 was the most frequently detected type in both adenocarcinoma and squamous cell carcinoma [43]. In our study, HPV 16 positivity was more common in adenocarcinomas ($p = 0.006$). These different results may be due to the prevalence of the histopathological type of cancer in the region, ethnicity, sample size of the study and other variables [3].

Furthermore, some studies revealed that HPV infections were more commonly detected in patients with EGFR mutations [22–25,45,46]. It is assumed that the EGFR/PI3K/AKT pathway may play an important role in HPV-associated lung carcinogenesis in EGFR-mutated patients [22,23,47]. In our study, EGFR mutation was detected in 6% (3/50) of the patients with cancer and all of the EGFR-mutated patients had a histopathological diagnosis of adenocarcinoma and multiple HPV infection with HPV types 16 and 51. There was no significant relationship between HPV positivity and the presence of EGFR mutations in the lung cancer cases ($p > 0.999$). This result may be due to the small number of EGFR-mutated patients detected in this study.

Moreover, p16, which is known as one of the regulators of the cell cycle, is found to be inhibited in several cancer types through methylation and deletion. In dysplastic and neoplastic cervical lesions, and oropharyngeal squamous cell carcinomas, the transcription of the p16 gene is inhibited by HPV, resulting in abnormal expression of the p16 protein, dysregulation of the cell cycle and tumorigenesis [48]. However, it is suggested that the well-established relationship between HPV and p16 in cervical and oropharyngeal cancer may not be the same in lung cancer. Not all HPV-infected patients who are expressing its oncoproteins exhibit significant changes in p16 expression [9,49,50]. One of the aims of our study was to search the relationship between HPV and p16 in lung cancer. We found that p16 expression was positive in 24% (12/50) of lung cancer patients and all (12/12) of the p16-positive patients were HPV-positive while none of the HPV-negative patients showed p16 expression and 30.8% (12/39) of the HPV-positive patients were p16-positive. In our study, there was no significant relationship between HPV status and p16 protein expression ($p = 0.05$) in consistent with the results some other studies in the literature [9,49,50].

There were also discrepant results concerning p16 expression in different types of lung tumors in the literature, with some studies reporting higher expression in adenocarcinomas while others found it to be higher in SCCs [9,10]. In our study, we found p16 expression to be higher in squamous cell carcinomas than adenocarcinomas. The number of patients, the distribution of the tumor types and the p16 detection method may be the reasons behind the discrepancy in the results.

Although there may be some possible limitations in our study, such as the small number of patients and lack of follow-up data for survival analysis, it contributes to the literature by providing information about the prevalence of HPV, the distribution of HPV types, and its relationship with p16 in lung cancer patients from the Mediterranean region of Turkey.

5. Conclusions

In conclusion, our study demonstrated the presence of HPV in lung cancer (39/50, 78%), but we think that more evidence is needed to prove the relationship between the presence of HPV and lung carcinogenesis. HPV infection may be one of the factors playing a role in the development of lung cancer. However, further studies using reliable methods to search for HPV in a larger number of lung cancer patients across different geographic regions are necessary to understand the role of HPV in lung cancer pathogenesis.

Author Contributions: Conceptualization, İ.A.K. and A.S.A.; data curation, İ.A.K.; methodology, İ.A.K. and A.S.A.; supervision, A.S.A.; writing—original draft, İ.A.K.; writing—review and editing, A.S.A. All authors have read and agreed to the published version of the manuscript.

Funding: This research received no external funding.

Institutional Review Board Statement: This study was performed in accordance with the Declaration of Helsinki and approved by the Ethics Committee of Health Sciences University, Antalya Education and Research Hospital (date and register number: 2019-242, 19/9).

Informed Consent Statement: Not applicable.

Data Availability Statement: Data are contained within the article.

Conflicts of Interest: The authors declare no conflicts of interest.

References

1. Sagerup, C.M.T.; Nymoen, D.A.; Halvorsen, A.R.; Iversen, M.L.; Helland, A.; Brustugun, O.T. Human papilloma virus detection and typing in 334 lung cancer patients. *Acta Oncol.* **2014**, *53*, 952–957. [CrossRef] [PubMed]
2. Shikova, E.; Ivanova, Z.; Alexandrova, D.; Shindov, M.; Lekov, A. Human papillomavirus prevalence in lung carcinomas in Bulgaria. *Microbiol. Immunol.* **2017**, *61*, 427–432. [CrossRef] [PubMed]
3. de Oliveira, T.H.A.; do Amaral, C.M.; de França São Marcos, B.; Nascimento, K.C.G.; de Miranda Rios, A.C.; Quixabeira, D.C.A.; Muniz, M.T.C.; Silva Neto, J.D.C.; de Freitas, A.C. Presence and activity of HPV in primary lung cancer. *J. Cancer Res. Clin. Oncol.* **2018**, *144*, 2367–2376. [CrossRef] [PubMed]

4. de Freitas, A.C.; Gurgel, A.P.; de Lima, E.G.; de França São Marcos, B.; do Amaral, C.M. Human papillomavirus and lung cancinogenesis: An overview. *J. Cancer Res. Clin. Oncol.* **2016**, *142*, 2415–2427. [CrossRef] [PubMed]
5. Klein, F.; Amin Kotb, W.F.; Petersen, I. Incidence of human papilloma virus in lung cancer. *Lung Cancer* **2009**, *65*, 13–18. [CrossRef] [PubMed]
6. Kotb, W.F.; Petersen, I. Morphology, DNA ploidy and HPV in lung cancer and head and neck cancer. *Pathol. Res. Pract.* **2012**, *208*, 1–8. [CrossRef] [PubMed]
7. Hussain, S.S.; Lundine, D.; Leeman, J.E.; Higginson, D.S. Genomic Signatures in HPV- Associated Tumors. *Viruses* **2021**, *13*, 1998. [CrossRef] [PubMed]
8. Gatta, L.B.; Balzarini, P.; Tironi, A.; Berenzi, A.; Benetti, A.; Angiero, F.; Grigolato, P.; Dessy, E. Human papillomavirus DNA and p16 gene in squamous cell lung carcinoma. *Anticancer Res.* **2012**, *32*, 3085–3089.
9. Zhou, Y.; Höti, N.; Ao, M.; Zhang, Z.; Zhu, H.; Li, L.; Askin, F.; Gabrielson, E.; Zhang, H.; Li, Q.K. Expression of p16 and p53 in non-small-cell lung cancer: Clinicopathological correlation and potential prognostic impact. *Biomark. Med.* **2019**, *13*, 761–771. [CrossRef]
10. São Marcos, B.F.; de Oliveira, T.H.A.; do Amaral, C.M.C.; Muniz, M.T.C.; Freitas, A.C. Correlation between HPV PCNA, p16, and p21 expression in lung cancer patients. *Cell. Microbiol.* **2022**, *8*, 1–13. [CrossRef]
11. Rubel, L.; Reynolds, R.E. Cytologic description of squamous cell papilloma of the respiratory tract. *Acta Cytol.* **1979**, *23*, 227–231. [PubMed]
12. Syrjänen, K.J. Condylomatous changes in neoplastic bronchial epithelium. *Respiration* **1979**, *38*, 299–304. [CrossRef]
13. Syrjänen, K.J. Epithelial lesions suggestive of a condylomatous origin found closely associated with invasive bronchial squamous cell carcinomas. *Respiration* **1980**, *40*, 150–160. [CrossRef]
14. Hu, Y.; Ren, S.; He, Y.; Wang, L.; Chen, C.; Tang, J.; Liu, W.; Yu, F. Possible Oncogenic Viruses Associated with Lung Cancer. *Onco Targets Ther.* **2020**, *13*, 10651–10666. [CrossRef]
15. Xiong, W.M.; Xu, Q.P.; Li, X.; Xiao, R.D.; Cai, L.; He, F. The association between human papillomavirus infection and lung cancer: A system review and meta-analysis. *Oncotarget* **2017**, *8*, 96419–96432. [CrossRef]
16. Hussen, B.M.; Ahmadi, G.; Marzban, H.; Azar, M.E.F.; Sorayyayi, S.; Karampour, R.; Nahand, J.S.; Hidayat, H.J.; Moghoofei, M. The role of HPV gene expression and selected cellular MiRNAs in lung cancer development. *Microb. Pathog.* **2021**, *150*, 104692. [CrossRef] [PubMed]
17. Carpagnano, G.E.; Koutelou, A.; Natalicchio, M.I.; Martinelli, D.; Ruggieri, C.; Di Taranto, A.; Antonetti, R.; Carpagnano, F.; Foschino-Barbaro, M.P. HPV in exhaled breath condensate of lung cancer patients. *Br. J. Cancer* **2011**, *105*, 1183–1190. [CrossRef] [PubMed]
18. Rezaei, M.; Shayan, M.; Aghaei, A.; Hosseini, N.; Darabi, H.; Nouri, M.; Etemadi, K.; O' Neill, A.; Nahand, J.S.; Mirzaei, H.; et al. The association between HPV gene expression, inflammatory agents and cellular genes involved in EMT in lung cancer tissue. *BMC Cancer* **2020**, *20*, 916. [CrossRef]
19. Yu, Y.; Yang, A.; Hu, S.; Yan, H. Correlation of HPV-16/18 infection of human papillomavirus with lung squamous cell carcinomas in Western China. *Oncol. Rep.* **2009**, *21*, 1627–1632. [CrossRef]
20. Gaur, P.; Bhattacharya, S.; Kant, S.; Kushwaha, R.A.S.; Singh, G.; Pandey, S. EGFR Mutation Detection and Its Association With Clinicopathological Characters of Lung Cancer Patients. *World J. Oncol.* **2018**, *9*, 151–155. [CrossRef]
21. Kumar, A.; Kumar, A. Non-small-cell lung cancer-associated gene mutations and inhibitors. *Adv. Cancer Biol. Metastasis* **2022**, *6*, 100076. [CrossRef]
22. Harabajsa, S.; Šefčić, H.; Klasić, M.; Milavić, M.; Židovec Lepej, S.; Grgić, I.; Zajc Petranović, M.; Jakopović, M.; Smojver-Ježek, S.; Korać, P. Infection with human cytomegalovirus, Epstein-Barr virus, and high-risk types 16 and 18 of human papillomavirus in EGFR-mutated lung adenocarcinoma. *Croat. Med. J.* **2023**, *64*, 84–92. [CrossRef] [PubMed]
23. Li, M.; Deng, F.; Qian, L.T.; Meng, S.P.; Zhang, Y.; Shan, W.L.; Zhang, X.L.; Wang, B.L. Association between human papillomavirus and EGFR mutations in advanced lung adenocarcinoma. *Oncol. Lett.* **2016**, *12*, 1953–1958. [CrossRef] [PubMed]
24. Karnosky, J.; Dietmaier, W.; Knuettel, H.; Freigang, V.; Koch, M.; Koll, F.; Zeman, F.; Schulz, C. HPV and lung cancer: A systematic review and meta-analysis. *Cancer Rep.* **2021**, *4*, e1350. [CrossRef] [PubMed]
25. Liang, H.; Pan, Z.; Cai, X.; Wang, W.; Guo, C.; He, J.; Chen, Y.; Liu, Z.; Wang, B.; He, J.; et al. The association between human papillomavirus presence and epidermal growth factor receptor mutations in Asian patients with non-small cell lung cancer. *Transl. Lung Cancer Res.* **2018**, *7*, 397–403. [CrossRef] [PubMed]
26. Zhai, K.; Ding, J.; Shi, H.Z. HPV and lung cancer risk: A meta-analysis. *J. Clin. Virol.* **2015**, *63*, 84–90. [CrossRef] [PubMed]
27. Argyri, E.; Tsimplaki, E.; Marketos, C.; Politis, G.; Panotopoulou, E. Investigating the role of human papillomavirus in lung cancer. *Papillomavirus Res.* **2017**, *3*, 7–10. [CrossRef] [PubMed]
28. Tsyganov, M.M.; Ibramigova, M.K.; Rodionov, E.O.; Cheremisina, O.V.; Miller, S.V.; Tuzikov, S.A.; Litvyakov, N.V. Human Papillomavirus in Non-Small Cell Lung Carcinoma: Assessing Virus Presence in Tumor and Normal Tissues and Its Clinical Relevance. *Microorganisms* **2023**, *11*, 212. [CrossRef] [PubMed]
29. Coissard, C.J.; Besson, G.; Polette, M.C.; Monteau, M.; Birembaut, P.L.; Clavel, C.E. Prevalence of human papillomaviruses in lung carcinomas: A study of 218 cases. *Mod. Pathol.* **2005**, *18*, 1606–1609. [CrossRef]
30. Syrjanen, K. Detection of human papillomavirus in lung cancer: Systematic review and meta-analysis. *Anticancer Res.* **2012**, *32*, 3235–3250.

31. Hasegawa, Y.; Ando, M.; Kubo, A.; Isa, S.; Yamamoto, S.; Tsujino, K.; Kurata, T.; Ou, S.H.; Takada, M.; Kawaguchi, T. Human papilloma virus in non-small cell lung cancer in never smokers: A systematic review of the literature. *Lung Cancer* **2014**, *83*, 8–13. [CrossRef] [PubMed]
32. Cheng, Y.W.; Chiou, H.L.; Sheu, G.T.; Hsieh, L.L.; Chen, J.T.; Chen, C.Y.; Su, J.M.; Lee, H. The association of human papillomavirus 16/18 infection with lung cancer among nonsmoking Taiwanese women. *Cancer Res.* **2001**, *61*, 2799–2803. [PubMed]
33. Fei, Y.; Yang, J.; Hsieh, W.C.; Wu, J.Y.; Wu, T.C.; Goan, Y.G.; Lee, H.; Cheng, Y.W. Different human papillomavirus 16/18 infection in Chinese non-small cell lung cancer patients living in Wuhan, China. *Jpn. J. Clin. Oncol.* **2006**, *36*, 274–279. [CrossRef] [PubMed]
34. Wang, Y.; Wang, A.; Jiang, R.; Pan, H.; Huang, B.; Lu, Y.; Wu, C. Human papillomavirus type 16 and 18 infection is associated with lung cancer patients from the central part of China. *Oncol. Rep.* **2008**, *20*, 333–339. [PubMed]
35. Lin, F.C.; Huang, J.Y.; Tsai, S.C.; Nfor, O.N.; Chou, M.C.; Wu, M.F.; Lee, C.T.; Jan, C.F.; Liaw, Y.P. The association between human papillomavirus infection and female lung cancer: A population-based cohort study. *Medicine* **2016**, *95*, e3856. [CrossRef] [PubMed]
36. Ragin, C.; Obikoya-Malomo, M.; Kim, S.; Chen, Z.; Flores-Obando, R.; Gibbs, D.; Koriyama, C.; Aguayo, F.; Koshiol, J.; Caporaso, N.E.; et al. HPV-associated lung cancers: An international pooled analysis. *Carcinogenesis* **2014**, *35*, 1267–1275. [CrossRef] [PubMed]
37. Zafer, E.; Ergun, M.A.; Alver, G.; Sahin, F.I.; Yavuzer, S.; Ekmekci, A. Detection and Typing of Human Papillomavirus in Non-Small Cell Lung Cancer. *Respiration* **2004**, *71*, 88–90. [CrossRef] [PubMed]
38. Kaya, H.; Kotiloğlu, E.; Inanli, S.; Ekicioğlu, G.; Bozkurt, S.U.; Tutkun, A.; Küllü, S. Prevalence of human papillomavirus (HPV) DNA in larynx and lung carcinomas. *Pathologica* **2001**, *93*, 531–534. [PubMed]
39. Buyru, N.; Altinisik, J.; Isin, M.; Dalay, N. p53 codon 72 polymorphism and HPV status in lung cancer. *Med. Sci. Monit.* **2008**, *14*, CR493–CR497.
40. Peña, N.; Carrillo, D.; Muñoz, J.P.; Chnaiderman, J.; Urzúa, U.; León, O.; Tornesello, M.L.; Corvalán, A.H.; Soto-Rifo, R.; Aguayo, F. Tobacco Smoke Activates Human Papillomavirus 16 p97 Promoter and Cooperates with High-Risk E6/E7 for Oxidative DNA Damage in Lung Cells. *PLoS ONE* **2015**, *10*, e0123029. [CrossRef]
41. Li, Y.J.; Tsai, Y.C.; Chen, Y.C.; Christiani, D.C. Human papilloma virus anf female lung adenocarcinoma. *Semin. Oncol.* **2009**, *36*, 542–552. [CrossRef] [PubMed]
42. Schabath, M.B.; Villa, L.L.; Lazcano-Ponce, E.; Salmerón, J.; Quiterio, M.; Giuliano, A.R.; HIM Study. Smoking and human papillomavirus (HPV) infection in the HPV in Men (HIM) study. *Cancer Epidemiol. Biomark. Prev.* **2012**, *21*, 102–110. [CrossRef]
43. Baba, M.; Castillo, A.; Koriyama, C.; Yanagi, M.; Matsumoto, H.; Natsugoe, S.; Shuyama, K.Y.; Khan, N.; Higashi, M.; Itoh, T.; et al. Human papillomavirus is frequently detected in gefitinib-responsive lung adenocarcinomas. *Oncol. Rep.* **2010**, *23*, 1085–1092. [CrossRef] [PubMed]
44. Hsu, N.Y.; Cheng, Y.W.; Chan, I.P.; Ho, H.C.; Chen, C.Y.; Hsu, C.P.; Lin, M.H.; Chou, M.C. Association between expression of human papillomavirus 16/18 E6 oncoprotein and survival in patients with stage I non-small cell lung cancer. *Oncol. Rep.* **2009**, *21*, 81–87.
45. Tung, M.C.; Wu, H.H.; Cheng, Y.W.; Wang, L.; Chen, C.Y.; Yeh, S.D.; Wu, T.C.; Lee, H. Association of epidermal growth factor receptor mutations with human papillomavirus 16/18 E6 oncoprotein expression in non-small cell lung cancer. *Cancer* **2013**, *119*, 3367–3376. [CrossRef] [PubMed]
46. Kato, T.; Koriyama, C.; Khan, N.; Samukawa, T.; Yanagi, M.; Hamada, T.; Yokomakura, N.; Otsuka, T.; Inoue, H.; Sato, M.; et al. EGFR mutations and human papillomavirus in lung cancer. *Lung Cancer* **2012**, *78*, 144–147. [CrossRef] [PubMed]
47. Wu, H.H.; Wu, J.Y.; Cheng, Y.W.; Chen, C.Y.; Lee, M.C.; Goan, Y.G.; Lee, H. cIAP2 upregulated by E6 oncoprotein via epidermal growth factor receptor/phosphatidylinositol 3-kinase/AKT pathway confers resistance to cisplatin in human papillomavirus 16/18-infected lung cancer. *Clin. Cancer Res.* **2010**, *16*, 5200–5210. [CrossRef] [PubMed]
48. Psyrri, A.; Dimaio, D. Human papillomavirus in cervical and head-and-neck cancer. *Nat. Clin. Pract. Oncol.* **2008**, *5*, 24–31. [CrossRef] [PubMed]
49. Anantharaman, D.; Gheit, T.; Waterboer, T.; Halec, G.; Carreira, C.; Abedi-Ardekani, B.; McKay-Chopin, S.; Zaridze, D.; Mukeria, A.; Szeszenia-Dabrowska, N.; et al. No causal association identified for human papillomavirus infections in lung cancer. *Cancer Res.* **2014**, *74*, 3525–3534. [CrossRef]
50. Lin, S.; Zhang, X.; Li, X.; Qin, C.; Zhang, L.; Lu, J.; Chen, Q.; Jin, J.; Wang, T.; Wang, F.; et al. Detection of human papillomavirus distinguishes second primary tumors from lung metastases in patients with squamous cell carcinoma of the cervix. *Thorac. Cancer* **2020**, *11*, 2297–2305. [CrossRef]

Disclaimer/Publisher's Note: The statements, opinions and data contained in all publications are solely those of the individual author(s) and contributor(s) and not of MDPI and/or the editor(s). MDPI and/or the editor(s) disclaim responsibility for any injury to people or property resulting from any ideas, methods, instructions or products referred to in the content.

Review

Relationship Between Human Papilloma Virus and Upper Gastrointestinal Cancers

Ömer Vefik Özozan [1,*], Hikmet Pehlevan-Özel [2], Veli Vural [3] and Tolga Dinç [2]

1 Ömer Özozan Private Clinic, Kadıköy, 34744 İstanbul, Türkiye
2 Department of General Surgery, Ankara Bilkent City Hospital, 06800 Ankara, Türkiye; hikmet.pehlevan@gmail.com (H.P.-Ö.); tolga_dr@hotmail.com (T.D.)
3 Department of General Surgery, Akdeniz University, 07070 Antalya, Türkiye; velivural1980@hotmail.com
* Correspondence: omerozozan@gmail.com; Tel.: +90-532-208-46-56

Abstract: The human papillomavirus (HPV) is an oncogenic DNA virus that is the most commonly transmitted sexually transmitted virus. There is substantial evidence that HPV is associated with different types of cancer. While the majority of studies have concentrated on urogenital system cancers and head and neck cancers, the relationship between HPV and gastrointestinal system cancers, particularly esophageal cancers, has also been the subject of investigation. Given that HPV is a disease that can be prevented through vaccination and treated with antiviral agents, identifying the types of cancers associated with the pathogen may inform the treatment of these cancers. This comprehensive review examines the relationship between HPV and cancers of the upper gastrointestinal tract, highlighting the oncogenic mechanisms of the virus and its reported prevalence. A deeper understanding of HPV's association with cancer is relevant to the further development of cancer therapies.

Keywords: HPV; human papillomavirus; esophagus cancer; gastric cancer

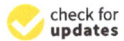

Academic Editors: Hossein H. Ashrafi and Mustafa Ozdogan

Received: 8 February 2025
Revised: 20 February 2025
Accepted: 26 February 2025
Published: 4 March 2025

Citation: Özozan, Ö.V.; Pehlevan-Özel, H.; Vural, V.; Dinç, T. Relationship Between Human Papilloma Virus and Upper Gastrointestinal Cancers. *Viruses* 2025, 17, 367. https://doi.org/10.3390/v17030367

Copyright: © 2025 by the authors. Licensee MDPI, Basel, Switzerland. This article is an open access article distributed under the terms and conditions of the Creative Commons Attribution (CC BY) license (https://creativecommons.org/licenses/by/4.0/).

1. Introduction

Infectious diseases are involved in the etiology of more than 50% of human cancers, and about 10% are caused by viral infection [1]. Cancer-inducing viruses can lead to cancer development by encoding several proteins in the target cell, reprogramming signals in the development, growth and apoptosis stages, or by the progression of inflammation caused by chronic viral infection [2]. Human papilloma virus (HPV) is one of the viruses known to cause cancer. HPV is one of the most common sexually transmitted viral infections worldwide, affecting both men and women. Among the most important cancer-causing infectious agents worldwide, Helicobacter pylori ranked first with 36.3% and HPV ranked second with 31.1% [3]. HPV has been identified as a causative agent of various types of infections, including those affecting the skin and mucosal surfaces. While it is predominantly associated with diseases in the genital area, there is growing evidence suggesting its role in infections and cancers affecting the head and neck region, as well as the gastrointestinal system. Recent years have seen an escalating focus on the link between HPV and upper gastrointestinal tract cancers, underscoring the need for further research and clinical monitoring in this area. HPVs infect stratified epithelium and can cause cervical (>90% associated), anal, vulvar, vaginal and vulvar anogenital carcinoma and are also causally associated with mucosal epithelial carcinomas, particularly oropharyngeal (4% association) [4]. Since HPV is a common type of oncogenic virus and can be silently present in the body for many years, its oncogenic properties, treatments and preventive methods such as vaccination are frequently the subject of research. In addition, due to its popularity and common occurrence, its relationship with other types of cancer has also been investigated. Studies have shown that HPV prevalence is associated with anal, colorectal, oral, pharyngeal and esophageal carcinogenesis [5]. The association of HPV prevalence with gastric carcinogenesis is controversial, and no study has shown an association with the duodenum. The aim of this study is to review studies on the relationship between HPV and esophageal, gastric and duodenal cancers.

2. HPV Virus

HPV is a DNA virus that does not encode for any enzyme or polymerase, requires a host cell for replication, can only infect actively dividing cells, and targets cutaneous or mucosal squamous epithelia [6]. The HPV genome has a circular DNA structure. There are three categories of genes: early genes (nonstructural proteins; E1 to E7), which facilitate viral genome expression and replication while also regulating host cell proliferation and differentiation; late genes (structural proteins; L1 and L2), which are involved in viral capsid formation; and transcriptional control region (long control region; LCR) [7,8]. There are more than 400 types of HPV [9]. HPV is divided into five groups: gamma, beta, mu, gamma and alpha; these are classified as cutaneous or mucosal. HPV8 (beta-cutaneous) and HPV16–18–31–33–35–39–45–51–52–52–5–5–58–59 (alpha-mucosal) subtypes are at high risk for invasive cancer, particularly cervical, anogenital, and oropharyngeal cancers [10]. Some cutaneous HPV types, such as HPV-8 (beta-cutaneous), have also been linked to non-melanoma skin cancers, particularly in immunocompromised individuals [9,10]. HPV is known to be transmitted through direct contact and through certain objects. Mucosal HPV is mainly transmitted by sexual contact, but vertical transmission from mother to child in the womb and more often perinatally is possible. HPV reaches the basal layer through a wound or microdamage in the epithelium, where it can infect only the dividing keratinocytes of the basal layer.

3. HPV Life Cycle

Human papillomaviruses (HPVs) are small, non-enveloped, double-stranded DNA viruses that infect epithelial cells and establish long-term infections without causing immediate cytopathic effects [11]. HPV transmission occurs primarily through direct contact, and infection is facilitated by microabrasions on the epithelial surface, allowing the virus to reach basal keratinocytes [12]. Once in a basal cell, HPV maintains its genome as an episome and replicates simultaneously with host DNA during cell division [11]. This episomal state allows the virus to persist in the host without triggering an immediate immune response.

HPV has an affinity for the squamocolumnar junctional tissue because basal cells are particularly accessible in the squamocolumnar transformation zone and are particularly susceptible to viral infection [13]. Progressive acid damage to the esophagus may increase the likelihood of mucosal breaks that allow virus entry into the basal layer of the transformation zone [13]. The SCJ is the transformation zone of the esophagus and resembles the transition zone of the uterine cervix, where nearly all high-grade cervical lesions and cancers arise [13]. The presence of HPV in these areas alone is not sufficient for cancer development; cancer development is multifactorial.

HPV exhibits a tightly regulated life cycle that depends on the differentiation of infected keratinocytes [14]. In basal cells, HPV replication is restricted, maintaining a low copy number of viral genomes, typically between 50 and 100 copies per cell, and viral oncogene expression is tightly controlled [11]. As infected basal cells differentiate and migrate toward the epithelial surface, the virus enters the productive phase. During this phase, viral genome replication increases to thousands of copies per cell, and structural proteins such as L1 and L2 are expressed, enabling the assembly of infectious virions [12].

The entire life cycle from initial infection to viral particle release takes approximately three weeks [11].

A key feature of the HPV life cycle is its ability to evade immune detection by restricting viral gene expression to differentiating keratinocytes that are not actively involved in immune surveillance [14]. Unlike many other viruses, HPV does not cause cell lysis; instead, virions are released via natural epithelial shedding, allowing transmission to continue without eliciting a strong immune response [11]. HPVs are often found integrated into host DNA in premalignant lesions and cancers, but this is not part of the viral life cycle. In fact, integration is the end for the virus because it can no longer form a circular genome [14].

HPVs are frequently detected to be integrated into host DNA in premalignant and malignant lesions, but integration is not part of the normal viral life cycle [14]. In fact, integration represents a dead end for the virus as it disrupts the circular structure of the viral genome, preventing further episomal replication and transmission [15]. However, integration is a crucial event in HPV-associated oncogenesis, as it often results in the deregulated expression of the viral oncogenes E6 and E7, leading to inactivation of the tumor suppressor proteins p53 and pRb, increased genetic instability, and malignant transformation [14].

The persistence of high-risk HPV types, particularly HPV16 and HPV18, is strongly associated with the development of cervical and other anogenital cancers [12]. Understanding the complex interplay between HPV replication, immune evasion, and oncogenic potential is essential to develop effective prevention and treatment strategies.

4. HPV and Cancer

HPV is a significant etiological factor in various types of cancer, particularly cervical, anogenital (anal, vulvar, vaginal, penile), and head and neck cancers (oropharyngeal). Among cancer-causing HPV types, the most common and researched types are HPV-16 and HPV-18, which are responsible for more than 80% of cervical cancers worldwide, while other types are HPV-31, HPV-33, HPV-45 and HPV-58, of which HPV-16 is the most common type [16].

The process of HPV-induced carcinogenesis involves a complex network of interactions between viral oncoproteins and host cellular pathways, resulting in genomic instability, deregulation of cell cycle control, and evasion of apoptosis. The primary drivers of these processes are the viral oncoproteins E5, E6, and E7.

HPV-associated lesions often become cancerous through damage to the viral genome resulting from integration into the host genome. HPV oncoproteins E1 and E2 are involved in initiation and regulation of HPV infection, E4 protein is mainly involved in viral release, transmission and post-translational modification, E5, E6 and E7 in cellular proliferation, invasion and metastasis, cell cycle arrest, angiogenesis, resistance to cell death, tumor-promoting inflammation, genomic instability, evasion of growth suppressors, dysregulation of cellular energy, escape from immune destruction and replicative immortality [17]. The E6 protein is known to promote the degradation of the tumor suppressor protein p53, whilst the E7 protein is capable of inactivating the retinoblastoma protein (pRb), a process that leads to uncontrolled cell proliferation and the avoidance of apoptosis. The E5 protein has been demonstrated to increase the activity of both the E6 and E7 proteins and is involved in the regulation of cell proliferation and apoptosis. These proteins have also been observed to contribute to the initiation and progression of malignancy by interacting with cellular signaling pathways, including PI3K/AKT, Wnt and Notch [7,18] (Table 1).

Table 1. HPV proteins and functions.

Region	Protein	Pathway	Function
Early Region	E1	NF-κB	Genome replication
	E2		Regulation of gene transcription Leas to cancer progression
	E4		Viral release
	E5	MAPK-ERK pathways	Major oncoprotein E6 and E7 modulation Suppression of p21 expression Angiogenesis, proliferation, evading cell death
	E6	PI3K, AKT, Wnt, Notch pathways	Degradation of p53 Degradation of apoptotic signaling cascade Downregulates tumor suppressor genes Genomic instability, proliferation, invasion, immortality, inhibition of apoptosis and DNA repair
	E7	PI3K, AKT pathways	Inactivates pRb Inactivation of p21 and p27 Overexpression of MMP-9 Immortality, invasion, metastasis, chronic inflammation, genomic instability
	E8		Repressor of transcription
Late Region	L1		Major capsid protein
	L2		Minor capsid protein
Long Control Region			Promotor elements, regulator region

NF-κB: Nuclear Factor kappa B, MAPK-ERK: mitogen activated protein kinase- extracellular-signal-regulated kinase, PI3K: phosphatidylinositol-3-kinase, AKT: protein kinase B, DNA: deoxyribonucleic acid, MMP-9: matrix metalloproteinase-9.

In addition to the abovementioned oncoproteins, the integration of HPV into the host genome has been demonstrated to result in the increased expression of oncogenes. This process has been shown to induce the disruption of normal chromatin interactions and to silence tumor suppressor genes, a critical step in the process of carcinogenesis that leads to genomic instability [9]. Proteases such as matrix metalloproteinases (MMPs) have been observed to be upregulated in HPV-mediated carcinogenesis. The function of these enzymes is to facilitate tumor invasion and metastasis by degrading components of the extracellular matrix. Protease inhibitors have been identified as potential prognostic markers for HPV-associated cancers, emphasizing their role in disease progression [7].

With HPV integration, the expression of E6 and E7 oncogenes is dysregulated, and carcinogenesis is initiated, but this integration is not essential [13]. HPV is responsible for more than 90% cervical cancers, and more than 70% of these are related to HPV16 and HPV18. While HPV 18 and HPV48 show their carcinogenic effects by integrating into the host DNA, HPV 16 integrates at a rate of 60–80%. In approximately 30% of HPV16-positive HPV-related cancers, HPV 16 does not integrate into the host DNA and leads to carcinogenesis by deletion and rearrangement [19].

The pathogenesis of HPV-related squamous cell carcinoma and adenocarcinoma of the cervix involves different mechanisms, although both are driven by HPV infection. These differences can be explained by differences in the DNA integration point of HPV (8q24.21 is integrated in adenocarcinoma, while 21p11.2 is integrated in squamous carcinoma), the involvement of different genomic areas (dysregulation of oncogenes such as STARD3 and ERBB2 is observed in adenocarcinoma, while expression of viral oncogenes is increased in aquatic carcinoma), and different molecular signatures (squamous carcinoma is associated with keratinization and glucose metabolism pathways, while adenocarcinoma uses different oncogenic pathways) [14,20].

In HPV-related cancers, a different mechanism operates compared to HPV-independent cancers of the same region. This has resulted in HPV-positive cancers having better prognosis; for example, in cervical cancer, HPV positivity increases radiosensitivity [16]. HPV-related cancers are more commonly associated with squamous-type cancer, whereas HPV-independent tumors are associated with both adenocarcinomas and squamous histological subtypes; they are associated with earlier-stage lymph node involvement, more distant metastasis, and generally worse oncologic outcomes [21].

5. HPV Detection

HPV screening tests are an important health screening that should be performed in individuals with certain risk factors, especially due to the known cancer-risk-increasing effects of HPV. HPV infections are mostly asymptomatic and in most cases are cleared spontaneously by the immune system. However, some high-risk HPV types (especially HPV 16 and HPV 18) can cause the development of cervical, anal and other types of cancer. Therefore, HPV screening can help detect cancer at an early stage. High-risk groups such as women, HIV-positive individuals, men who have anal sex and those with weakened immune systems are the people who would benefit most from HPV screening tests.

The known tests for HPV diagnosis today are cervical screening and diagnostic tests. Tests for other body parts are still under development. Oral HPV tests and anal HPV tests are known tests, and genital tests for men are also under development. HPV DNA screening tests can be performed with swab samples, liquid-based cytology or tissue samples taken from areas such as the perianal region, oropharyngeal region, or skin. HPV is not a hematological virus; therefore, it cannot be screened using serum samples. However, there are studies that utilize antibodies, circular DNA, or fragments produced by HPV for screening purposes.

HPV is a virus that does not grow in cell culture and therefore requires molecular tests for diagnosis. HPV tests can be classified into three categories for cervical smear tests: (1) nucleic acid amplification assays, (2) nucleic acid hybridization assays, (3) signal amplification assays (Table 2) [22].

Table 2. Classification of HPV tests for cervical specimens.

Classification of HPV Tests	
Nucleic Acid Amplification Assays	Micoarray PapilloCheck Polymerase Chain Reaction COBASE 4800 HPV Genome Sequencing CLART HPV2 INNO-LIPA
Nucleic Acid Hybridization Assays	Southern blot In situ hybridization Dot blot hybridization
Signal Amplification Assays	Cervista HPV Hyrid Capture 2

The recommended test for the diagnosis of HPV-associated oropharyngeal squamous cancer in the College of American Pathologists (CAP) and American Society of Clinical Oncology (ASCO) guidelines is p16 immunohistochemistry [23].

Anal area screening tests include a smear test and HPV DNA screening, just as in the cervical area. In addition, biopsies taken from HPV-induced lesions such as warts can also be diagnosed by HPV DNA screening.

It has been established that in numerous forms of cancer, DNA fragments, such as circulating tumor DNA (ctDNA), are released into the blood. In HPV-associated cancers, human papillomavirus (HPV) DNA can also be released into the blood following integration into the host genome. Consequently, the presence of circulating HPV-DNA fragments has the potential to serve as a marker for these cancers [24].

Next-generation sequencing (NGS) offers a non-invasive approach for the detection of circulating tumor DNA (ctDNA) in HPV-associated cancers, offering significant advantages over traditional methods such as droplet digital PCR (ddPCR) and quantitative real-time PCR (qPCR), particularly in terms of sensitivity, specificity and the ability to provide comprehensive genomic information, providing a non-invasive approach for diagnosis, monitoring and prognosis.

6. HPV and Geographic–Epidemiological Insights

The prevalence of HPV exhibits significant variation across geographic and demographic contexts, thereby influencing its correlation with upper gastrointestinal cancers and other HPV-associated malignancies. This variation is crucial for understanding the broader implications of HPV in cancer epidemiology.

The prevalence of HPV was found to be 11.7% worldwide, in a meta-analysis conducted by Bruni et al., which included 194 studies and more than 1 million women [22]. HPV is associated with 4.5% of all cancers worldwide and is responsible for 8.6% of cancers in women and 0.8% in men [25].

It is reported that 90% of cervical and anal cancers, 70% of vulvar and vaginal cancers, 60% of penile cancers and 70% of oropharyngeal cancers are attributable to HPV infection [26,27]. Approximately 60% of occurrences of oropharyngeal cancer (OPC) in the United States have been associated with HPV, compared to 31% in Europe and 4% in Brazil [28]. In contrast, India reports a high incidence of 38.4% of HPV-related OPCs, in contrast to the low rates observed in many African countries [29].

HPV represents the most significant etiological agent in the development of cervical cancer in women; nevertheless, it is also associated with anal and oropharyngeal cancers in men, and HPV-associated cancer rates are elevated in younger age groups, especially in areas exhibiting low vaccination rates [30].

The development of gastrointestinal cancers is often multifactorial, and HPV is one of several risk factors; in particular, the association of HPV with esophageal squamous cell carcinoma is very strong, but the evidence is insufficient for gastric or colorectal cancer [31]. Research indicates that the prevalence of HPV is elevated in patients diagnosed with oropharyngeal and gastrointestinal cancers, thereby suggesting a potential association between HPV 16 and 18 and the development of gastrointestinal system oncogenesis [31].

7. HPV and Esophagus

Esophageal cancer is the eighth most common cancer and the sixth most common cause of death [32]. There are two main histologic subtypes of esophageal cancer: squamous cell carcinoma (ESCC), 88% of cases, and adenocarcinoma (EAC), 12% of cases [33]. The most commonly known etiologies of ESCC are drinking, smoking, heredity, hot drinks, HPV infection and achalasia [34]. Recent studies have begun to investigate the mechanisms by which specific high-risk HPV types, particularly HPV 16 and HPV 18, may contribute to the development of esophageal cancer, leading to novel preventive strategies and therapeutic approaches targeting HPV.

HPV is a virus transmitted through contact and reaches the esophagus through orosexual contact. The relationship between HPV and ESCC was first demonstrated by Syrjänen in 1982, and as a result of the studies that followed, it is now known that the most common types are HPV 16 and HPV 18 [35,36]. HPV-associated ESCC of the esophagus occurs between 0 and 78% depending on geography, study design and method of HPV detection, and in regions with high incidence of ESCC such as Iran and Northern China, HPV incidence ranges between 32.8 and 63.6%, while in Europe and the USA where there is low incidence of ESCC, HPV incidence is 15.6% and 16.6% [33].

The results of a meta-analysis and review conducted by Petrelli et al. indicate that the association between HPV and ESCC is not as strong as that observed in cervical and oropharyngeal cancers [37]. Furthermore, there is no definitive correlation between HPV and p53 expression, a weak association with p16, and evidence suggests that ESCC environmental factors may be a more significant risk factor [33,37]. In a study reported by Feng et al. on Asian races, the oncogenic HPV E6 and E7 genes were shown to be involved in the pathogenesis of ESCC by upregulating susceptible HLA-DQB1 by DNA demethylation [38]. HPV-16 E6 contributes to EC carcinogenesis by downregulating microRNA-125b, a negative regulator of the Wnt/β-catenin signaling pathway [39]. Zhang et al. reported that HPV-infected ESCC tumor tissue, compared with HPV-negative tissue, contained longer telomeres due to the DNA methylation status of telomerase reverse transcriptase, indicating a relationship with poor prognosis [40].

Barrett's esophagus (BE) is a metaplastic change in the esophageal epithelium, whereby the squamous cells are replaced by columnar cells. BE is the greatest risk factor for esophageal adenocarcinoma (EAC). The risk factors for BE include gastroesophageal reflux disease, smoking, obesity, hiatal hernia, male gender, white, and the sixth to seventh decade of life, and the risk factors for EAC include BE, hiatal hernia, and smoking [41]. Barrett's esophagus affects about 5% of people in the US and about 1% worldwide, and first-line treatment consists of proton pump inhibitors for control of reflux symptoms [42]. There are some studies associated with HPV infection in EAC and BE, and it has been suggested that HPV may cause EAC and BE due to abnormalities in the p53 and retinoblastoma protein pathways, but these studies are very limited [1]. In a 2017 French study, 180 patients were studied, 61 of whom had BE, and no association between BE and HPV was found [43]. Although there are some studies showing a negative association between HPV and EAC and BE, the quality of the studies, geography, race and inappropriate tissue samples may have contributed to this result, but it is now recognized that approximately 25% of patients with EAC and BE are associated with HPV 16 and 18 [33]. The majority of HPV-positive BE and EAC samples show downregulation of pRb due to cleavage of pRb by the E7 oncoprotein, upregulation of p16INK4a, and overexpression of p53 due to inactivation by the E6 oncoprotein [44].

8. HPV and Stomach

Gastric cancer (GC) is the fifth most common type of cancer and the fourth most common cause of cancer-related death [45]. GC has a complex etiology that is influenced by a multifactorial genetic and environmental basis. The most well-established risk factors include smoking, alcohol consumption, family history, dietary habits, infection with the Epstein–Barr virus (EBV), and Helicobacter pylori (H. pylori). HPV is recognized for its association with cervical cancer; however, recent research suggests a potential link between HPV infection and gastric cancer. Understanding the biological pathways through which

HPV may contribute to gastric carcinogenesis is essential to uncover potential preventive strategies and therapeutic targets.

In 2007, the International Agency for Research on Cancer analyzed and discussed previous studies and could not suggest an association between HPV infection and GC [46]. Studies on the association between HPV and GC are contradictory. It is considered that these differences are related to factors such as the year in which the studies were conducted, the design, the materials used and the test methods. In general, studies conducted in China show that there is a relationship between HPV and GC, and as a result of large meta-analyses conducted in recent years, it is seen that there is a positive relationship between HPV and GC, especially HPV 16 [33,47,48]. HPV positivity in gastric cardia cancers varies between 0 and 68% with the influence of factors such as geography, ethnicity and gender, and it is known that the HPV association is stronger than in non-cardia gastric cancers [49]. Although the presence of HPV in gastric cancer tissues has been shown in studies, the molecular relationship between HPV and carcinogenesis has not yet been clearly demonstrated.

Researchers have also examined the relationship between H. pylori, which is a known etiological factor of gastric cancer, and HPV. Studies have demonstrated a correlation between HPV positivity and H. pylori positivity in gastric cancer, with one potential interaction pathway being correlation of HPV 16 and H. pylori Cag A positivity, the development of dysplasia and adenocarcinoma due to HPV chronic infection, or HPV and H. pylori coinfection [5,50]. EBV is the second most important viral factor in the etiology of GC and accounts for approximately 10% of all gastric carcinomas. Similarly to EBV infection, HPV may play a role in carcinogenesis by stimulating the NFκB signaling pathway, which is critical for the proliferation and survival of cancer cells [51]. It has been established that HPV infection accelerates the carcinogenic process through various epigenetic mechanisms, including DNA methylation, histone modifications and changes in microRNA expression. HPV oncoproteins E6 and E7, for instance, have been demonstrated to promote a positive feedback loop by inhibiting histone acetyl transferase p300, thereby increasing their own expression and further contributing to malignancy through the process of epigenetic alteration [52].

A meta-analysis demonstrated an association between HPV 16 and gastric cancer (GC), with a reported prevalence of HPV of 23.6%. Although HPV screening with serologic tests is a reliable marker, the relationship between GC and HPV is more clearly evident in gastric tissue samples. It was hypothesized that HPV may play a role in oncogenesis by infecting gastric epithelial cells through oral entry, particularly by evading immune system mechanisms [47].

9. HPV and Duodenum

Small bowel cancers constitute 3% of all gastrointestinal system cancers [53]. Duodenal adenocarcinomas account for only 0.5% of all gastrointestinal tract cancers [54]. The molecular abnormalities observed in small bowel adenocarcinomas are prevalent in colon adenocarcinomas, but some occur with varying rates. There are no clearly defined environmental risk factors for small bowel adenocarcinomas, but approximately 20% are associated with predisposing diseases such as Crohn's disease, Lynch syndrome, familial adenomatous polyposis, Peutz–Jeghers syndrome, and celiac disease [55]. There are studies showing that HPV is effective in colorectal carcinogenesis by inactivating p53 via the E6 oncoprotein. Considering the similarity of the molecular pathogenesis of small bowel cancers to the molecular pathogenesis of colorectal cancers, HPV may also be effective in small bowel cancers, but there is no study in the literature showing this relationship [51]. A study showing a relationship between HPV and duodenal cancer has not been seen in previous studies. However, it has been observed that cervical cancer and head and neck cancer may involve the duodenum through metastasis [56,57]. However, the association of HPV with cancer and metastasis in these patients has not been established.

10. Vaccine Status

HPV can cause cervical, vaginal, vulvar, penile, anal or oropharyngeal cancers, usually clearing within 2 years, but with the development of persistent infection, especially in types with a high risk of cancerization, such as HPV 16. HPV vaccines target the HPV types that cause most HPV-associated cancers, and studies have shown that vaccines are highly effective in preventing HPV-associated precancerous lesions and cancers [58].

It is recommended that HPV vaccines be administered at the age of 11–12 years. These vaccines have demonstrated strong efficacy against anogenital diseases and associated cancers, and they also have the advantage of potentially halting disease progression by preventing the spread of HPV in individuals being treated for HPV-related diseases [59].

HPV vaccines comprise three categories, all of which utilize DNA recombinant technology and L1 protein purification, a process which has been demonstrated to activate the immune system (Table 3) [60,61]. HPV vaccines are highly immunogenic, producing high concentrations of neutralizing antibodies against the antigen HPV L1 protein and activating both humoral and cellular immune responses. Numerous randomized clinical trials have demonstrated almost 100% efficacy in preventing HPV subtype-specific precancerous cervical cell changes, but vaccination does not provide protection in women already infected with HPV-16 or HPV-18 [62,63].

Table 3. HPV vaccine types.

Vaccine Type	HPV Type
Bivalent vaccine	HPV 16-18
Quadrivalent vaccine	HPV 9-11-16-18
Nonavalent vaccine	HPV9-11-16-18-33-35-4-52-58

The increase in HPV-associated head and neck cancers, along with the demonstration of efficacy in different cancer types, such as ESCC, underscores the importance of HPV vaccination. The incidence of HPV-associated ESCC may be reduced through prophylactic HPV vaccination.

11. HPV-Related Treatment

HPV-related cancers may create differences and some advantages in treatment due to viral pathogenesis. In HPV-associated cervical cancers, when HPV is detected by a smear test to prevent the disease, cancer development can be prevented with minimal surgical treatments such as conization and cauterization in the precancerous period. Cervical, oropharyngeal and vulvar cancers are more radiosensitive when HPV-associated than when not, and this facilitates treatment [64]. In addition, preclinical and clinical studies for the treatment of HPV viral oncogenesis are ongoing. TALENs and CRISPR/Cas9 gene editing techniques, which aim to disrupt viral oncogenes by targeting E6 and E7 oncoproteins, the most important oncoproteins in HPV-associated cancers, and thus inhibit tumor growth and progression, are being investigated [65]. Another promising preclinical study in the treatment of HPV-associated cancers aimed to induce CD8+ T cell responses and kill tumor cells with customized viral immunotherapy targeting E6 and E7 proteins [66]. Oncolytic viruses are genetically modified or naturally occurring viruses that aim to induce an immune response against the tumor and, to do so, selectively infect and kill cancer cells while sparing normal cells. In HPV-associated cancers such as cervical cancer and head and neck squamous cell carcinoma, oncolytic viruses can be used more effectively as it is easier to recognize cancerous cells due to the nature of the cancer. Oncolytic HSV, especially genetically modified versions such as T-01, have been shown to inhibit the growth of cancer cells in HPV-related cervical cancer models by restricting the spread of the virus to tumors, leading to tumor cell death and immune response activation [67].

12. Future Research Directions

The role of HPV in the oncogenesis of upper gastrointestinal system cancers remains to be fully substantiated; however, there exist significant data indicating a correlation between the two. The multifaceted interactions among genetic, environmental, and viral factors in cancer development hinder a definitive evaluation of this relationship. In order to understand the pathogenesis and oncogenesis of HPV and to reveal its relationship with upper gastrointestinal system cancers, disciplines such as pathology, virology, oncology, surgery and gastroenterology should work together and create a common perspective.

Current prophylactic vaccines target specific high-risk HPV types but do not cover all oncogenic strains. Research is ongoing to develop vaccines that provide broader protection. One promising approach involves the use of the minor capsid protein L2, which is highly conserved across multiple HPV genotypes. Improving the immunogenicity of L2 by linking short amino acid sequences from different oncogenic HPV types or by displaying L2 peptides on more immunogenic carriers may lead to pan-HPV vaccines. Additionally, there is considerable interest in therapeutic vaccines aimed at eliciting immune responses against established HPV infections and associated malignancies. These vaccines primarily target the E6 and E7 oncoproteins that are consistently expressed in HPV-associated cancers. A variety of platforms are being investigated in clinical trials, including protein-based, viral vector, bacterial vector, and lipid-encapsulated mRNA vaccines [68].

One of the most challenging issues in HPV-related diseases is the lack of standardization in HPV diagnosis. In addition to tissue screening, the development of new diagnostic and screening tests from specimens such as blood and urine will pave the way for improvements in the diagnosis and treatment of HPV and related cancers. Early detection of HPV-associated lesions is crucial for effective intervention. New technologies such as DNA methylation triage, HPV integration detection, liquid biopsies, and AI-assisted diagnostics have the potential to augment traditional screening methods such as cytology and HPV nucleic acid testing. These innovations aim to increase sensitivity and specificity, reduce false-positive rates, and enable more personalized risk assessments. Further research is needed to validate and integrate these approaches into clinical practice [69].

Despite the proven efficacy of HPV vaccines, global immunization efforts face challenges such as low vaccination coverage, vaccine hesitancy, and inequalities in access to healthcare in low- and middle-income countries. Research focused on understanding the underlying causes of vaccine hesitancy, developing targeted education campaigns, and implementing policies to improve vaccine availability is critical. Additionally, exploring alternative vaccination strategies, such as single-dose regimens or needle-free delivery systems, may increase acceptance and coverage [70].

The heterogeneity of HPV-associated cancers necessitates personalized treatment approaches. Identification of biomarkers that predict response to treatment or disease progression may inform personalized treatment strategies. Research into the tumor microenvironment, immune response profiles, and genetic alterations associated with HPV-associated malignancies will aid in the development of personalized medicine approaches and potentially improve patient outcomes.

As HPV vaccination programs mature, long-term studies assessing the durability of vaccine-induced immunity and monitoring potential adverse events are essential. Such studies will inform booster vaccination programs when necessary and ensure continued safety and efficacy of vaccination programs.

13. Conclusions

The human papilloma virus (HPV) is one of the well-documented oncogenic viruses and has been the subject of extensive research. The fact that the source of cancer is a viral pathogen makes the disease both preventable through vaccination and treatable with antiviral therapy. Consequently, researchers are aiming to investigate viral diseases that may be causative agents in diseases such as cancer, which have poor prophylaxis, diagnosis, treatment, and prognosis. The objective is to make the disease less concerning by identifying these viral pathogens. The objective of this study was to synthesize the existing literature on the relationship between HPV and upper gastrointestinal tract cancers. We believe that further investigation into the relationship between HPV and ESCC, EAC, and GC is justified. Should the relationship and its underlying pathogenesis be elucidated through further study, it would have significant implications for the treatment of these cancers.

Author Contributions: All authors have contributed to every stage of this review. All authors have read and agreed to the published version of the manuscript.

Funding: This research received no external funding.

Data Availability Statement: No new data were created or analyzed in this study. Data sharing is not applicable to this article.

Conflicts of Interest: The authors declare no conflicts of interest.

References

1. Yamashina, T.; Shimatani, M.; Takeo, M.; Sasaki, K.; Orino, M.; Saito, N.; Matsumoto, H.; Kasai, T.; Kano, M.; Horitani, S.; et al. Viral Infection in Esophageal, Gastric, and Colorectal Cancer. *Healthcare* **2022**, *10*, 1626. [CrossRef] [PubMed]
2. Hewavisenti, R.V.; Arena, J.; Ahlenstiel, C.L.; Sasson, S.C. Human Papillomavirus in the Setting of Immunodeficiency: Pathogenesis and the Emergence of Next-Generation Therapies to Reduce the High Associated Cancer Risk. *Front. Immunol.* **2023**, *14*, 1112513. [CrossRef] [PubMed]
3. Szymonowicz, K.A.; Chen, J. Biological and Clinical Aspects of HPV-Related Cancers. *Cancer Biol. Med.* **2020**, *17*, 864–878. [CrossRef] [PubMed]
4. Schiller, J.T.; Lowy, D.R. An Introduction to Virus Infections and Human Cancer. *Recent. Results Cancer Res.* **2021**, *217*, 1–11. [CrossRef]
5. Zeng, Z.M.; Luo, F.F.; Zou, L.X.; He, R.Q.; Pan, D.H.; Chen, X.; Xie, T.-T.; Li, Y.-Q.; Peng, Z.-G.; Chen, G.; et al. Human Papillomavirus as a Potential Risk Factor for Gastric Cancer: A Meta-Analysis of 1917 Cases. *OncoTargets Ther.* **2016**, *9*, 7105–7114. [CrossRef]
6. Cosper, P.F.; Bradley, S.; Luo, L.; Kimple, R.J. Biology of HPV Mediated Carcinogenesis and Tumor Progression. *Semin. Radiat. Oncol.* **2021**, *31*, 265–273. [CrossRef]
7. Vieira, G.V.; Somera dos Santos, F.; Lepique, A.P.; da Fonseca, C.K.; Innocentini, L.M.; Braz-Silva, P.H.; Quintana, S.M.; Sales, K.U. Proteases and HPV-Induced Carcinogenesis. *Cancers* **2022**, *14*, 3038. [CrossRef]
8. Kajitani, N.; Satsuka, A.; Kawate, A.; Sakai, H. Productive Lifecycle of Human Papillomaviruses that Depends Upon Squamous Epithelial Differentiation. *Front. Microbiol.* **2012**, *3*, 152. [CrossRef]
9. Porter, V.L.; Marra, M.A. The Drivers, Mechanisms, and Consequences of Genome Instability in HPV-Driven Cancers. *Cancers* **2022**, *14*, 4623. [CrossRef]
10. Soheili, M.; Keyvani, H.; Soheili, M.; Nasseri, S. Human Papilloma Virus: A Review Study of Epidemiology, Carcinogenesis, Diagnostic Methods, and Treatment of All HPV-Related Cancers. *Med. J. Islam. Repub. Iran* **2021**, *35*, 65. [CrossRef]
11. Stanley, M.A. Epithelial Cell Responses to Infection with Human Papillomavirus. *Clin. Microbiol. Rev.* **2012**, *25*, 215–222. [CrossRef] [PubMed]
12. Schiffman, M.; Doorbar, J.; Wentzensen, N.; de Sanjosé, S.; Fakhry, C.; Monk, B.J.; Franceschi, S. Carcinogenic Human Papillomavirus Infection. *Nat. Rev. Dis. Primers* **2016**, *2*, 16086. [CrossRef] [PubMed]
13. Rajendra, P.S. Transforming human papillomavirus infection and the esophageal transformation zone: Prime time for total excision/ablative therapy? *Dis. Esophagus* **2019**, *32*, doz008. [CrossRef]

14. McBride, A.A.; Warburton, A. The Role of Integration in Oncogenic Progression of HPV-Associated Cancers. *PLoS Pathog.* **2017**, *13*, e1006211. [CrossRef]
15. Bi, Y.; Hu, J.; Zeng, L.; Chen, G.; Cai, H.; Cao, H.; Ma, Q.; Wu, X. Characteristics of HPV Integration in Cervical Adenocarcinoma and Squamous Carcinoma. *J. Cancer Res. Clin. Oncol.* **2023**, *149*, 17973–17986. [CrossRef]
16. Pešut, E.; Đukić, A.; Lulić, L.; Skelin, J.; Šimić, I.; Milutin Gašperov, N.; Tomaić, V.; Sabol, I.; Grce, M. Human Papillomaviruses-Associated Cancers: An Update of Current Knowledge. *Viruses* **2021**, *13*, 2234. [CrossRef]
17. Khan, I.; Harshithkumar, R.; More, A.; Mukherjee, A. Human Papilloma Virus: An Unraveled Enigma of Universal Burden of Malignancies. *Pathogens* **2023**, *12*, 564. [CrossRef]
18. Bhattacharjee, R.; Das, S.S.; Biswal, S.S.; Nath, A.; Das, D.; Basu, A.; Malik, S.; Kumar, L.; Kar, S.; Singh, S.K.; et al. Mechanistic role of HPV-associated early proteins in cervical cancer: Molecular pathways and targeted therapeutic strategies. *Crit. Rev. Oncol./Hematol.* **2022**, *174*, 103675. [CrossRef] [PubMed]
19. Rossi, N.M.; Dai, J.; Xie, Y.; Wangsa, D.; Heselmeyer-Haddad, K.; Lou, H.; Boland, J.F.; Yeager, M.; Orozco, R.; Freites, E.A.; et al. Extrachromosomal Amplification of Human Papillomavirus Episomes Is a Mechanism of Cervical Carcinogenesis. *Cancer Res.* **2023**, *83*, 1768–1781. [CrossRef]
20. Song, Q.; Yang, Y.; Jiang, D.; Qin, Z.; Xu, C.; Wang, H.; Huang, J.; Chen, L.; Luo, R.; Zhang, X.; et al. Proteomic Analysis Reveals Key Differences Between Squamous Cell Carcinomas and Adenocarcinomas Across Multiple Tissues. *Nat. Commun.* **2022**, *13*, 4167. [CrossRef]
21. Fernandes, A.; Viveros-Carreño, D.; Hoegl, J.; Ávila, M.; Pareja, R. Human Papillomavirus-Independent Cervical Cancer. *Int. J. Gynecol. Cancer* **2022**, *32*, 1–7. [CrossRef] [PubMed]
22. Abreu, A.L.P.; Souza, R.P.; Gimenes, F.; Consolaro, M.E.L. A Review of Methods for Detecting Human Papillomavirus Infection. *Virol. J.* **2012**, *9*, 262. [CrossRef] [PubMed]
23. Williams, J.; Kostiuk, M.; Biron, V.L. Molecular Detection Methods in HPV-Related Cancers. *Front. Oncol.* **2022**, *12*, 864820. [CrossRef]
24. Bryan, S.J.; Lee, J.; Gunu, R.; Jones, A.; Olaitan, A.; Rosenthal, A.N.; Cutts, R.J.; Garcia-Murillas, I.; Turner, N.; Lalondrelle, S.; et al. Circulating HPV DNA as a Biomarker for Pre-Invasive and Early Invasive Cervical Cancer: A Feasibility Study. *Cancers* **2023**, *15*, 2590. [CrossRef]
25. Bruni, L.; Diaz, M.; Castellsagué, M.; Ferrer, E.; Bosch, F.X.; de Sanjosé, S. Cervical Human Papillomavirus Prevalence in Five Continents: Meta-Analysis of 1 Million Women with Normal Cytological Findings. *J. Infect. Dis.* **2010**, *202*, 1789–1799. [CrossRef]
26. Roman, B.R.; Aragones, A. Epidemiology and Incidence of HPV-Related Cancers of the Head and Neck. *J. Surg. Oncol.* **2021**, *124*, 920–922. [CrossRef]
27. Jensen, J.E.; Becker, G.L.; Jackson, J.B.; Rysavy, M.B. Human Papillomavirus and Associated Cancers: A Review. *Viruses* **2024**, *16*, 680. [CrossRef]
28. Anantharaman, D.; Abedi-Ardekani, B.; Beachler, D.C.; Gheit, T.; Olshan, A.F.; Wisniewski, K.; Wunsch-Filho, V.; Toporcov, T.N.; Tajara, E.H.; Levi, J.E.; et al. Geographic Heterogeneity in the Prevalence of Human Papillomavirus in Head and Neck Cancer. *Int. J. Cancer* **2017**, *140*, 1968–1975. [CrossRef]
29. Singhavi, H.R.; Chaturvedi, P.; Nair, D. The Human Papillomavirus Enigma: A Narrative Review of Global Variations in Oropharyngeal Cancer Epidemiology and Prognosis. *Indian J. Public Health* **2024**, *68*, 268–275. [CrossRef]
30. Chaturvedi, A.K. Beyond Cervical Cancer: Burden of Other HPV-Related Cancers Among Men and Women. *J. Adolesc. Health* **2010**, *46* (Suppl. 4), S20–S26. [CrossRef]
31. Deniz, Z.; Uraz, S.; Holem, R.; Ozaras, R.; Tahan, V. Human Papillomavirus Infection and Oropharyngeal and Gastrointestinal Cancers: A Causal Relationship? *Diseases* **2022**, *10*, 94. [CrossRef] [PubMed]
32. Zhou, B.; Bie, F.; Zang, R.; Zhang, M.; Song, P.; Liu, L.; Peng, Y.; Bai, G.; Huai, Q.; Li, Y.; et al. Global Burden and Temporal Trends in Incidence and Mortality of Oesophageal Cancer. *J. Adv. Res.* **2023**, *50*, 135–144. [CrossRef] [PubMed]
33. Rajendra, K.; Sharma, P. Viral Pathogens in Oesophageal and Gastric Cancer. *Pathogens* **2022**, *11*, 476. [CrossRef] [PubMed]
34. Liu, Z.; Su, R.; Ahsan, A.; Liu, C.; Liao, X.; Tian, D.; Su, M. Esophageal Squamous Cancer from 4NQO-Induced Mice Model: CNV Alterations. *Int. J. Mol. Sci.* **2022**, *23*, 14304. [CrossRef]
35. Gao, S.; Zhang, Z.; Sun, K.; Li, M.X.; Qi, Y.J. Upper Gastrointestinal Tract Microbiota with Oral Origin in Relation to Oesophageal Squamous Cell Carcinoma. *Ann. Med.* **2023**, *55*, 2295401. [CrossRef]
36. Syrjänen, K.J. HPV Infections and Oesophageal Cancer. *J. Clin. Pathol.* **2002**, *55*, 721–728. [CrossRef]
37. Petrelli, F.; De Santi, G.; Rampulla, V.; Ghidini, A.; Mercurio, P.; Mariani, M.; Manara, M.; Rausa, E.; Lonati, V.; Viti, M.; et al. Human Papillomavirus (HPV) Types 16 and 18 Infection and Esophageal Squamous Cell Carcinoma: A Systematic Review and Meta-Analysis. *J. Cancer Res. Clin. Oncol.* **2021**, *147*, 3011–3023. [CrossRef]
38. Feng, B.; Awuti, I.; Deng, Y.; Li, D.; Niyazi, M.; Aniwar, J.; Sheyhidin, I.; Lu, G.; Li, G.; Zhang, L. Human Papillomavirus Promotes Esophageal Squamous Cell Carcinoma by Regulating DNA Methylation and Expression of HLA-DQB1. *Asia Pac. J. Clin. Oncol.* **2014**, *10*, 66–74. [CrossRef]

39. Zang, B.; Huang, G.; Wang, X.; Zheng, S. HPV-16 E6 Promotes Cell Growth of Esophageal Cancer via Downregulation of miR-125b and Activation of Wnt/β-Catenin Signaling Pathway. *Int. J. Clin. Exp. Pathol.* **2015**, *8*, 13687–13694.
40. Zhang, D.H.; Chen, J.Y.; Hong, C.Q.; Yi, D.Q.; Wang, F.; Cui, W. High-Risk Human Papillomavirus Infection Associated with Telomere Elongation in Patients with Esophageal Squamous Cell Carcinoma with Poor Prognosis. *Cancer* **2014**, *120*, 2673–2683. [CrossRef]
41. Fabian, T.; Leung, A. Epidemiology of Barrett's Esophagus and Esophageal Carcinoma. *Surg. Clin. N. Am.* **2021**, *101*, 381–389. [CrossRef] [PubMed]
42. Sharma, P. Barrett Esophagus: A Review. *JAMA* **2022**, *328*, 663–671. [CrossRef] [PubMed]
43. Brochard, C.; Ducancelle, A.; Pivert, A.; Bodin, M.; Ricard, A.; Coron, E.; Couffon, C.; Dib, N.; Luet, D.; Musquer, N.; et al. Human Papillomavirus Does Not Play a Role in the Barrett Esophagus: A French Cohort. *Dis. Esophagus* **2017**, *30*, 1–7. [CrossRef] [PubMed]
44. Rajendra, S.; Pavey, D.; McKay, O.; Merrett, N.; Gautam, S.D. Human Papillomavirus Infection in Esophageal Squamous Cell Carcinoma and Esophageal Adenocarcinoma: A Concise Review. *Ann. N. Y. Acad. Sci.* **2020**, *1482*, 36–48. [CrossRef]
45. Sung, H.; Ferlay, J.; Siegel, R.L.; Laversanne, M.; Soerjomataram, I.; Jemal, A.; Bray, F. Global Cancer Statistics 2020: GLOBOCAN Estimates of Incidence and Mortality Worldwide for 36 Cancers in 185 Countries. *CA Cancer J. Clin.* **2021**, *71*, 209–249. [CrossRef]
46. IARC Working Group on the Evaluation of Carcinogenic Risks to Humans. Human Papillomaviruses. *IARC Monogr. Eval. Carcinog. Risks Hum.* **2007**, *90*, 1–636.
47. Wang, H.; Chen, X.L.; Liu, K.; Bai, D.; Zhang, W.H.; Chen, X.Z.; Hu, J.K.; SIGES Research Group. Associations Between Gastric Cancer Risk and Virus Infection Other Than Epstein-Barr Virus: A Systematic Review and Meta-analysis Based on Epidemiological Studies. *Clin. Transl. Gastroenterol.* **2020**, *11*, e00201. [CrossRef]
48. Bae, J.M. Human Papillomavirus Infection and Gastric Cancer Risk: A Meta-epidemiological Review. *World J. Virol.* **2021**, *10*, 209–216. [CrossRef]
49. Ding, G.C.; Ren, J.L.; Chang, F.B.; Li, J.L.; Yuan, L.; Song, X.; Zhou, S.L.; Guo, T.; Fan, Z.M.; Zeng, Y.; et al. Human Papillomavirus DNA and P16(INK4A) Expression in Concurrent Esophageal and Gastric Cardia Cancers. *World J. Gastroenterol.* **2010**, *16*, 5901–5906. [CrossRef]
50. Wang, Z.J.; Zhang, Y.Q.; Zhang, Y.T. Analysis of Relationship of the Infection of Human Papillomavirus 16, H. pylori cagA Gene, and ureA Gene in Gastric Carcinogenesis. *J. Pract. Med. Tech.* **2013**, *20*, 1061–1064.
51. Baj, J.; Forma, A.; Dudek, I.; Chilimoniuk, Z.; Dobosz, M.; Dobrzyński, M.; Teresiński, G.; Buszewicz, G.; Flieger, J.; Portincasa, P. The Involvement of Human Papilloma Virus in Gastrointestinal Cancers. *Cancers* **2022**, *14*, 2607. [CrossRef] [PubMed]
52. MacLennan, S.A.; Marra, M.A. Oncogenic Viruses and the Epigenome: How Viruses Hijack Epigenetic Mechanisms to Drive Cancer. *Int. J. Mol. Sci.* **2023**, *24*, 9543. [CrossRef] [PubMed]
53. Mousavi, S.E.; Ilaghi, M.; Mahdavizadeh, V.; Ebrahimi, R.; Aslani, A.; Yekta, Z.; Nejadghaderi, S.A. A Population-Based Study on Incidence Trends of Small Intestine Cancer in the United States from 2000 to 2020. *PLoS ONE* **2024**, *19*, e0307019. [CrossRef] [PubMed]
54. Meijer, L.L.; Alberga, A.J.; de Bakker, J.K.; van der Vliet, H.J.; Le Large, T.Y.; van Grieken, N.C.; de Vries, R.; Daams, F.; Zonderhuis, B.M.; Kazemier, G. Outcomes and Treatment Options for Duodenal Adenocarcinoma: A Systematic Review and Meta-Analysis. *Ann. Surg. Oncol.* **2018**, *25*, 2681–2692. [CrossRef]
55. Aparicio, T.; Pachev, A.; Laurent-Puig, P.; Svrcek, M. Epidemiology, Risk Factors, and Diagnosis of Small Bowel Adenocarcinoma. *Cancers* **2022**, *14*, 2268. [CrossRef]
56. Chen, Y.; Zhang, H.; Zhou, Q.; Lu, L.; Lin, J. Metastases to Duodenum in Cervical Squamous Cell Carcinoma: A Case Report and Review of the Literature. *Medicine* **2022**, *101*, e28526. [CrossRef]
57. Sanchez-Cordero, M.M.; Troia, F.R.; Villa, F.J.; Villa, F.J., Jr. Duodenal Squamous Cell Carcinoma from Metastatic Spread of Head and Neck Cancer: A Case Report. *Cureus* **2024**, *16*, e69826. [CrossRef]
58. Markowitz, L.E.; Unger, E.R. Human Papillomavirus Vaccination. *N. Engl. J. Med.* **2023**, *388*, 1790–1798. [CrossRef]
59. Karaoğlan, B.B.; Ürün, Y. Unveiling the Role of Human Papillomavirus in Urogenital Carcinogenesis: A Comprehensive Review. *Viruses* **2024**, *16*, 667. [CrossRef]
60. Garbuglia, A.R.; Lapa, D.; Sias, C.; Capobianchi, M.R.; Del Porto, P. The Use of Both Therapeutic and Prophylactic Vaccines in the Therapy of Papillomavirus Disease. *Front. Immunol.* **2020**, *11*, 188. [CrossRef]
61. Rosalik, K.; Tarney, C.; Han, J. Human Papilloma Virus Vaccination. *Viruses* **2021**, *13*, 1091. [CrossRef] [PubMed]
62. Petrosky, E.; Bocchini, J.A., Jr.; Hariri, S.; Chesson, H.; Curtis, C.R.; Saraiya, M.; Unger, E.R.; Markowitz, L.E.; Centers for Disease Control and Prevention (CDC). Use of 9-Valent Human Papillomavirus (HPV) Vaccine: Updated HPV Vaccination Recommendations of the Advisory Committee on Immunization Practices. *MMWR Morb. Mortal. Wkly. Rep.* **2015**, *64*, 300–304. [PubMed]

63. Paavonen, J.; Naud, P.; Salmeron, J.; Wheeler, C.M.; Chow, S.N.; Apter, D.; Kitchener, H.; Castellsague, X.; Teixeira, J.C.; Skinner, S.R.; et al. Efficacy of Human Papillomavirus (HPV)-16/18 AS04-Adjuvanted Vaccine Against Cervical Infection and Precancer Caused by Oncogenic HPV Types (PATRICIA): Final Analysis of a Double-Blind, Randomized Study in Young Women. *Lancet* **2009**, *374*, 301–314. [CrossRef] [PubMed]
64. Li, W.; Zhai, L.; Zhu, Y.; Lou, F.; Liu, S.; Li, K.; Chen, L.; Wang, H. Effects of Radiation Treatment on HPV-Related Vulvar Cancer: A Meta-Analysis and Systematic Review. *Front. Oncol.* **2024**, *14*, 1400047. [CrossRef]
65. Lu, Z.; Haghollahi, S.; Afzal, M. Potential Therapeutic Targets for the Treatment of HPV-Associated Malignancies. *Cancers* **2024**, *16*, 3474. [CrossRef]
66. Atherton, M.J.; Stephenson, K.B.; Pol, J.; Wang, F.; Lefebvre, C.; Stojdl, D.F.; Nikota, J.K.; Dvorkin-Gheva, A.; Nguyen, A.; Chen, L.; et al. Customized Viral Immunotherapy for HPV-Associated Cancer. *Cancer Immunol. Res.* **2017**, *5*, 847–859. [CrossRef]
67. Kagabu, M.; Yoshino, N.; Murakami, K.; Kawamura, H.; Sasaki, Y.; Muraki, Y.; Baba, T. Treatment of HPV-Related Uterine Cervical Cancer with a Third-Generation Oncolytic Herpes Simplex Virus in Combination with an Immune Checkpoint Inhibitor. *Int. J. Mol. Sci.* **2023**, *24*, 1988. [CrossRef]
68. Wang, R.; Huang, H.; Yu, C.; Li, X.; Wang, Y.; Xie, L. Current Status and Future Directions for the Development of Human Papillomavirus Vaccines. *Front. Immunol.* **2024**, *15*, 1362770. [CrossRef]
69. Xu, M.; Cao, C.; Wu, P.; Huang, X.; Ma, D. Advances in Cervical Cancer: Current Insights and Future Directions. *Cancer Commun.* **2024**, *45*, 77–109. [CrossRef]
70. Branda, F.; Pavia, G.; Ciccozzi, A.; Quirino, A.; Marascio, N.; Gigliotti, S.; Matera, G.; Romano, C.; Locci, C.; Azzena, I.; et al. Human Papillomavirus (HPV) Vaccination: Progress, Challenges, and Future Directions in Global Immunization Strategies. *Vaccines* **2024**, *12*, 1293. [CrossRef]

Disclaimer/Publisher's Note: The statements, opinions and data contained in all publications are solely those of the individual author(s) and contributor(s) and not of MDPI and/or the editor(s). MDPI and/or the editor(s) disclaim responsibility for any injury to people or property resulting from any ideas, methods, instructions or products referred to in the content.

Review

Unveiling the Role of Human Papillomavirus in Urogenital Carcinogenesis a Comprehensive Review

Beliz Bahar Karaoğlan [1,2] and Yüksel Ürün [1,2,*]

1. Department of Medical Oncology, Ankara University Faculty of Medicine, 06620 Ankara, Türkiye; bbaharulas@gmail.com
2. Faculty of Medicine, Department of Internal Medicine, Division of Internal Medicine, Ankara University Cancer Research Institute, 06620 Ankara, Türkiye
* Correspondence: yuksel.urun@ankara.edu.tr; Tel.: +90-312-595-71-12

Abstract: Human papillomavirus (HPV), an oncogenic DNA virus, is the most common sexually transmitted virus and significant public health concern globally. Despite the substantial prevalence of HPV infection among men, routine testing remains elusive due to the lack of approved HPV tests and the complexity of detection methods. Various studies have explored the link between HPV and genitourinary cancers, revealing different associations influenced by geographic variation, histological subtype and methodological differences. These findings underscore the importance of further research to elucidate the role of HPV in male urogenital cancers. This comprehensive review delves into the intricate relationship between HPV and male genitourinary cancers, shedding light on the virus's oncogenic mechanisms and its reported prevalence. A deeper understanding of HPV's implications for male health is essential for advancing public health initiatives and reducing the burden of urogenital cancers worldwide.

Keywords: anal cancer; bladder cancer; HPV; Human papillomavirus; kidney cancer; male health; oncogenic virus; penile cancer; prostate cancer; renal cell carcinoma; testicular cancer; urogenital cancers; vaccine

1. Introduction

Human papillomavirus (HPV) is an oncogenic virus that primarily infects epithelium or mucous membranes. Mucosal HPVs, transmitted through sexual contact, is the most common sexually transmitted infection worldwide [1]. The prevalence of genital HPV infection among men is significant, with approximately one-third of men worldwide being infected by at least one type of genital HPV [2]. High-risk HPV types can lead to precancerous lesions and are responsible for about 10% of cancers globally, including over 90% of cervical cancers, most anal cancers, and some vulvar, vaginal, penile, and head and neck cancers [1]. HPV infection can persist for years before progressing to invasive cancer. Understanding these mechanisms is crucial for developing effective treatments and preventive measures against HPV-related cancers.

In recent years, there has been growing interest in the high prevalence of HPV in men and its potential role in the etiology of urogenital cancers. There are two hypotheses regarding the link between HPV and male genitourinary cancers. The first suggests an anatomical basis, as the urethra serves as a reservoir and direct link between the urinary and genital area, providing a natural route for viral migration. The second hypothesis pertains to the natural affinity of HPV for epithelial cells. Typically, these viruses infect epithelial cells with a strong preference for squamous epithelium, indicating a propensity for urethral and bladder epithelium as well [3]. The aim of this study is to elucidate the potential role of HPV in the etiology of male urogenital cancers, by examining its oncogenic effects and reported frequency, within the context of current scientific evidence.

2. HPV Types and Oncogenesis

HPV-DNA is a circular, double-stranded molecule surrounded by a protein coat. It contains eight genes, split into early (E) and late (L) stages. E1 and E2 handle replication, transcription, and cell regulation. E4 assists in cell cycle control and virion assembly. E5 controls cell growth and virus modulation. E6 and E7 inhibit apoptosis and regulate cell cycling.

HPV types fall into two categories: cutaneous and mucosal. Mucosal HPVs, transmitted through sexual contact, include high- and low-risk oncogenic strains. Low-risk types like 6 and 11 cause genital warts and recurrent respiratory papillomatosis, which seldom progress to cancer. In contrast, persistent infection with high-risk types like 16, 18, 31, 33, 45, 52, and 58 can lead to precancerous lesions and are responsible for about 10% of cancers globally, including over 90% of cervical cancers, most anal cancers, and some vulvar, vaginal, penile and head and neck cancers [1].

3. Human Papillomavirus (HPV) and Its Role in Carcinogenesis

The most well-known mechanism of HPV in cancer development involves its oncoproteins E6 and E7 (Figure 1).

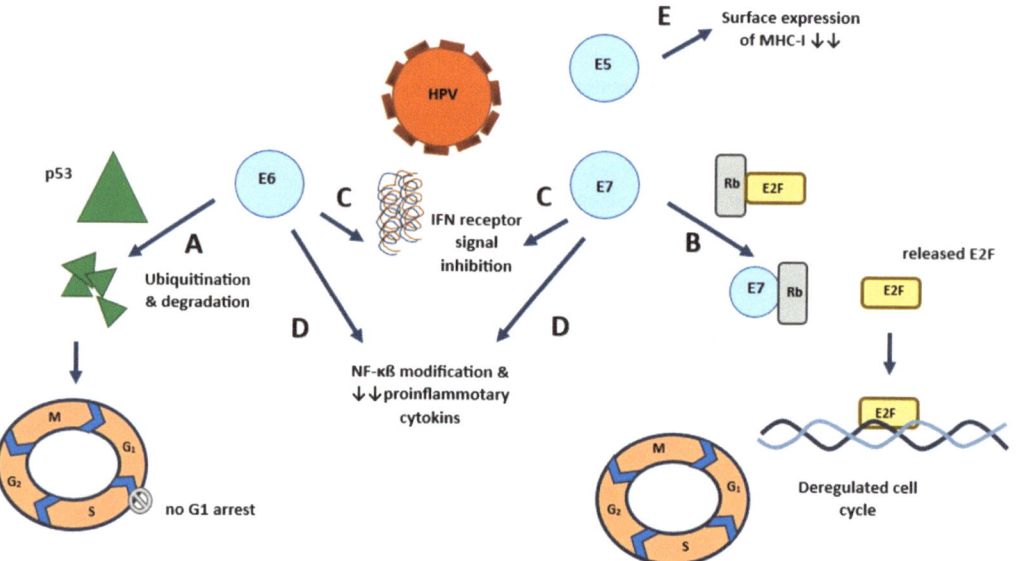

Figure 1. Effects of HPV on host cells. HPV disrupts cell cycle regulation post-infection through two main mechanisms: (A) Firstly, the E6 oncoprotein binds to P53, triggering proteolysis via the ubiquitination pathway, activating the CDK cycle and cell cycle. (B) Secondly, the E7 oncoprotein binds to Rb and other associated proteins, releasing the E2F transcription factor complex and activating the cell cycle. (C) HPV inhibits type 1 IFN-γ receptor with E6 and E7 oncoproteins, and it inhibits type 2 IFN-γ receptor signaling with E7 oncoproteins. (D) E6 and E7 oncoproteins also inhibit NF-κB signaling. (E) E5 and E7 prevent surface expression of MHC molecules. E5 binds to MHC-I and MHC-II in the Golgi and ER, inhibiting their transport to the cell surface. Abbreviations: CDK: Cyclin-dependent kinase, ER: Endoplasmic reticulum, HPV: Human papillomavirus, IFN-γ: interferon-gamma, NF-κB: Nuclear Factor kappa B.

When HPV DNA integrates into the host genome, E6 and E7 inactivate tumor suppressor proteins such as p53 and Rb. High-risk HPV E6 proteins can activate telomerase, a key enzyme for maintaining telomere length and ensuring cell immortality [4]. Additionally, E6 can hinder DNA repair by binding and inhibiting DNA repair proteins, leading to an accumulation of mutations in the host genome [5]. Meanwhile, the E7 protein can disrupt centrosome duplication by affecting cyclin E/cyclin-dependent kinase 2 (CDK2) complexes, causing genomic instability and aneuploidy [6]. All these proccess leads to increased cell proliferation, apoptosis resistance, and malignant transformation. Additionally, HPV triggers chronic inflammation in prostate tissue, contributing to the oncogenic process [7–9]. Another mechanism involves HPV disrupting the activity of the protective enzyme APOBEC3B against viral infections. It's believed that this process resulting in genomic instability and oncogenesis is due to the indirect effect of HPV [10,11]. Persistent infection with high-risk HPVs and progression from latent infection to invasive cancer can take years to decades [4,12].

4. Immune Response to HPV Infection

Host defense mechanisms effectively control initial HPV infections in most individuals, with only a subset progressing to invasive cancer. Physical barriers like mucous membranes blocks virus entry, virus innate immunity recognizes HPV DNA through pathogen sensors. HPV alters host gene expression to evade virus responses by deregulating DNA methylation, histone modification, and nuclear factor kappa B (NF-κB) signaling. The virus interacts with host proteins to inhibit virus responses, impairing antigen presentation and promoting virus suppression. HPV manipulates protein functions to evade virus responses by disrupting protein-protein interactions, inhibiting IFN signaling, and inducing proteasome-mediated degradation of cytokines. The virus also interferes with MHC molecule trafficking and antigen presentation [11].

5. Detection of HPV

Determining the link between exposure and outcome relies on accurately identifying the exposure. Various methods are used in different studies to detect HPV, each with its own strengths and limitations.

While the role of HPV in women's health is well understood and extensively studied through various screening and research programs, men have been significantly less involved in these efforts. This is partly because HPV-related diseases affect and result in fatalities among women more frequently than men [13]. Although there's been increased focus on HPV infection in males in recent years, awareness and understanding of HPV-related issues in men still lag behind that in women. Currently, there isn't a universally accepted and validated test for screening HPV in males [14]. The lack of routine screening for HPV in men can be attributed to inconsistent results observed in testing. Obtaining samples from penile skin poses challenges due to its anatomical structure, which is less permeable compared to that of women. As a result, the efficacy of HPV testing methods in men remains uncertain.

While obtaining samples for HPV detection in men isn't as straightforward as cervical smear collection, optimal sampling site for HPV testing in men remains unknown. Penoscopy may be useful for detecting warts and carriers but has limited sensitivity for flat lesions. Urethroscopy is recommended only for condylomas in the urethral meatus [15]. Other methods include investigating HPV presence in body fluids like urine and semen. Serological methods that detect antibodies against HPV in serum have low sensitivity due to the virus's weak immune response in many cases and may not provide information about infection activity or localization [16].

Morphological changes such as papillomatosis, hypergranulosis, acanthosis, and koilocytosis in cancerous tissues indicate HPV infection but with low sensitivity. Immunohistochemical (IHC) methods for detecting HPV capsid proteins are highly specific but have low sensitivity. Over the past decades, there has been significant advancement in the methods used to detect HPV infection. Earlier techniques like hybridization/blotting have been replaced by more efficient signal amplification assays, particularly quantitative polymerase chain reaction (qPCR), which can identify individual HPV genotypes. These qPCR tests have become the primary approach for HPV screening and clinical diagnosis [17,18].

Next-generation sequencing (NGS) offers a highly sensitive method for HPV detection, capable of identifying low-copy-number types, novel variants, and even those that may evade detection by standard molecular methods. Whole-genome NGS, covering the entire HPV genome, allows for precise identification of variants and subvariants beyond genotype level.

Recent studies utilizing NGS have provided more accurate estimates of HPV's contribution to cervical cancer compared to traditional PCR techniques [19–21]. Discrepancies in HPV testing methodologies across countries and studies primarily arise from differences in sample types and the scientific resources at their disposal. This situation often leads to methodological inconsistencies in studies aiming to evaluate the relationship between HPV and organ-associated cancers, thereby compromising the reliability of the data. With NGS technology becoming more cost-effective and robust, it is poised to rival existing HPV-DNA tests. Furthermore, NGS holds promise in elucidating the genotype-phenotype relationships in HPV-associated malignancies such as male urogenital cancers, offering insights into the underlying molecular mechanisms of these diseases.

6. Penile Cancer

Penile cancer, with an average annual incidence of 1 per 100,000 men, is a rare malignancy [22]. Despite its rarity and the curative potential of early-stage surgical intervention, the physical and psychosocial morbidity associated with the disease and its treatment is significant. Etiological factors are HPV infection, poor hygiene, lack of circumcision, inflammatory conditions, lichen sclerosis, immunosuppression, and smoking [23]. It typically arises from mucosal surfaces and the most common localizations are glans penis and inner prepuce [24]. Squamous cell cancer (SCC) is the most common type and carious subtypes of SCC exist, including usual, papillary, condylomatous (warty), basaloid, verrucous, and sarcomatoid [25,26]. Penile SCC mainly impacts older men, with the highest incidence occurring in their sixties [27]. Recent observations suggest a rise in cases among younger individuals, possibly linked to changes in sexual behaviors leading to increased exposure to sexually transmitted diseases and higher rates of HPV infection [28].

Studies suggest approximately 40% of penile cancers are HPV-positive [29,30]. In a retrospective analysis of over 1200 penile cancer cases by Backes et al., HPV positivity was observed in 48% of patients, with the highest risk of HPV-related penile cancer development reported in Asia [31]. HPV types 16 and 18 are the most commonly detected in penile cancer cases, with both types present together in about one-third of cases [30,32,33]. The prevalence of HPV positivity varies among different SCC subtypes, with higher rates observed in basaloid and condylomatous types [31,34].

In penile intraepithelial neoplasia (PeIN), known as a precursor lesion of penile SCC, HPV positivity rate increases with higher grades of dysplasia [30]. PeINs are now classified as HPV-independent or HPV-associated according to the 2022 World Health Organization (WHO) classification [35].

Uncircumcised men have higher HPV prevalence and it seem like circumcision protects against HPV and HPV-related penile cancer [27,36]. The prognostic significance of HPV in penile cancer, which is well-established in head and neck cancers [37], remains an area of research interest. Studies suggest that HPV presence is associated with a favorable prognosis in penile cancer [38,39], while a few suggests a poorer prognosis [40]. A better understanding of HPV-related oncogenic mechanisms will likely shed light on the prognostic significance of HPV in penile cancer.

In conclusion, penile cancer, though rare, warranting attention to preventive measures and early detection strategies. HPV infection, among other factors, plays a pivotal role in its etiology, with HPV-positive cases exhibiting varying prognostic implications.

7. Anal Cancer

Anal cancer is a relatively rare malignancy, but its incidence has been rising steadily over the past few decades [22]. Anal squamous cell carcinoma (ASCC) is the most common histologic type. HPV infection has emerged as a significant risk factor for the development of ASCC. High-risk HPV has been detected in 90% of ASCCs, with HPV-16 is the most common type [41,42]. Anal intercourse and a high number of sexual partners throughout life elevate the risk of persistent HPV infection, leading to subsequent high-grade squamous intraepithelial neoplasia (HSIL) and ASCC. Additionally, factors such as immunosuppression resulting from HIV infection or the use of immunosuppressants post-solid organ transplantation, hematologic malignancies, prior HPV-related cancers, autoimmune disorders, low socio-economic status, and smoking history are also associated with an increased risk of ASCC [43].

ASCC is considered to share similarities in its biology and natural history with cervical cancer, including association with high-risk HPV infection to precancerous lesions to cancer. Similar to the cervical transformation zone, the virus targets actively dividing basal cells located in the transition zone, situated within the rectal columnar mucosa distal to the dentate line, and spreads towards the squamocolumnar junction. Anal Papanicolaou (Pap) smears involve cytological examination beyond the squamocolumnar junction but this method lacks utility as a screening tool in high-risk populations. The gold standard is high-resolution anoscopy (HRA), which involves examining the squamocolumnar junction, anal canal, and perianal skin under magnification using an anoscope [44].

Anal HPV prevalence varies substantially by HIV-status and sexual orientation in men, which is considered to increase HPV prevalence at the anal site [45]. A recent systematic review, encompassing a large cohort of nearly thirty thousand men, assessed the prevalence of anal HPV and HSIL, stratified by HIV status and sexual orientation. Among HIV-negative men who have sex with women (MSW), the prevalence of anal HR-HPV was found to be at 6.9%. In contrast, among HIV-positive MSW, the prevalence rates were notably higher at 26.9% for HR-HPV. Among HIV-negative MSM, the prevalence was 41.2%, while among HIV-positive MSM, the prevalence rates were substantially elevated at 74.3% [46].

Findings from the U.S. Anal Cancer HSIL Outcomes Research (ANCHOR) study revealed that treating anal precancers notably diminishes the risk of progressing to anal cancer, particularly among people living with HIV aged 35 years and older [47]. These outcomes emphasize the urgency of identifying effective methods for detecting anal precancers that can be promptly treated to avert further progression. Guidelines recommend the implementation of screening programs utilizing anal cytology and high-resolution anoscopy for high-risk populations, such as gay, bisexual, and other MSM, as well as HIV-negative women with a history of anal intercourse or other HPV-related anogenital malignancies. These recommendations draw inspiration from the successes observed in cervical cytology screening. However, the absence of randomized controlled studies demonstrating the preventive efficacy of screening in these high-risk populations precludes its routine endorsement at present [43].

The high prevalence of anal HPV among young MSM underscores the importance of gender-neutral HPV vaccination prior to sexual debut, compared to catch-up vaccination efforts. Additionally, HIV-positive MSM represent a priority group for ASCC screening initiatives [46]. Consistent with these findings, another study investigating the efficacy of HPV vaccines in preventing anal precancerous lesions and ASCC revealed compelling evidence supporting the substantial effectiveness of vaccination in reducing anal HPV infection and HSIL among HIV-negative individuals vaccinated at or before the age of 26. Importantly, the limited impact observed in individuals HIV-positive beyond this age suggests that vaccines may confer greater benefits in populations with lower levels of sexual exposure to anal HPV [48].

The presence of HPV infection significantly impacts the prognosis of ASCC. Individuals with HPV-negative tumors are less likely to respond to CRT than those with HPV-positive tumors [49,50]. A meta-analysis has shown that patients with HPV-positive/p16-positive tumors have improved survival outcomes compared with patients with either HPV-negative/p16-positive or HPV-positive/p16-negative tumors [51].

In an NGS study of HPV in ASCC, samples with viral integration had higher PIK3CA-activating mutation rates, which is an APOBEC editing signature in HPV-positive HNSCC were associated with increased mutational burden, suggesting immunogenicity and suitability for immune therapy [52].

In conclusion, the escalating incidence of anal cancer, primarily attributable to HPV infection, necessitates a multifaceted approach for effective management. While HPV vaccination represents a crucial preventive strategy, screening programs utilizing anal cytology and HPV testing hold promise, particularly for high-risk groups.

8. Prostate Cancer

Prostate cancer (PCa) is the most common solid tumor in men and ranks high among cancer-related deaths [53]. Alongside known factors like age, family history, and genetic risk; modifiable risk factors such as smoking, diet, obesity, and reduced physical activity play a role in PCa etiology [54–56].

Prostate tissue is predominantly glandular in origin, it also contains a transition zone similar to the cervix. However, only about a quarter of PCa cases originate from this zone [57]. Although squamous metaplasia can occasionally occur in PCa tissues, it is known to be hormonally driven. Glandular structures are dominant in PCa [58–60]. While it could be speculated that squamous metaplasia observed in the prostate may be HPV-related, it could also serve as a potential reservoir for HPV.

HPV presence in prostate tissue was first identified by McNicol and Dodd using PCR method [61]. Subsequent studies showing koilocytosis in PCa tissues suggest a potential role for HPV in PCa etiology [62,63]. Most studies investigating the relationship between HPV and PCa use tissues from patients with benign prostatic hyperplasia (BPH) as the control group [63–67]. While understandable due to the quantitative advantage over normal prostate tissues, this approach can lead to confusion considering that pre-cancerous lesions are often evaluated under the umbrella of BPH. A meta-analysis, conducted by Tsydenova IA et al., included 27 studies and 3122 tissue samples, focusing solely on studies using PCR-based methods, showed a significant association between HPV and PCa in normal tissues, although among the studies using BPH tissues as controls, there was no significant relationship between HPV presence and PCa. These results highlighted how even the choice of control tissue can influence outcomes [68].

The most comprehensive review examining the relationship between PCa and HPV included 60 studies, with 51 studies investigating HPV presence in tissues and 13 studies in blood, using various methods including PCR, ELISA, hybridization, and IHC. Among the included studies, 11 (18%) showed a positive association between HPV presence and PCa development [69].

Research exploring the potential role of HPV in PCa pathogenesis has utilized various methodologies, yet findings remain inconclusive. Traditional PCR-based techniques, commonly employed in prior studies, may lack the sensitivity required to detect past HPV infections, limiting their ability to elucidate the HPV-PCa relationship [63–67,70]. In contrast, a study by Khoury et al., utilizing NGS methods on the Human Genome Atlas database, found no HPV presence in 53 PCa cases [71]. Given the high sensitivity and specificity of the method employed, this study stands out with a high level of evidence compared to many others with different methodologies. Further studies using similar methodology are crucial to investigate the relationship between HPV and Pca.

The timing of human papillomavirus (HPV) involvement in the oncogenic process is another unresolved problem. Although HPV is implicated in both cervical cancer formation and progression, its role in PCa is thought to involve a 'hit and run' phenomenon, wherein HPV triggers early malignant transformation in prostate cells and then becomes cleared, explaining the absence of viral genome detection in PCa tissues [72–76]. Some studies propose HPV's effectiveness in later stages of oncogenesis, associating HPV presence with a high Gleason score, contradicting the 'hit and run' hypothesis [65]. However, many studies have not confirmed this relationship [72,77]. These inconsistencies underscore the need for further research to elucidate the complex interplay between HPV and PCa development. Additionally, the potential impact of HPV vaccination on PCa risk remains uncertain, warranting future studies to explore preventive measures in PCa carcinogenesis.

In conclusion, existing studies on the association between HPV and PCa are hindered by methodological variations and diverse control groups, resulting in insufficient evidence to conclusively establish the role of HPV in PCa etiology. Despite suggestive findings, the current body of literature lacks robustness, emphasizing the inadequacy of available data to firmly support the involvement of HPV in PCa carcinogenesis. Conflicting results and differing interpretations underscore the necessity for more comprehensive investigations in this field. Moreover, as all studies to date have been observational in nature, the potential impact of HPV vaccination on PCa risk remains uncertain and warrants further exploration.

9. Bladder Cancer

Bladder cancer (BC) ranks as the tenth most common cancer globally [53]. It originates from the urothelium, which is a waterproof protective barrier against urinary tract infections. It undergoes rapid shedding and regeneration in response to acute injury or infection.

Histologically, BC is categorized into different types, including urothelial carcinoma (UC), squamous-cell carcinoma (SCC), and adenocarcinoma. UC constitutes about 95% of BC cases, encompassing various differentiated and histologic subtypes. BC can be further classified based on invasion depth into muscle-infiltrating BC (MIBC) and non-muscle-infiltrating BC (NMIBC). NMIBC affects around 75% of patients [78].

Smoking remains a significant independent risk factor for BC development, with persistent smokers having a threefold higher risk compared to non-smokers. Schistosomiasis is recognized as a notable cause of SCC. Other factors contributing to BC occurrence include exposure to occupational carcinogens, genetic predisposition, and dietary habits [79]. Lately, there's been a focus on the link between BC and infections like HPV and similar viruses [80–82].

Numerous investigations have explored how HPV infection impacts the bladder epithelium. Furthermore, HPV DNA has been identified in urine and washing specimens from individuals with BC, along with BC tissues [83]. Additionally, there's a positive correlation between high-risk HPV infection and tumor advancement, with the latter often linked to p53 mutation [84].

In a meta-analysis conducted by Sun J. et al., comprising 6065 BC patients, the prevalence of HPV was found to be 16% (11–21%). Studies indicated that HPV increases the risk of BC (OR: 3.35, 95% CI: 1.75–6.43) and its recurrence (OR:1.87, 95% CI: 1.24–2.82), which showed the latent prognostic effect of the virus [85]. In a meta-analysis conducted by Muresu et al., a HPV prevalence of 19% was reported. HPV types 16 and 18 were most commonly detected in BC samples, and HPV was shown to increase the risk of BC by more than sevenfold (OR: 7.84, 95% CI: 4.34–14.15) [86]. Studies have also found that the virus is associated with muscle invasion, high grade, and advanced stage disease in patients with BC [87,88]. However, these results were influenced by heterogeneous variables such as region, the method used to detect HPV (PCR vs. others), sample (e.g., FFPE, fresh tissue), and BC histology.

Asia has the highest prevalence of HPV, with reported HPV positivity reaching up to 45% in studies [85]. The difference in prevalence between continents may be attributed to factors such as genetic differences, cultural disparities, and sexual habits, in addition to the method used to detect HPV. Furthermore, analysis of studies conducted in Asia indicates that the presence of HPV increases the risk of BC by more than sixfold (OR: 6.2, 95% CI: 2.167–18.250) [89].

The relationship between HPV and BC varies according to the histological subtypes. Due to the predominant histological subtype being UC, many studies have indicated an association between HPV and UC, while data showing an increased risk for SCC are limited [58,59]. Interestingly, in patients with UC, squamous differentiation associated with HPV has been shown to negatively affect prognosis [90,91].

While the exact connection between HPV infection and the development and advancement of BC isn't fully understood, a comprehensive review of existing literature indicates that there is a positive link between HPV infection (especially high-risk types) and BC, particularly UC, although some studies suggest that HPV may not be a direct cause [92–94].

10. Renal Cell Carcinoma

Renal cell carcinoma (RCC) is one of the common cancers in men, with an incidence rate of 4.4% reported worldwide [95]. The predominant histological type, clear cell RCC, accounts for the majority of cases. Risk factors for RCC are advanced age, male gender [96], genetic factors (e.g., von Hippel-Lindau syndrome) [97,98], smoking [99], diet, hypertension [100], obesity [101], and environmental exposures (e.g., cadmium and asbestos) [102,103].

The potential role of HPV in RCC etiology was first studied in the early 1990s [104]. Subsequent research has explored whether this virus, commonly found in the male genital system, contributes to RCC risk. In a study by Farhadi et al., HPV was detected in 30% of tumor tissues from RCC patients. The absence of HPV's L1 capsid protein and cellular changes associated with the virus, such as koilocytosis, in RCC patients led to the interpretation that HPV's life cycle is disrupted in advanced stages. The presence of HPV was also associated with high-grade tumors in this study [105]. Another study showed a 14.3% prevalence of HR-HPV in RCC samples using PCR, while HPV was not found in any healthy renal tissue in the control group, suggesting a potential role for HPV in RCC etiology [106]. Additionally, a study using ISH demonstrated a 52% positivity rate for HPV-DNA in RCC tissues [107]. However, a comprehensive study by Khoury et al. using data from the Human Genome Atlas did not establish a relationship between RCC and HPV [71]. Similarly, another study involving various histological types of RCC found no association between HPV and RCC [108]. Apart from case reports and case-control studies, there is a lack of extensive research on this topic. Given the heterogeneity of methods used to detect HPV-DNA and the conflicting results of studies, it is not possible to definitively conclude that HPV plays a role in RCC etiology based on current evidence. Further large-scale studies using standardized methods are needed to investigate this relationship.

11. Testicular Cancer

Testicular cancer (TC) is the most common solid tumor in men aged 20–40 years, comprising approximately 1–2% of all cancers. It is histologically classified into germ cell tumors (TGCT) and non-germ cell tumors. Risk factors for TC include cryptorchidism, genetic predisposition, and substance use [109,110]. The similarity in age of onset between TC and diseases caused by sexually transmitted infections raises the possibility of infectious agents playing a role in the etiology of TC.

In a case-control study investigating HPV presence in semen samples using PCR and FISH, HPV was detected in 9.7% of patients diagnosed with TGCT and 2.4% of healthy controls [111]. Another study by Stricker et al. evaluated HPV antibody levels in 39 TC patients using ELISA, revealing a 5% HPV positivity rate, although HPV presence in malignant tissues of these patients was not examined [112]. This finding is not sufficient to demonstrate an association between HPV presence and TC. Indeed, studies evaluating HPV in tissues using PCR have not found HPV presence in either patients or control groups [113,114].

Recent studies have highlighted the potential role of HPV in male infertility by directly infecting male gametes, leading to decreased fertility due to increased sperm DNA damage and abnormal chromosome numbers. HPV is believed to attach to sperm cells at specific sites on their heads, similar to other viruses that infect sperm [115,116]. With increasing evidence suggesting a link between HPV and male infertility, questions have arisen about its role in TC. But when assessing the correlation between testicular germ cell neoplasms and HPV, it is crucial to consider that HPV exhibits a predilection for epithelial tissues, whereas testicular germ cell neoplasms originate from non-epithelial sources. Further research of high quality is required to better understand this relationship.

12. HPV Vaccination

The optimal long-term approach for mitigating the risks associated with HPV-related cancers is vaccination. Vaccines consist of virus-like particles (VLPs) designed to elicit immunity against specific HPV types included in the vaccine formulation. The initial efficacy trials focused on quadrivalent (4vHPV) vaccine, containing HPV-16, HPV-18, HPV-6, and HPV-11 VLPs and bivalent vaccine (2vHPV), containing HPV-16, HPV-18, HPV-6, and HPV-11 VLPs. There is also nine-valent HPV vaccine (9vHPV), provides additional protection against HPV-31, 33, 45, 52, and 58. The Centers for Disease Control (CDC) recommends HPV vaccination for individuals aged 11 to 12 years, with females up to the age of 26 years, boys up to the age of 21 years, and specific populations up to the age of 26 years recommended for catch-up immunization [117]. 9vHPV vaccine is also indicated for preventing anogenital lesions in both men and women up to the age of 45, as well as oropharyngeal and other head and neck cancers caused by select HPV types [117].

HPV vaccination elicits robust levels of HPV-type-specific antibodies, particularly in children under 16 years, compared to older age groups [118]. Despite the demonstrated efficacy of HPV vaccination in males, several countries have yet to implement routine vaccination for boys, resulting in notably low vaccination coverage among males. Efforts to enhance medical awareness regarding the benefits of male HPV vaccination may enhance disease management and increase vaccine acceptance among parents and boys. A systematic review assessing HPV vaccination efficacy in male populations found significant effectiveness against HPV-related anogenital diseases, with the highest efficacy observed against anal intraepithelial neoplasia (AIN) and genital condyloma [119].

The era of prophylactic vaccination underscores the importance of updating the potential individual benefits for boys receiving the HPV vaccine, especially in light of the rising frequency of head and neck HPV-associated cancers. Lechner et al. highlighted key points indicating that the incidence of HPV-associated oropharyngeal cancer is expected to rise until the benefits of gender-neutral prophylactic HPV vaccination become evident [120]. Also, individuals living with HIV and MSM face elevated risks of HPV-related diseases due to HIV-induced immunosuppression. Although vaccinating women can confer indirect protection to heterosexual men, MSM and bisexual men do not benefit from this herd immunity [119].

Although the existing vaccines are primarily preventive, they have shown advantages in individuals undergoing treatment for HPV-related conditions such as cervical intraepithelial neoplasia (CIN), genital warts, anal neoplasia, and recurrent respiratory papillomatosis (RRP). The mechanism behind inhibiting further disease progression is believed to involve halting the spread of HPV [121,122].

Another area of research pertains to the protective efficacy of single-dose HPV vaccination. In a randomized, multicenter, double-blind, controlled trial conducted in Kenya in 2022, involving women aged 15–20 years, single-dose administration of 9vHPV or 2vHPV vaccines revealed that a single dose effectively prevented incident persistent oncogenic HPV infection, demonstrating comparable efficacy to multidose regimens assessed over an 18-month period [122]. However, evidence regarding the effectiveness of a single dose of HPV vaccine in boys is currently lacking.

Young cancer survivors have a higher risk of developing HPV-related malignancies compared to the general population, often due to underimmunization [123,124]. HPV vaccines are effective in these individuals, with timing based on individual risk factors and no need for prior HPV testing [125].

13. Conclusions and Future Directions

Unraveling the complex interplay between HPV and genitourinary cancers in men requires further research. While evidence suggests a potential link, inconsistencies and methodological limitations necessitate a multifaceted approach (Figure 2). Standardizing HPV detection methods across healthcare settings is essential to ensure consistency and reliability in diagnosis. Longitudinal studies are needed to track HPV progression over time and understand its evolution into cancer.

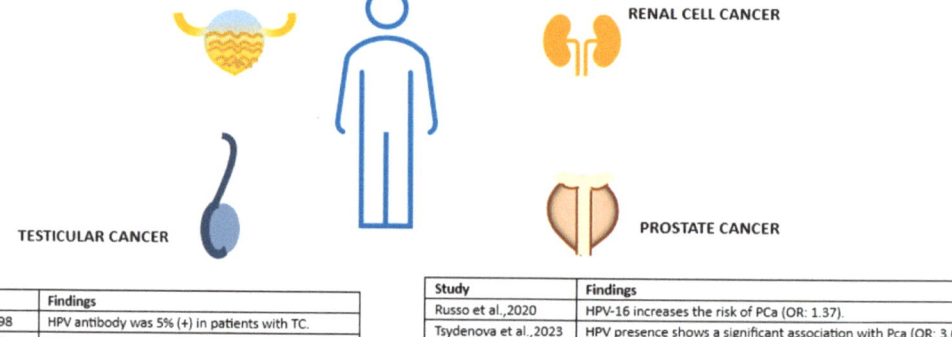

Figure 2. Unraveling Possible Male Urogenital Cancers Linked to HPV: Summary of findings. References cited in the figure: [85–89,91] for BC, [71,105–108] for RCC, [111,112,114] for TC and [68–71] for PCa. Abbreviations: BC: Bladder cancer, HPV: Human papillomavirus, PCa: Prostate cancer, RCC: Renal cell carcinoma, TC: Testicular cancer.

Evaluating the impact of HPV vaccination on cancer incidence will provide valuable insights into the effectiveness of vaccination programs. Deciphering the oncogenic mechanisms of HPV in genitourinary tissues is crucial for identifying potential therapeutic targets. Identifying high-risk populations and developing targeted interventions can help tailor prevention and screening strategies. Additionally, developing specific diagnostic tools for early detection and conducting comprehensive epidemiological surveys are essential for global mapping and informed public health policies. Promoting vaccination and safe sex practices through targeted public health campaigns can increase vaccine uptake and reduce HPV transmission. Evaluating the feasibility and benefits of routine HPV testing in clinical settings is necessary for effective screening programs. Lastly, investigating the efficacy of existing and novel therapies for HPV-positive cancers will improve treatment outcomes and patient survival. By prioritizing these research avenues, we can enhance our understanding of the HPV-genitourinary cancer link and achieve significant advancements in public health.

Author Contributions: Both authors have been contributed to every stage of this review. All authors have read and agreed to the published version of the manuscript.

Funding: No funding was received for conducting this study.

Conflicts of Interest: The authors declare no conflicts of interest.

References

1. Narisawa-Saito, M.; Kiyono, T. Basic mechanisms of high-risk human papillomavirus-induced carcinogenesis: Roles of E6 and E7 proteins. *Cancer Sci.* **2007**, *98*, 1505–1511. [CrossRef] [PubMed]
2. Bruni, L.; Albero, G.; Rowley, J.; Alemany, L.; Arbyn, M.; Giuliano, A.R.; Markowitz, L.E.; Broutet, N.; Taylor, M. Global and regional estimates of genital human papillomavirus prevalence among men: A systematic review and meta-analysis. *Lancet Glob. Health* **2023**, *11*, e1345–e1362. [CrossRef] [PubMed]
3. Egawa, N.; Egawa, K.; Griffin, H.; Doorbar, J. Human Papillomaviruses; Epithelial Tropisms, and the Development of Neoplasia. *Viruses* **2015**, *7*, 3863–3890. [CrossRef]
4. Moody, C.A.; Laimins, L.A. Papanicolau smear Human papillomavirus oncoproteins: Pathways to transformation. *Nat. Rev. Cancer* **2010**, *10*, 550–560. [CrossRef]
5. Iftner, T.; Elbel, M.; Schopp, B.; Hiller, T.; Loizou, J.I.; Caldecott, K.W.; Stubenrauch, F. Interference of papillomavirus E6 protein with single-strand break repair by interaction with XRCC1. *EMBO J.* **2002**, *21*, 4741–4748. [CrossRef]
6. Korzeniewski, N.; Spardy, N.; Duensing, A.; Duensing, S. Genomic instability and cancer: Lessons learned from human papillomaviruses. *Cancer Lett.* **2011**, *305*, 113–122. [CrossRef] [PubMed]
7. Zhang, L.; Wang, Y.; Qin, Z.; Gao, X.; Xing, Q.; Li, R.; Wang, W.; Song, N.; Zhang, W. Correlation between Prostatitis, Benign Prostatic Hyperplasia and Prostate Cancer: A systematic review and Meta-analysis. *J. Cancer* **2020**, *11*, 177–189. [CrossRef]
8. Jain, P.; Ghosh, A.; Jana, D.; Pal, D.K. Chronic pelvic pain syndrome/chronic prostatitis: Is it related to human papillomavirus infection? A case-control study from Eastern India. *Urol. J.* **2020**, *87*, 137–141. [CrossRef]
9. La Vignera, S.; Condorelli, R.A.; Cannarella, R.; Giacone, F.; Mongioi', L.; Scalia, G.; Favilla, V.; Russo, G.I.; Cimino, S.; Morgia, G.; et al. High rate of detection of ultrasound signs of prostatitis in patients with HPV-DNA persistence on semen: Role of ultrasound in HPV-related male accessory gland infection. *J. Endocrinol. Investig.* **2019**, *42*, 1459–1465. [CrossRef]
10. Smith, N.J.; Fenton, T.R. The APOBEC3 genes and their role in cancer: Insights from human papillomavirus. *J. Mol. Endocrinol.* **2019**, *62*, R269–R287. [CrossRef]
11. Westrich, J.A.; Warren, C.J.; Pyeon, D. Evasion of host immune defenses by human papillomavirus. *Virus Res.* **2017**, *231*, 21–33. [CrossRef] [PubMed]
12. Graham, S.V. The human papillomavirus replication cycle, and its links to cancer progression: A comprehensive review. *Clin. Sci.* **2017**, *131*, 2201–2221. [CrossRef] [PubMed]
13. Lenzi, A.; Mirone, V.; Gentile, V.; Bartoletti, R.; Ficarra, V.; Foresta, C.; Mariani, L.; Mazzoli, S.; Parisi, S.G.; Perino, A.; et al. Rome consensus conference—statement; human papilloma virus diseases in males. *BMC Public Health* **2013**, *13*, 117. [CrossRef]
14. STD Facts—HPV and Men. Available online: https://www.cdc.gov/std/HPV/STDFact-HPV-and-men.htm (accessed on 15 February 2024).
15. Cai, T.; Di Vico, T.; Durante, J.; Tognarelli, A.; Bartoletti, R. Human papilloma virus and genitourinary cancers: A narrative review. *Minerva Urol. Nefrol.* **2018**, *70*, 579–587. [CrossRef]
16. Dunne, E.F.; Nielson, C.M.; Stone, K.M.; Markowitz, L.E.; Giuliano, A.R. Prevalence of HPV Infection among Men: A Systematic Review of the Literature. *J. Infect. Dis.* **2006**, *194*, 1044–1057. [CrossRef] [PubMed]
17. Vives, A.; Cosentino, M.; Palou, J. The role of human papilloma virus test in men: First exhaustive review of literature. *Actas Urol. Esp.* **2020**, *44*, 86–93. [CrossRef]
18. Lorincz, A.; Wheeler, C.M.; Cuschieri, K.; Meijer, C.J.L.M.; Quint, W. Developing and Standardizing Human Papillomavirus Tests. In *Human Papillomavirus Proving and Using a Viral Cause for Cancer*; Jenkins, D., Bosch, F.X., Eds.; Academic Press: Cambridge, MA, USA, 2019; pp. 111–130.
19. Arroyo, L.S.; Smelov, V.; Bzhalava, D.; Eklund, C.; Hultin, E.; Dillner, J. Next generation sequencing for human papillomavirus genotyping. *J. Clin. Virol.* **2013**, *58*, 437–442. [CrossRef]
20. Nilyanimit, P.; Chansaenroj, J.; Poomipak, W.; Praianantathavorn, K.; Payungporn, S.; Poovorawan, Y. Comparison of Four Human Papillomavirus Genotyping Methods: Next-generation Sequencing, INNO-LiPA, Electrochemical DNA Chip, and Nested-PCR. *Ann. Lab. Med.* **2018**, *38*, 139–146. [CrossRef]
21. Clifford, G.M.; Tenet, V.; Georges, D.; Alemany, L.; Pavón, M.A.; Chen, Z.; Yeager, M.; Cullen, M.; Boland, J.F.; Bass, S.; et al. Human papillomavirus 16 sub-lineage dispersal and cervical cancer risk worldwide: Whole viral genome sequences from 7116 HPV16-positive women. *Papillomavirus Res.* **2019**, *7*, 67–74. [CrossRef]
22. Siegel, R.L.; Giaquinto, A.N.; Jemal, A. Cancer statistics, 2024. *CA Cancer J. Clin.* **2024**, *74*, 12–49. [CrossRef]
23. Douglawi, A.; Masterson, T.A. Updates on the epidemiology and risk factors for penile cancer. *Transl. Androl. Urol.* **2017**, *6*, 785–790. [CrossRef]
24. Barnholtz-Sloan, J.S.; Maldonado, J.L.; Pow-Sang, J.; Giuliano, A.R. Incidence trends in primary malignant penile cancer. *Urol. Oncol.* **2007**, *25*, 361–367. [CrossRef]
25. Brouwer, O.R.; Albersen, M.; Parnham, A.; Protzel, C.; Pettaway, C.A.; Ayres, B.; Antunes-Lopes, T.; Barreto, L.; Campi, R.; Crook, J.; et al. European Association of Urology-American Society of Clinical Oncology Collaborative Guideline on Penile Cancer: 2023 Update. *Eur. Urol.* **2023**, *83*, 548–560. [CrossRef]

26. Sanchez, D.F.; Soares, F.; Alvarado-Cabrero, I.; Cañete, S.; Fernández-Nestosa, M.J.; Rodríguez, I.M.; Barreto, J.; Cubilla, A.L. Pathological factors, behavior, and histological prognostic risk groups in subtypes of penile squamous cell carcinomas (SCC). *Semin. Diagn. Pathol.* **2015**, *32*, 222–231. [CrossRef] [PubMed]
27. Thomas, A.; Necchi, A.; Muneer, A.; Tobias-Machado, M.; Tran, A.T.H.; Van Rompuy, A.-S.; Spiess, P.E.; Albersen, M. Penile cancer. *Nat. Rev. Dis. Prim.* **2021**, *7*, 11. [CrossRef]
28. Hansen, B.T.; Orumaa, M.; Lie, A.K.; Brennhovd, B.; Nygård, M. Trends in incidence, mortality and survival of penile squamous cell carcinoma in Norway 1956–2015. *Int. J. Cancer* **2018**, *142*, 1586–1593. [CrossRef]
29. Anic, G.M.; Giuliano, A.R. Genital HPV infection and related lesions in men. *Prev. Med.* **2011**, *53* (Suppl. S1), S36–S41. [CrossRef] [PubMed]
30. Alemany, L.; Cubilla, A.; Halec, G.; Kasamatsu, E.; Quirós, B.; Masferrer, E.; Tous, S.; Lloveras, B.; Hernández-Suarez, G.; Lonsdale, R.; et al. Role of Human Papillomavirus in Penile Carcinomas Worldwide. *Eur. Urol.* **2016**, *69*, 953–961. [CrossRef] [PubMed]
31. Backes, D.M.; Kurman, R.J.; Pimenta, J.M.; Smith, J.S. Systematic review of human papillomavirus prevalence in invasive penile cancer. *Cancer Causes Control.* **2009**, *20*, 449–457. [CrossRef]
32. Olesen, T.B.; Sand, F.L.; Rasmussen, C.L.; Albieri, V.; Toft, B.G.; Norrild, B.; Munk, C.; Kjær, S.K. Prevalence of human papillomavirus DNA and p16INK4a in penile cancer and penile intraepithelial neoplasia: A systematic review and meta-analysis. *Lancet Oncol.* **2019**, *20*, 145–158. [CrossRef]
33. Chaux, A.; Cubilla, A.L. The role of human papillomavirus infection in the pathogenesis of penile squamous cell carcinomas. *Semin. Diagn. Pathol.* **2012**, *29*, 67–71. [CrossRef]
34. Chaux, A.; Velazquez, E.F.; Algaba, F.; Ayala, G.; Cubilla, A.L. Developments in the pathology of penile squamous cell carcinomas. *Urology* **2010**, *76* (Suppl. S1), S7–S14. [CrossRef]
35. Moch, H.; Amin, M.B.; Berney, D.M.; Compérat, E.M.; Gill, A.J.; Hartmann, A.; Menon, S.; Raspollini, M.R.; Rubin, M.A.; Srigley, J.R.; et al. The 2022 World Health Organization Classification of Tumours of the Urinary System and Male Genital Organs—Part A: Renal, Penile, and Testicular Tumours. *Eur. Urol.* **2022**, *82*, 458–468. [CrossRef]
36. Albero, G.; Castellsagué, X.; Giuliano, A.R.; Bosch, F.X. Male circumcision and genital human papillomavirus: A systematic review and meta-analysis. *Sex Transm. Dis.* **2012**, *39*, 104–113. [CrossRef]
37. Ang, K.K.; Harris, J.; Wheeler, R.; Weber, R.; Rosenthal, D.I.; Nguyen-Tân, P.F.; Westra, W.H.; Chung, C.H.; Jordan, R.C.; Lu, C.; et al. Human Papillomavirus and Survival of Patients with Oropharyngeal Cancer. *N. Engl. J. Med.* **2010**, *363*, 24–35. [CrossRef]
38. Lont, A.P.; Kroon, B.K.; Horenblas, S.; Gallee, M.P.; Berkhof, J.; Meijer, C.J.; Snijders, P.J. Presence of high-risk human papillomavirus DNA in penile carcinoma predicts favorable outcome in survival. *Int. J. Cancer* **2006**, *119*, 1078–1081. [CrossRef]
39. Djajadiningrat, R.S.; Jordanova, E.S.; Kroon, B.K.; Van Werkhoven, E.; De Jong, J.; Pronk, D.T.; Snijders, P.J.; Horenblas, S.; Heideman, D.A. Human Papillomavirus Prevalence in Invasive Penile Cancer and Association with Clinical Outcome. *J. Urol.* **2015**, *193*, 526–531. [CrossRef]
40. Lopes, A.; Bezerra, A.L.R.; Pinto, C.A.L.; Serrano, S.V.; de MellO, C.A.; Villa, L.L. p53 as a New Prognostic Factor for Lymph Node Metastasis in Penile Carcinoma: Analysis of 82 Patients Treated with Amputation and Bilateral Lymphadenectomy. *J. Urol.* **2002**, *168*, 81–86. [CrossRef]
41. de Martel, C.; Plummer, M.; Vignat, J.; Franceschi, S. Worldwide burden of cancer attributable to HPV by site, country and HPV type. *Int. J. Cancer* **2017**, *141*, 664–670. [CrossRef]
42. Hoots, B.E.; Palefsky, J.M.; Pimenta, J.M.; Smith, J.S. Human papillomavirus type distribution in anal cancer and anal intraepithelial lesions. *Int. J. Cancer* **2009**, *124*, 2375–2383. [CrossRef]
43. Rao, S.; Guren, M.; Khan, K.; Brown, G.; Renehan, A.; Steigen, S.; Deutsch, E.; Martinelli, E.; Arnold, D. Anal cancer: ESMO Clinical Practice Guidelines for diagnosis, treatment and follow-up. *Ann. Oncol.* **2021**, *32*, 1087–1100. [CrossRef]
44. Krzowska-Firych, J.; Lucas, G.; Lucas, C.; Lucas, N.; Pietrzyk, Ł. An overview of Human Papillomavirus (HPV) as an etiological factor of the anal cancer. *J. Infect. Public Health* **2019**, *12*, 1–6. [CrossRef]
45. Clarke, M.A.; Deshmukh, A.A.; Suk, R.; Roberts, J.; Gilson, R.; Jay, N.; Stier, E.A.; Wentzensen, N. A systematic review and meta-analysis of cytology and HPV-related biomarkers for anal cancer screening among different risk groups. *Int. J. Cancer* **2022**, *151*, 1889–1901. [CrossRef]
46. Wei, F.; Gaisa, M.M.; D'Souza, G.; Xia, N.; Giuliano, A.R.; E Hawes, S.; Gao, L.; Cheng, S.-H.; Donà, M.G.; E Goldstone, S.; et al. Epidemiology of anal human papillomavirus infection and high-grade squamous intraepithelial lesions in 29 900 men according to HIV status, sexuality, and age: A collaborative pooled analysis of 64 studies. *Lancet HIV* **2021**, *8*, e531–e543. [CrossRef]
47. Palefsky, J.M.; Lee, J.Y.; Jay, N.; Goldstone, S.E.; Darragh, T.M.; Dunlevy, H.A.; Rosa-Cunha, I.; Arons, A.; Pugliese, J.C.; Vena, D.; et al. Treatment of Anal High-Grade Squamous Intraepithelial Lesions to Prevent Anal Cancer. *N. Engl. J. Med.* **2022**, *386*, 2273–2282. [CrossRef]
48. Wei, F.; Alberts, C.J.; Albuquerque, A.; Clifford, G.M. Impact of Human Papillomavirus Vaccine Against Anal Human Papillomavirus Infection, Anal Intraepithelial Neoplasia, and Recurrence of Anal Intraepithelial Neoplasia: A Systematic Review and Meta-analysis. *J. Infect. Dis.* **2023**, *228*, 1496–1504. [CrossRef]
49. Meulendijks, D.; Tomasoa, N.B.; Dewit, L.; Smits, P.H.M.; Bakker, R.; van Velthuysen, M.-L.F.; Rosenberg, E.H.; Beijnen, J.H.; Schellens, J.H.M.; Cats, A. HPV-negative squamous cell carcinoma of the anal canal is unresponsive to standard treatment and frequently carries disruptive mutations in TP53. *Br. J. Cancer* **2015**, *112*, 1358–1366. [CrossRef]

50. Serup-Hansen, E.; Linnemann, D.; Skovrider-Ruminski, W.; Høgdall, E.; Geertsen, P.F.; Havsteen, H. Human Papillomavirus Genotyping and p16 Expression As Prognostic Factors for Patients With American Joint Committee on Cancer Stages I to III Carcinoma of the Anal Canal. *J. Clin. Oncol.* **2014**, *32*, 1812–1817. [CrossRef]
51. Sun, G.; Dong, X.; Tang, X.; Qu, H.; Zhang, H.; Zhao, E. The prognostic value of HPV combined p16 status in patients with anal squamous cell carcinoma: A meta-analysis. *Oncotarget* **2017**, *9*, 8081–8088. [CrossRef]
52. Morel, A.; Neuzillet, C.; Wack, M.; Lameiras, S.; Vacher, S.; Deloger, M.; Servant, N.; Veyer, D.; Péré, H.; Mariani, O.; et al. Mechanistic Signatures of Human Papillomavirus Insertions in Anal Squamous Cell Carcinomas. *Cancers* **2019**, *11*, 1846. [CrossRef]
53. Sung, H.; Ferlay, J.; Siegel, R.L.; Laversanne, M.; Soerjomataram, I.; Jemal, A.; Bray, F. Global Cancer Statistics 2020: GLOBOCAN Estimates of Incidence and Mortality Worldwide for 36 Cancers in 185 Countries. *CA Cancer J. Clin.* **2021**, *71*, 209–249. [CrossRef] [PubMed]
54. Leitzmann, M.F.; Rohrmann, S. Risk factors for the onset of prostatic cancer: Age, location, and behavioral correlates. *Clin. Epidemiol.* **2012**, *4*, 1–11. [CrossRef] [PubMed]
55. Gandaglia, G.; Leni, R.; Bray, F.; Fleshner, N.; Freedland, S.J.; Kibel, A.; Stattin, P.; Van Poppel, H.; La Vecchia, C. Epidemiology and Prevention of Prostate Cancer. *Eur. Urol. Oncol.* **2021**, *4*, 877–892. [CrossRef] [PubMed]
56. Bruner, D.W.; Moore, D.; Parlanti, A.; Dorgan, J.; Engstrom, P. Relative risk of prostate cancer for men with affected relatives: Systematic review and meta-analysis. *Int. J. Cancer* **2003**, *107*, 797–803. [CrossRef] [PubMed]
57. McNeal, J.E.; Redwine, E.A.; Freiha, F.S.; Stamey, T.A. Zonal distribution of prostatic adenocarcinoma. Correlation with histologic pattern and direction of spread. *Am. J. Surg. Pathol.* **1988**, *12*, 897–906. [CrossRef] [PubMed]
58. Quintanal-Villalonga, Á.; Chan, J.M.; Yu, H.A.; Pe'er, D.; Sawyers, C.L.; Sen, T.; Rudin, C.M. Lineage plasticity in cancer: A shared pathway of therapeutic resistance. *Nat. Rev. Clin. Oncol.* **2020**, *17*, 360–371. [CrossRef]
59. Kwon, O.-J.; Zhang, L.; Ittmann, M.M.; Xin, L. Prostatic inflammation enhances basal-to-luminal differentiation and accelerates initiation of prostate cancer with a basal cell origin. *Proc. Natl. Acad. Sci. USA* **2013**, *111*, E592–E600. [CrossRef]
60. Egevad, L.; Delahunt, B.; Furusato, B.; Tsuzuki, T.; Yaxley, J.; Samaratunga, H. Benign mimics of prostate cancer. *Pathology* **2021**, *53*, 26–35. [CrossRef] [PubMed]
61. McNicol, P.J.; Dodd, J.G. High Prevalence of Human Papillomavirus in Prostate Tissues. *J. Urol.* **1991**, *145*, 850–853. [CrossRef]
62. Whitaker, N.J.; Glenn, W.K.; Sahrudin, A.; Orde, M.M.; Delprado, W.; Lawson, J.S. Human papillomavirus and Epstein Barr virus in prostate cancer: Koilocytes indicate potential oncogenic influences of human papillomavirus in prostate cancer. *Prostate* **2013**, *73*, 236–241. [CrossRef]
63. Medel-Flores, O.; Valenzuela-Rodríguez, V.A.; Ocadiz-Delgado, R.; Castro-Muñoz, L.J.; Hernández-Leyva, S.; Lara-Hernández, G.; Silva-Escobedo, J.-G.; Vidal, P.G.; Sánchez-Monroy, V. Association between HPV infection and prostate cancer in a Mexican population. *Genet. Mol. Biol.* **2018**, *41*, 781–789. [CrossRef] [PubMed]
64. Aydin, M.; Bozkurt, A.; Cikman, A.; Gulhan, B.; Karabakan, M.; Gokce, A.; Alper, M.; Kara, M. Lack of evidence of HPV etiology of prostate cancer following radical surgery and higher frequency of the Arg/Pro genotype in turkish men with prostate cancer. *Int. Braz. J. Urol.* **2017**, *43*, 36–46. [CrossRef] [PubMed]
65. Singh, N.; Hussain, S.; Kakkar, N.; Singh, S.K.; Sobti, R.C.; Bharadwaj, M. Implication of high risk Human papillomavirus HR-HPV infection in prostate cancer in Indian population—A pioneering case-control analysis. *Sci. Rep.* **2015**, *5*, 7822. [CrossRef]
66. Ghasemian, E.; Monavari, S.H.R.; Irajian, G.R.; Nodoshan, M.R.J.; Roudsari, R.V.; Yahyapour, Y. Evaluation of Human Papillomavirus Infections in Prostatic Disease: A Cross-Sectional Study in Iran. *Asian Pac. J. Cancer Prev.* **2013**, *14*, 3305–3308. [CrossRef]
67. Yin, S.-H.; Chung, S.-D.; Hung, S.-H.; Liu, T.-C.; Lin, H.-C. Association of prostate cancer with human papillomavirus infections: A case-control study. *Prostate Cancer Prostatic Dis.* **2023**. [CrossRef] [PubMed]
68. Tsydenova, I.A.; Ibragimova, M.K.; Tsyganov, M.M.; Litviakov, N.V. Human papillomavirus and prostate cancer: Systematic review and meta-analysis. *Sci. Rep.* **2023**, *13*, 16597. [CrossRef]
69. Opeyemi Bello, R.; Willis-Powell, L.; James, O.; Sharma, A.; Marsh, E.; Ellis, L.; Gaston, K.; Siddiqui, Y. Does Human Papillomavirus Play a Causative Role in Prostate Cancer? A Systematic Review Using Bradford Hill's Criteria. *Cancers* **2023**, *15*, 3897. [CrossRef]
70. Russo, G.I.; Calogero, A.E.; Condorelli, R.A.; Scalia, G.; Morgia, G.; La Vignera, S. Human papillomavirus and risk of prostate cancer: A systematic review and meta-analysis. *Aging Male* **2020**, *23*, 132–138. [CrossRef]
71. Khoury, J.D.; Tannir, N.M.; Williams, M.D.; Chen, Y.; Yao, H.; Zhang, J.; Thompson, E.J.; Meric-Bernstam, F.; Medeiros, L.J.; Weinstein, J.N.; et al. Landscape of DNA Virus Associations across Human Malignant Cancers: Analysis of 3,775 Cases Using RNA-Seq. *J. Virol.* **2013**, *87*, 8916–8926. [CrossRef]
72. Korodi, Z.; Dillner, J.; Jellum, E.; Lumme, S.; Hallmans, G.; Thoresen, S.; Hakulinen, T.; Stattin, P.; Luostarinen, T.; Lehtinen, M.; et al. Human papillomavirus 16, 18, and 33 infections and risk of prostate cancer: A Nordic nested case-control study. *Cancer Epidemiol. Biomark. Prev.* **2005**, *14*, 2952–2955. Available online: https://pubmed.ncbi.nlm.nih.gov/16365015/ (accessed on 20 February 2024). [CrossRef]
73. Sutcliffe, S.; Giovannucci, E.; Gaydos, C.A.; Viscidi, R.P.; Jenkins, F.J.; Zenilman, J.M.; Jacobson, L.P.; De Marzo, A.M.; Willett, W.C.; Platz, E.A. Plasma Antibodies against *Chlamydia trachomatis*, Human Papillomavirus, and Human Herpesvirus Type 8 in Relation to Prostate Cancer: A Prospective Study. *Cancer Epidemiol. Biomark. Prev.* **2007**, *16*, 1573–1580. [CrossRef]

74. Sutcliffe, S.; Viscidi, R.P.; Till, C.; Goodman, P.J.; Hoque, A.M.; Hsing, A.W.; Thompson, I.M.; Zenilman, J.M.; De Marzo, A.M.; Platz, E.A. Human Papillomavirus Types 16, 18, and 31 Serostatus and Prostate Cancer Risk in the Prostate Cancer Prevention Trial. *Cancer Epidemiol. Biomark. Prev.* **2010**, *19*, 614–618. [CrossRef]
75. Dillner, J.; Knekt, P.; Boman, J.; Lehtinen, M.; Geijersstam, V.A.; Sapp, M.; Schiller, J.; Maatela, J.; Aromaa, A. Sero-epidemiologal association between human-papillomavirus infection and risk of prostate cancer. *Int. J. Cancer* **1998**, *75*, 564–567. [CrossRef]
76. Glenn, W.K.; Ngan, C.C.; Amos, T.G.; Edwards, R.J.; Swift, J.; Lutze-Mann, L.; Shang, F.; Whitaker, N.J.; Lawson, J.S. High risk human papillomaviruses (HPVs) are present in benign prostate tissues before development of HPV associated prostate cancer. *Infect. Agents Cancer* **2017**, *12*, 46. [CrossRef]
77. Carozzi, F.; Lombardi, F.; Zendron, P.; Confortini, M.; Sani, C.; Bisanzi, S.; Pontenani, G.; Ciatto, S. Association of Human Papillomavirus with Prostate Cancer: Analysis of a Consecutive Series of Prostate Biopsies. *Int. J. Biol. Markers* **2004**, *19*, 257–261. [CrossRef]
78. Babjuk, M.; Burger, M.; Capoun, O.; Cohen, D.; Compérat, E.M.; Escrig, J.L.D.; Gontero, P.; Liedberg, F.; Masson-Lecomte, A.; Mostafid, A.H.; et al. European Association of Urology Guidelines on Non–muscle-invasive Bladder Cancer (Ta, T1, and Carcinoma in Situ). *Eur. Urol.* **2022**, *81*, 75–94. [CrossRef]
79. Saginala, K.; Barsouk, A.; Aluru, J.S.; Rawla, P.; Padala, S.A.; Barsouk, A. Epidemiology of Bladder Cancer. *Med. Sci.* **2020**, *8*, 15. [CrossRef]
80. Yao, X.; Xu, Z.; Duan, C.; Zhang, Y.; Wu, X.; Wu, H.; Liu, K.; Mao, X.; Li, B.; Gao, Y.; et al. Role of human papillomavirus and associated viruses in bladder cancer: An updated review. *J. Med. Virol.* **2023**, *95*, e29088. [CrossRef]
81. Rao, N.; Starrett, G.J.; Piaskowski, M.L.; Butler, K.E.; Golubeva, Y.; Yan, W.; Lawrence, S.M.; Dean, M.; Garcia-Closas, M.; Baris, D.; et al. Analysis of Several Common APOBEC-type Mutations in Bladder Tumors Suggests Links to Viral Infection. *Cancer Prev. Res.* **2023**, *16*, 561–570. [CrossRef]
82. Hrbáček, J.; Hanáček, V.; Kadlečková, D.; Cirbusová, A.; Čermák, P.; Tachezy, R.; Zachoval, R.; Saláková, M. Urinary shedding of common DNA viruses and their possible association with bladder cancer: A qPCR-based study. *Neoplasma* **2023**, *70*, 311–318. [CrossRef]
83. Nakagawa, T.; Shigehara, K.; Kato, Y.; Kawaguchi, S.; Nakata, H.; Nakano, T.; Izumi, K.; Kadono, Y.; Mizokami, A. Are bladder washing samples suitable for investigation of HPV infection in urinary bladder? Comparison in HPV prevalence between urine and washing samples. *J. Med. Virol.* **2023**, *95*, e28110. [CrossRef]
84. Moonen, P.M.J.; Bakkers, J.M.J.E.; Kiemeney, L.A.L.M.; Schalken, J.A.; Melchers, W.J.G.; Witjes, J.A. Human Papilloma Virus DNA and p53 Mutation Analysis on Bladder Washes in Relation to Clinical Outcome of Bladder Cancer. *Eur. Urol.* **2007**, *52*, 464–468. [CrossRef]
85. Sun, J.; Xu, J.; Liu, C.; An, Y.; Xu, M.; Zhong, X.; Zeng, N.; Ma, S.; He, H.; Hu, J.; et al. The association between human papillomavirus and bladder cancer: Evidence from meta-analysis and two-sample mendelian randomization. *J. Med. Virol.* **2022**, *95*, e28208. [CrossRef]
86. Muresu, N.; Di Lorenzo, B.; Saderi, L.; Sechi, I.; Del Rio, A.; Piana, A.; Sotgiu, G. Prevalence of Human Papilloma Virus Infection in Bladder Cancer: A Systematic Review. *Diagnostics* **2022**, *12*, 1759. [CrossRef]
87. Javanmard, B.; Barghi M reza Amani, D.; Fallah-Karkan, M.; Mazloomfard, M.M. Human papilloma virus DNA in tumor tissue and urine in different stage of bladder cancer. *Urol. J.* **2019**, *16*, 352–356. [CrossRef]
88. Moghadam, S.O.; Mansori, K.; Nowroozi, M.R.; Afshar, D.; Abbasi, B.; Nowroozi, A. Association of human papilloma virus (HPV) infection with oncological outcomes in urothelial bladder cancer. *Infect. Agents Cancer* **2020**, *15*, 52. [CrossRef]
89. Khatami, A.; Salavatiha, Z.; Razizadeh, M.H. Bladder cancer and human papillomavirus association: A systematic review and meta-analysis. *Infect. Agents Cancer* **2022**, *17*, 3. [CrossRef]
90. Jørgensen, K.R.; Høyer, S.; Jakobsen, J.K.; Jensen, T.K.; Marcussen, N.; Lam, G.W.; Hasselager, T.; Thind, P.O.; Toft, B.G.; Steinche, T.; et al. Human papillomavirus and squamous cell carcinoma of the urinary bladder: DaBlaCa-10 study. *Scand. J. Urol.* **2018**, *52*, 371–376. [CrossRef]
91. Musangile, F.Y.; Matsuzaki, I.; Okodo, M.; Shirasaki, A.; Mikasa, Y.; Iwamoto, R.; Takahashi, Y.; Kojima, F.; Murata, S. Detection of HPV infection in urothelial carcinoma using RNAscope: Clinicopathological characterization. *Cancer Med.* **2021**, *10*, 5534–5544. [CrossRef]
92. Yavuzer, D.; Karadayi, N.; Salepci, T.; Baloglu, H.; Bilici, A.; Sakirahmet, D. Role of human papillomavirus in the development of urothelial carcinoma. *Med. Oncol.* **2011**, *28*, 919–923. [CrossRef]
93. Yıldızhan, M.; Koçak, İ.; Kırdar, S.; Çulhacı, N. Detection of Human Papillomavirus using polymerase chain reaction methods in transitional urothelial bladder cancer. *Ann. Clin. Anal. Med.* **2021**, *12*, 353–357. [CrossRef]
94. Khatami, A.; Nahand, J.S.; Kiani, S.J.; Khoshmirsafa, M.; Moghoefei, M.; Khanaliha, K.; Tavakoli, A.; Emtiazi, N.; Bokharaei-Salim, F. Human papilloma virus (HPV) and prostate cancer (PCa): The potential role of HPV gene expression and selected cellular MiRNAs in PCa development. *Microb. Pathog.* **2022**, *166*, 105503. [CrossRef] [PubMed]
95. Cancer Site Ranking. Available online: https://gco.iarc.who.int/media/globocan/factsheets/cancers/29-kidney-fact-sheet.pdf (accessed on 22 February 2024).
96. Siegel, R.L.; Miller, K.D.; Wagle, N.S.; Jemal, A. Cancer statistics, 2023. *CA Cancer J. Clin.* **2023**, *73*, 17–48. [CrossRef] [PubMed]
97. Bodmer, D.; Van Den Hurk, W.; Van Groningen, J.J.M.; Eleveld, M.J.; Martens, G.J.M.; Weterman, M.A.J.; van Kessel, A.G. Understanding familial and non-familial renal cell cancer. *Hum. Mol. Genet.* **2002**, *11*, 2489–2498. [CrossRef] [PubMed]

98. Tang, J.; Baba, M. MiT/TFE Family Renal Cell Carcinoma. *Genes* **2023**, *14*, 151. [CrossRef] [PubMed]
99. Cumberbatch, M.G.; Rota, M.; Catto, J.W.F.; La Vecchia, C. The Role of Tobacco Smoke in Bladder and Kidney Carcinogenesis: A Comparison of Exposures and Meta-analysis of Incidence and Mortality Risks. *Eur. Urol.* **2016**, *70*, 458–466. [CrossRef] [PubMed]
100. Hidayat, K.; Du, X.; Zou, S.Y.; Shi, B.M. Blood pressure and kidney cancer risk: Meta-analysis of prospective studies. *J. Hypertens.* **2017**, *35*, 1333–1344. [CrossRef] [PubMed]
101. Pischon, T.; Lahmann, P.H.; Boeing, H.; Tjønneland, A.; Halkjær, J.; Overvad, K.; Klipstein-Grobusch, K.; Linseisen, J.; Becker, N.; Trichopoulou, A.; et al. Body size and risk of renal cell carcinoma in the European Prospective Investigation into Cancer and Nutrition (EPIC). *Int. J. Cancer* **2006**, *118*, 728–738. [CrossRef] [PubMed]
102. Whitney Lee, F.-S.; Chen, Y.-H.; Dang Tran, N.; Lin, C.-K.; An Pham, L. Association between Asbestos Exposure and the Incidence of Kidney Cancer: A Weight-of-Evidence Evaluation and Meta-analysis. *Curr. Environ. Health Rep.* **2023**, *10*, 394–409. [CrossRef]
103. Mandel, J.S.; McLaughlin, J.K.; Schlehofer, B.; Mellemgaard, A.; Helmert, U.; Lindblad, P.; McCredie, M.; Adami, H. International renal-cell cancer study. IV. Occupation. *Int. J. Cancer* **1995**, *61*, 601–605. [CrossRef]
104. Rotola, A.; Monini, P.; di Luca, D.; Savioli, A.; Simone, R.; Secchiero, P.; Reggiani, A.; Cassai, E. Presence and physical state of HPV DNA in prostate and urinary-tract tissues. *Int. J. Cancer* **1992**, *52*, 359–365. [CrossRef] [PubMed]
105. Farhadi, A.; Behzad-Behbahani, A.; Geramizadeh, B.; Sekawi, Z.; Rahsaz, M.; Sharifzadeh, S. High-risk human papillomavirus infection in different histological subtypes of renal cell carcinoma. *J. Med. Virol.* **2014**, *86*, 1134–1144. [CrossRef] [PubMed]
106. Salehipoor, M.; Khezri, A.; Behzad-Behbahani, A.; Geramizadeh, B.; Rahsaz, M.; Aghdaei, M.; Afrasiabi, M.A. Role of viruses in renal cell carcinoma. *Saudi J. Kidney Dis. Transpl.* **2012**, *23*, 53–57. [PubMed]
107. Kamel, D.; Turpeenniemi-Hujanen, T.; Vähäkangas, K.; Pääkkö, P.; Soini, Y. Proliferating cell nuclear antigen but not p53 or human papillomavirus DNA correlates with advanced clinical stage in renal cell carcinoma. *Histopathology* **1994**, *25*, 339–347. [CrossRef] [PubMed]
108. Hodges, A.; Talley, L.M.; Gokden, N. Human Papillomavirus DNA and P16INK4A are not Detected in Renal Tumors With Immunohistochemistry and Signal-amplified In Situ Hybridization in Paraffin-embedded Tissue. *Appl. Immunohistochem. Mol. Morphol.* **2006**, *14*, 432–435. [CrossRef] [PubMed]
109. Boccellino, M.; Vanacore, D.; Zappavigna, S.; Cavaliere, C.; Rossetti, S.; D'aniello, C.; Chieffi, P.; Amler, E.; Buonerba, C.; Di Lorenzo, G.; et al. Testicular cancer from diagnosis to epigenetic factors. *Oncotarget* **2017**, *8*, 104654–104663. [CrossRef] [PubMed]
110. King, J.; Adra, N.; Einhorn, L.H. Testicular Cancer: Biology to Bedside. *Cancer Res* **2021**, *81*, 5369–5376. [CrossRef] [PubMed]
111. Garolla, A.; Pizzol, D.; Bertoldo, A.; Ghezzi, M.; Carraro, U.; Ferlin, A.; Foresta, C. Testicular cancer and HPV semen infection. *Front. Endocrinol.* **2012**, *3*, 172. [CrossRef] [PubMed]
112. Strickler, H.D.; Schiffman, M.H.; Shah, K.V.; Rabkin, C.S.; Schiller, J.T.; Wacholder, S.; Clayman, B.; Viscidi, R.P. A survey of human papillomavirus 16 antibodies in patients with epithelial cancers. *Eur. J. Cancer Prev.* **1998**, *7*, 305–313. [CrossRef]
113. Meyts, E.R.; Hørding, U.; Nielsen, H.W.; Skakkebæk, N.E. Human papillomavirus and Epstein-Barr virus in the etiology of testicular germ cell tumours. *Apmis* **1994**, *102*, 38–42. [CrossRef]
114. Bertazzoni, G.; Sgambato, A.; Migaldi, M.; Grottola, A.; Sabbatini, A.M.T.; Nanni, N.; Farinetti, A.; Iachetta, F.; Giacobazzi, E.; Pecorari, M.; et al. Lack of evidence for an association between seminoma and human papillomavirus infection using GP5+/GP6+ consensus primers. *J. Med. Virol.* **2013**, *85*, 105–109. [CrossRef] [PubMed]
115. Foresta, C.; Patassini, C.; Bertoldo, A.; Menegazzo, M.; Francavilla, F.; Barzon, L.; Ferlin, A. Mechanism of Human Papillomavirus Binding to Human Spermatozoa and Fertilizing Ability of Infected Spermatozoa. *PLoS ONE* **2011**, *6*, e15036. [CrossRef] [PubMed]
116. Sucato, A.; Buttà, M.; Bosco, L.; Di Gregorio, L.; Perino, A.; Capra, G. Human Papillomavirus and Male Infertility: What Do We Know? *Int. J. Mol. Sci.* **2023**, *24*, 17562. [CrossRef] [PubMed]
117. HPV Vaccination Recommendations | CDC [Internet]. Available online: https://www.cdc.gov/vaccines/vpd/hpv/hcp/recommendations.html (accessed on 26 February 2024).
118. Aldakak, L.; Huber, V.M.; Rühli, F.; Bender, N. Sex difference in the immunogenicity of the quadrivalent Human Papilloma Virus vaccine: Systematic review and meta-analysis. *Vaccine* **2021**, *39*, 1680–1686. [CrossRef] [PubMed]
119. Rosado, C.; Fernandes, R.; Rodrigues, A.G.; Lisboa, C. Impact of Human Papillomavirus Vaccination on Male Disease: A Systematic Review. *Vaccines* **2023**, *11*, 1083. [CrossRef] [PubMed]
120. Lechner, M.; Liu, J.; Masterson, L.; Fenton, T.R. HPV-associated oropharyngeal cancer: Epidemiology, molecular biology and clinical management. *Nat. Rev. Clin. Oncol.* **2022**, *19*, 306–327. [CrossRef]
121. Eriksen, D.O.; Jensen, P.T.; Schroll, J.B.; Hammer, A. Human papillomavirus vaccination in women undergoing excisional treatment for cervical intraepithelial neoplasia and subsequent risk of recurrence: A systematic review and meta-analysis. *Acta Obstet. Gynecol. Scand.* **2022**, *101*, 597–607. [CrossRef]
122. Barnabas, R.V.; Brown, E.R.; Onono, M.A.; Bukusi, E.A.; Njoroge, B.; Winer, R.L.; Galloway, D.A.; Pinder, L.F.; Donnell, D.; Wakhungu, I.; et al. Efficacy of Single-Dose Human Papillomavirus Vaccination among Young African Women. *NEJM Évid.* **2022**, *1*, EVIDoa2100056. [CrossRef]
123. Teepen, J.C.; Kremer, L.; Ronckers, C.M.; van Leeuwen, F.E.; Hauptmann, M.; Dulmen-Den Broeder, V.; Van Der Pal, H.J.; Jaspers, M.W.; Tissing, W.J.; Den Heuvel-Eibrink, V. Long-term risk of subsequent malignant neoplasms after treatment of childhood cancer in the DCOG LATER study cohort: Role of chemotherapy. *J. Clin. Oncol.* **2017**, *35*, 2288–2298. [CrossRef]

124. York, J.M.; Klosky, J.L.; Chen, Y.; Connelly, J.A.; Wasilewski-Masker, K.; Giuliano, A.R.; Robison, L.L.; Wong, F.L.; Hudson, M.M.; Bhatia, S.; et al. Patient-Level Factors Associated With Lack of Health Care Provider Recommendation for the Human Papillomavirus Vaccine Among Young Cancer Survivors. *J. Clin. Oncol.* **2020**, *38*, 2892–2901. [CrossRef]
125. Kamboj, M.; Bohlke, K.; Baptiste, D.M.; Dunleavy, K.; Fueger, A.; Jones, L.; Kelkar, A.H.; Law, L.Y.; LeFebvre, K.B.; Ljungman, P.; et al. Vaccination of Adults with Cancer: ASCO Guideline. *J. Clin. Oncol.* **2024**, JCO2400032. [CrossRef] [PubMed]

Disclaimer/Publisher's Note: The statements, opinions and data contained in all publications are solely those of the individual author(s) and contributor(s) and not of MDPI and/or the editor(s). MDPI and/or the editor(s) disclaim responsibility for any injury to people or property resulting from any ideas, methods, instructions or products referred to in the content.

Communication

HPV-Associated Sexually Transmitted Infections in Cervical Cancer Screening: A Prospective Cohort Study

Miriam Latorre-Millán [1,*], Alexander Tristancho-Baró [1], Natalia Burillo [1], Mónica Ariza [1], Ana María Milagro [1], Pilar Abad [1], Laura Baquedano [2], Amparo Borque [2] and Antonio Rezusta [1]

1. Research Group on Infections Difficult to Diagnose and Treat, Institute for Health Research Aragón, Miguel Servet University Hospital, 50009 Zaragoza, Spain; aitristancho@salud.aragon.es (A.T.-B.); nburillon@salud.aragon.es (N.B.); mparizas@salud.aragon.es (M.A.); amilagro@salud.aragon.es (A.M.M.); mpa.alejaldre@gmail.com (P.A.); arezusta@salud.aragon.es (A.R.)
2. Gynaecology Department, Miguel Servet University Hospital, 50009 Zaragoza, Spain; lbaquedano@salud.aragon.es (L.B.); aborqueib@salud.aragon.es (A.B.)
* Correspondence: mlatorre@iisaragon.es

Abstract: High-risk human papillomavirus (HR-HPV) and other sexually transmitted infections (STIs-O) are promoters to the development of cervical cancer (CC), especially when they co-exist. This study aims to determine the prevalence of the major STIs-O and the rate of co-infection in women previously diagnosed with HR-HPV infection. For this observational study, 254 women aged 25–65 years who were being followed up for HR-HPV infection (without a CC history) were recruited at a hospital's Gynaecology Department from February 2024 to November 2024. Their endocervical specimens were collected and processed for HR-HPV, *Chlamydia trachomatis*, *Neisseria gonorrhoeae*, *Mycoplasma genitalium*, and *Trichomonas vaginalis* detection by RT-PCR using commercially available reagents and equipment. The overall rate of infection was 38.6% for HPV and 4.3% for ITSs-O (3.8% in HPV-negative women and 5.1% in HPV-positive women). The presence of ITSs-O in women aged 25–34 was higher in those with a persistent positive result for HR-HPV (20.0% vs. 4.2%). Diverse multiple co-infections were found in HPV-positive women, whilst some single STIs-O were found in HPV-negative women. These results support the benefits of STI-O screening beyond an HR-HPV positive result, especially in those women under 35 years old.

Keywords: sexually transmitted infections; human papillomavirus; cervical cancer screening

1. Introduction

Cervical cancer (CC) represents the second most prevalent oncological disease among women worldwide, with a significant impact on quality of life and economic costs. In Spain, estimates for 2023 indicate that 2047 women were diagnosed with CC and 664 deaths were attributed to this disease [1]. Nevertheless, there is substantial scientific evidence that preventive measures against CC can be both feasible and effective. Firstly, although not typically fatal, the disease predominantly affects young, sexually active women. Secondly, it is associated with modifiable environmental risk factors. Thirdly, it is frequently preceded by progressive cell dysplasia. Finally, the cervix is easily accessible for diagnostic procedures, specimen collection, and indirect observation.

In relation to the aforementioned environmental risk factors, a number of microorganisms have been identified as contributing to the development of alterations and malignancies that lead to CC by altering the cellular environment [2]. However, the Spanish

CC screening programme, apart from smear tests, only include high-risk human papillomavirus (HR-HPV) detection [3–5], despite the fact that HPV infections are encountered by over 80% of women during their lifetime, with less than 2% developing CC [6] and the majority of infections being cleared by the host [7,8].

In fact, the risk of developing CC and/or cervical intraepithelial neoplasia (CIN) as well as the incidence and persistence of HR-HPV and other sexually transmitted infections (STI-O) have been found to be increased in the presence of vaginal dysbiosis and vaginosis (symptomatic vaginal dysbiosis) [9–11]. Conversely, the absence of STI-O in addition to HR-HPV is associated with a reduced likelihood of histological abnormalities. Furthermore, certain microorganisms have been found to be associated with the appearance of CIN even with a higher OR for CC than HR-HPV. This is exemplified by *Chlamydia trachomatis* (CT), the most prevalent STI in western countries: its co-infection with HR-HPV increases the OR for high-grade squamous intraepithelial lesion (HGSIL) and CC even further [10,12]. Indeed, screening for CT is recommended in sexually active women under 25 years of age and in sexually active women over 25 years old when at increased risk, such as those having new partners, multiple partners, or a partner who has an STI [13].

Moreover, in addition to CC, STIs can impact personal wellbeing, mental health, and relationships and lead to significant complications "including pelvic inflammatory disease, ectopic pregnancy, postpartum endometriosis, infertility, and chronic abdominal pain in women; adverse pregnancy outcomes, including abortion, intrauterine death, and premature delivery; neonatal and infant infections and blindness; urethral strictures and epididymitis in men" and other extra-gynaecological malignancies depending on the specific pathogen involved, such as arthritis secondary to gonorrhoea and chlamydia [14]. Therefore, it is of the utmost importance that diagnosis and treatment be promptly initiated in order to ensure optimal medical care [13,14]. The greatest risk factor for an STI is a previous diagnosis of another STI. This is due in part to the fact that the subsequent oxidative stress and/or chronic inflammation serves as a facilitator for new pathogens to exert damage, thereby increasing the risk of co-infections, chronic infections, and further disorders. Despite the focus on HR-HPV infection's role in the development of CC, it is crucial to recognise that HPV is the most frequent STI worldwide and should be treated as such. This entails assessing for co-infection, establishing a window of opportunity for treatment and promoting HPV clearance.

There is considerable variation in the prevalence of STIs-O between countries; however, it is higher in women who are HR-HPV positive. Hence, numerous studies have emphasised the necessity for routine screening and monitoring of HR-HPV co-infection with STIs-O [15–18], aligning with the viewpoint that this approach is cost-effective when the rate of co-infection exceeds 3% [19,20]. In this regard, it is well documented that the prevalence of CT exceeds 3% in women up to 40 years of age in other countries [21]. However, the presence of HR-HPV and STIs-O, as well as the rates of co-infection, remain insufficiently documented in our setting. Furthermore, a unifying criterion is currently being established at the national level to provide a standardised guideline for CC prevention programmes, which have previously been implemented at the discretion of each Autonomous Community [3,22]. Consequently, new local insights are essential to inform public health guidelines regarding screening, diagnosis, and treatment of HR-HPV infection and STIs-O, with the aim of reducing their contribution to the burden of disease.

Therefore, the present study aims to determine the presence of the major STIs (*Chlamydia trachomatis* (CT), *Trichomonas vaginalis* (TV), *Neisseria gonorrhoeae* (NG), and *Mycoplasma genitalium* (MG)) and the rate of co-infection with HR-HPV in women previously diagnosed with HR-HPV infection in a Spanish setting.

2. Materials and Methods

2.1. Study Setting and Design

A prospective cross-sectional observational study was conducted in the Miguel Servet University Hospital, a Spanish tertiary care hospital located in Zaragoza, which serves a total catchment area of over 400,000 people. Samples were collected from February 2024 to November 2024.

2.2. Participants and Sample Collection

All women attending the hospital's Gynaecology Department for the CC screening programme, who met the eligibility criteria listed below and signed the informed consent form, were recruited to participate in this study. The following inclusion criteria were applied: participants had to be followed up for HR-HPV infection detected in the last year and be aged between 18 and 65 years old. As exclusion criteria, participants had to have no history of CC, and they could not have been treated for an STI-O or enrolled in an HPV vaccine study in the previous year.

Their endocervical specimens were collected by a trained gynaecologist and preserved in transport medium (PreservCyt® solution, Hologic, MA, USA) for transfer to the laboratory on the same day. They were stored at room temperature until the next day, when they were analysed in accordance with the routine procedure.

2.3. Laboratory Testing and Outcomes of Interest

The samples were processed at the hospital microbiology laboratory for the detection of HR-HPV, and those with a positive result were subjected to further analysis to determine the presence of CT, NG, MG, and TV. All analyses were conducted using real-time PCR (polymerase chain reaction) on the cobas® 5800 System with the use of cobas® HPV, cobas® CT/NG, and cobas® TV/MG reagents (Roche Diagnostics, IN, USA).

The results were classified in accordance with the manufacturer's specifications as either negative or positive. In cases where the initial classification was inconclusive, a second test was conducted to provide further clarification. In instances where uncertainty persisted, a new sample from the participant was analysed.

The results obtained from the cobas® 5800 System software regarding the HR-HPV, CT, NG, TC, and MG tests were exported as a tab-separated values file from the instrument and converted into a spreadsheet for analysis. The designated investigator extracted the results for data storage and analysis, and the age of each participant at the time of sample collection was added as an additional outcome of interest.

2.4. Statistical Analysis

A descriptive analysis of the clinical results was conducted. The rates of STI co-infection were determined by calculating the ratio of the total number of cases to the number of positive results. Further analyses of the data were conducted using descriptive and inferential statistics. Categorical variables were presented as absolute and relative frequencies (n, %), and age was presented as the median and interquartile range. Group-wise comparisons by age were performed using Student's t-test or Chi-square (χ^2) test. A two-tailed p value was considered statistically significant when $p \leq 0.05$. All analyses and graphs were conducted using the open-source software Jamovi 2.2.5, MS Excel 2016 (Microsoft, Redmond, WA, USA), MS PowerPoint 2016 (Microsoft, Redmond, WA, USA), and MS Word 2016 (Microsoft, Redmond, WA, USA).

2.5. Ethics

This study was conducted in accordance with the Declaration of Helsinki and its subsequent modifications. Prior to sample collection, all participants provided written informed consent. The protocol was approved by the Ethics Committee of Aragon and by the hospital management.

3. Results

A total of 254 women were selected for the present analysis, with a median age of 40.5 years (interquartile range 35.0–48.0). Supplementary Figure S1 shows that there were HR-HPV-positive cases included 23 (9.1%) HPV16, 12 (4.7%) HPV18, and 73 (28.7%) other HR-HPV cases; STIs-O-positive cases included 7 (2.8%) CT, 3 (1.2%) MG, 2 (0.8%) TV, and 1 (0.4%) NG cases.

Table 1 shows the overall infection rates, which were 38.6% for HR-HPV and 4.3% for ITSs-O (3.8% in HR-HPV-negative women and 5.1% in HR-HPV-positive women). Additionally, ITSs-O rates were shown according to age group. A higher rate of ITSs-O was found among women under 35 years of age with a HR-HPV positive result, in comparison to those with a negative HR-HPV result (20.0% vs. 4.2%). Furthermore, in this age group, the odds ratio for an ITS-O positive result in HR-HPV-positive women was 5.6 when compared to HR-HPV-negative women (p = 0.05). In the case of the eldest women, no STIs were found after 48 years of age (the positive ITS results found in those HR-HPV-negative women over the age of 45 belong to women aged between 47 and 48).

Table 1. STIs rates by HR-HPV test result.

	HR-HPV-Positive	STI-O in HR-HPV-Positive 98/254 (38.6%)	STI-O in HR-HPV-Negative 156/254 (61.4%)	Raw OR (CI 95%)	p Value
Overall	98/254 (38.6%)	5/98 (5.1%)	6/156 (3.8%)	1.34 (0.4–4.5)	0.63
Age (years)					
25–34	15 (24.2%)	3/15 (20.0%)	2/47 (4.2%)	5.6 (0.8–37.6)	0.05
35–44	43 (43.0%)	2/43 (4.6%)	2/57 (3.5%)	1.3 (0.2–9.9)	0.78
45–54	27 (45.8%)	0/27 (0.0%)	2/32 (6.2%)	0.22 (0.0–4.8)	0.19
55–65	13 (39.4%)	0/13 (0.0%)	0/20 (0.0%)	-	-

Note. HR-HPV: high-risk human papillomavirus, STI-O: sexually transmitted infection other than HR-HPV, OR: odds ratio.

Supplementary Figure S2 illustrates the distribution of age according to the HR-HPV and ITS-O results. The distribution of age differs significantly according to the ITS-O result in both HR-HPV-positive and -negative women. No older women from 55 to 64 years of age tested positive for ITS-O (independently of the HR-HPV result), and only two (33%) women between 45 and 54 years tested positive for ITS-O among those with a negative HR-HPV result.

Supplementary Figure S3 depicts the values for age according to the presence or absence of each ITS. The age of women with a positive result for MG was found to be lower (31.0 (interquartile range 29.5–32.5)) than that of women with a negative result (41.0 (interquartile range 35.0–48.0)). Conversely, the age of women with a positive result for overall HR-HPV was higher (39.5 (interquartile range 33.0–47.3)) than that of women with a negative result (42.0 (interquartile range 37.0–48.8)). Both p values are $\leq$ 0.05.

Figure 1 and Table 2 shows the microorganisms involved in ITS co-infections. Figure 1 depicts a total of 104 infected specimens, representing 40.9% of the total number tested. Of these, 4 (1.6%) were triple infections, 9 (3.5%) were double infections, and 91 (35.8%) were single infections. HR-HPV (in particular those differing from HPV16 and HPV18) were the microorganisms most frequently involved (100% in triple and double infection and 93.4% in single infection), being followed by CT (present in 25.0%, 22.2%, and 4.4%, respectively) and MG (present in 50.0%, 0.0%, and 1.1%, respectively), as Table 2 shows. In addition, in women with HR-HPV positivity, one case was identified with MG and CT and another with MG and NG. The remaining cases were identified as co-infections between different types of HR-HPV. Eight specimens with multiple HR-HPV co-infections were found. These included five cases of co-infection with HPV16 and other HR-HPVs, one case of co-infection with HPV18 and other HR-HPVs, and two cases of co-infection with HPV16, HPV18, and other HR-HPVs. In samples from women negative for HR-HPV, only single ITS cases were found: CT was found in four samples, MG in one, and TV in another.

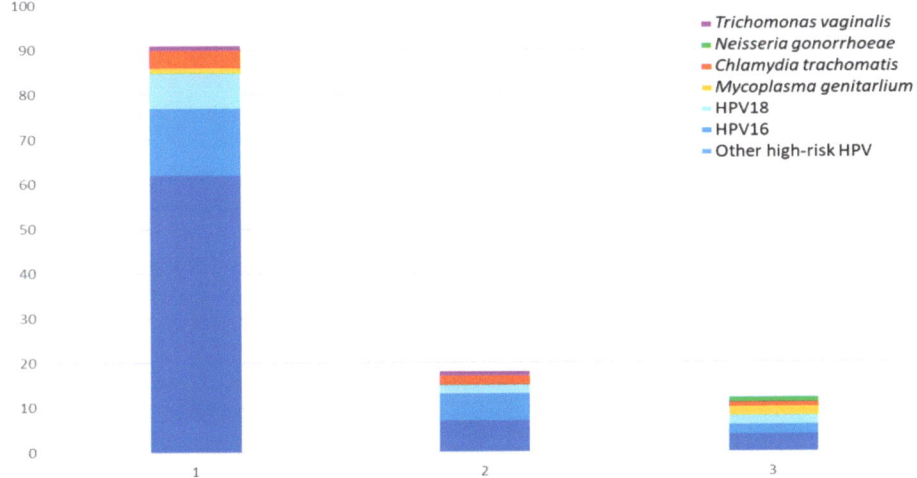

Figure 1. ITS rate by number of co-infections (single, double, and triple).

Table 2. Major microorganisms involved in double and triple STIs co-infection.

No. of Involved Microorganisms	*Chlamydia trachomatis*	*Neisseria gonorrhoeae*	*Mycoplasma genitalium*	*Trichomonas vaginalis*	HPV-16	HPV-18	Other HR-HPV	No. HR-HPV
3	0	0	0	0	1	1	1	3
3	0	0	0	0	1	1	1	3
3	1	0	1	0	0	0	1	1
3	0	1	1	0	0	0	1	1
2	0	0	0	0	1	0	1	2
2	0	0	0	0	1	0	1	2
2	0	0	0	0	1	0	1	2
2	0	0	0	0	0	1	1	2
2	0	0	0	0	1	0	1	2
2	1	0	0	0	0	0	1	1
2	1	0	0	0	0	1	0	1
2	0	0	0	1	1	0	0	1

Note. HR-HPV: high-risk human papillomavirus, HPV: human papillomavirus, No.: number, and STIs: sexually transmitted infections.

4. Discussion

In women participating in a CC screening program who had a previous HR-HVP positive result in the last year, the following rates were documented: a persistent positive result for HR-HPV (38.6%), an any-ITS rate (40.9%), and a multiple infection rate (5.1%) involving at least one HR-HPV (in 100%) and one ITS-O (in 38.5%). Furthermore, a significantly higher presence of ITS-O was observed in women under 35 years old with a persistent positive HR-HPV result when compared to women with a negative HR-HPV result (20% vs. 4.2%).

The present findings are in alignment with those of several studies from various countries, which also identified a simultaneous presence of HR-HPV with the STI-O [10,12,15,19,21]. However, it should be noted that the rates vary according to the specific population and methods under study. For instance, a study conducted in our city in 2005 found HR-HPV in the 8.4% of their total population, compared to our 38.6%, and this rate differed significantly according to age (10.6% vs. 24.2% in 25–35 years, 4.4% vs. 43.0% in 35–44 years, 5% vs. 45.8% in 45–54 years, and 0% vs. 39.4% in 55–64 years), but all these differences could be explained by the fact that their participants were not identified as having a previous HR-HPV positive result [23]. Likewise, a study on female sex workers in Galicia, published in 2012, found that HR-HPV presence was associated with bacterial vaginosis, including TV and *Candida* spp. [24]. Moreover, a large European study (with notable Spanish contributions) identified a positive correlation between the number of identified STIs and the risk for CC development [25]. To the best of our knowledge, however, the present study is the first to assess several STI-O regarding HR-VPH presence in our city and region.

Notwithstanding the unavailability of a framework for the comparison of studies, it is anticipated that our findings will contribute to the scientific evidence that the prevailing guidelines for CC screening should be observed to ensure their continued utility. Indeed, the Spanish CC screening programme is currently under review [26], and nowadays it includes a cytology every three years for those between 25 and 34 years of age and a HR-HPV test every five years for the rest under 65 years, except in case of a positive result for HR-HPV, for which cytology is conditionally performed and the frequency of HR-HPV testing is reduced to one year. Although Spanish guidelines already recognised that co-infection with some STI-O is one of the risk factors for VPH persistence and CIN and CC development [23], this concern is not currently incorporated in the general protocol, but it is asserted that specific action protocols should be implemented for women who meet the high-risk criteria for their individual risk assessment and follow-up [26].

In this regard, the findings of the present study suggest that the routine indication for ITS-O screening should be considered as conditional on a HR-HPV positive result for Spanish women, as it is aligned with the criteria described in the Spanish CC screening programme consensus [26], and it is evident that it would be cost-effective at the rates observed here [19,20]. In this context, it is important to note that the cost-effectiveness of STI screening varies according to the approach adopted [27]; however, most researchers agree that interventions should be justified based on the prevalence of STIs in each population, with a lower threshold of 3.1% suggested in a previous review of this assessment [20]. Furthermore, it is crucial to recognise that the cost-effectiveness of STI screening is often underestimated, as many studies fail to account for the long-term complications of STIs or the associated intersectoral or social costs, such as the impact on patients and their families, informal care, and work productivity [28]. Consequently, experts recommend implementing STI screening interventions at least in high-risk populations (where STI prevalence is higher), while also considering their cost-effectiveness in the general population, encompassing key aspects such as self-sampling, tailored strategies, and accessibility improvement [29]. Regarding this matter, self-sampling has been shown to reduce both costs and disparities in access to cervical swab testing, though professionals are still required to address the psychological impact of co-infection diagnoses and to establish effective treatments, especially given the stigma surrounding STIs, which may act as a barrier to healthcare access [30]. In response, experts advocate for reducing stigma by integrating sexual health services within a broader healthcare framework; this approach would also provide patients with opportunities for additional STI testing, including HIV screening, partner notification, and access to pre-exposure prophylaxis for HIV prevention (if appropriate), as well as other essential services [29]. Moreover, extending testing for STIs-O by using the same unique sample and extracting with a similar PCR technique by using multiplex kits (as enabled by Roche Diagnostic reagents, instruments, and platforms) would facilitate implementation into the laboratory routine contributing to improved cost-effectiveness.

In fact, given the imminent adoption of population-based CC screening in Spain in accordance with a European Commission directive [31], and the assertion that HR-HPV detection would serve as the most suitable primary screening test for vaccinated women (basically the younger women) due to its sensitivity and predictive value surpasses that of cytology [32], in which a higher frequency of STI detection is also observed for this population group, this particular scenario offers an opportunity for screening STI-O by PCR conditional on the primary HR-HPV result. This approach would be highly valuable for this population group, not only in terms of CC prevention but also in addressing some of the issues associated with STI-O testing in Spain [33].

However, it is important to recognise the limitations of this study. Its cross-sectional design does not allow for causality or other longitudinal effects to be observed. The potential for bias arising from the desire to participate could not be assessed. Moreover, the relatively small size of our sample limits the statistical power of our results and may give rise to type 1 error, particularly in the context of segmented analyses. However, this issue can be overcome by increasing the sample size through further recruitment, which is planned for the continuation of the present study. This will also allow for the identification of additional related findings.

Furthermore, it is evident that the local nature of this study means that findings should be interpreted with caution when attempting to extrapolate them to other populations or healthcare settings, in which the presence of potential confounders (e.g., sexual behaviour, vaccination status, immunosuppression, smoking, alcohol consumption, or socio-economic status) may impact both HR-HPV and STIs-O rates in different ways [34]. In this sense, it is noteworthy to acknowledge that the incidence and prevalence rates of cervical cancer in Zaragoza are consistent with those of Spain (5 and 31 per 100,000 inhabitants, respectively) [1] and are among the lowest in the European Union (EU) [22]. Comparing with the EU rates, the Spanish CC screening participation is lower (access disparities related to education and income groups are present), and the proportion of daily smokers and individuals with excess of weight is higher; however, alcohol consumption is lower, and HPV vaccination among 15-year-old girls is among the highest [22]. Furthermore, the employment of different diagnostic methods used for identifying STIs or microorganisms may potentially lead to misclassification of infection status, depending on their level of sensitivity and specificity [35].

On the other hand, the present study focuses on the major STIs, in accordance with the research priorities of the WHO 2022–2030 agenda for STI diagnosis and prevention [36]. However, cervicovaginal dysbiosis, characterised by a decrease in lactobacilli populations and an increase in both alpha and beta diversity, has also been found to be associated with different stages of CC development and other related gynaecological conditions, involving additional microorganism species through mechanisms and relationships that are beginning to be elucidated [2,34,37–40]: bacteria such as *Gardnerella vaginalis*, *Atopobium vaginae*, *Sneathia amnii*, *Lactobacillus iners*, *Prevotella* spp., and *Ureaplasma* spp., fungus such as *Sporidiobolaceae*, *Saccharomyces*, *Candida* spp., and *Malassezia*, and viruses such as herpes simplex 2 and anelloviruses. Likewise, several host endogenous risk factors for CC, such as nutritional or genetic features, could be considered for the management of CC prevention [34]. Therefore, further studies are required to explore the usefulness of additional microorganism determinations and other biomarkers in order to improve future preventive screening.

5. Conclusions

The findings of the present study support the benefits of implementing STI screening in Spanish women under 50 years old previously diagnosed with a HR-HPV infection, especially in those under 35.

Given the potential benefits and projected cost-effectiveness of incorporating STI-O testing into preventive CC screening, policymakers should consider implementing evidence-based interventions in this manner, particularly among high-risk and younger populations. Further research is encouraged to identify and optimise the most effective approaches.

Supplementary Materials: The following supporting information can be downloaded at https://www.mdpi.com/article/10.3390/v17020247/s1: Figure S1: Relative frequency of HR-HPV and other sexually transmitted infections (ITS-O); Figure S2: Distribution of age according to the HR-HPV and other sexually transmitted infection (STIS-O) results; Figure S3: Age by STI result.

Author Contributions: Conceptualisation, A.R., A.T.-B. and M.L.-M.; methodology, A.T.-B. and M.L.-M.; validation, P.A. and A.M.M.; formal analysis, M.L.-M., N.B. and M.A.; investigation, M.L.-M. and A.T.-B.; resources, A.R., L.B. and A.B.; data curation, M.L.-M.; writing—original draft preparation, M.L.-M.; writing—review and editing, M.L.-M., N.B., M.A., A.T.-B., A.M.M., P.A., L.B., A.B. and A.R.; visualisation, M.L.-M. and A.T.-B.; supervision, A.R.; project administration, A.R., A.T.-B. and M.L.-M.; funding acquisition, A.R. All authors have read and agreed to the published version of the manuscript.

Funding: This research was funded by ROCHE DIAGNOSTICS GmbH (Sanhofer Str. 116 68305 Mannheim, Germany), which provided the PCR reagents (cobas® CT/NG and cobas® TV/MG) for performing the tests included in the present study, contract signed 30/07/2024 (internal code F24-096).

Institutional Review Board Statement: This study was conducted in accordance with the Declaration of Helsinki and was approved by the Ethics Committee of the Autonomous Community of Aragon (CEICA) (protocol code PI23/530 and date of approval 20 December 2023).

Informed Consent Statement: Informed consent was obtained from all subjects involved in this study.

Data Availability Statement: The original contributions presented in this study are included in this article/Supplementary Materials. An anonymised raw dataset is openly available as a Supplementary File. Further inquiries can be directed to the corresponding author.

Acknowledgments: We would like to express our gratitude to the participants who kindly allowed us to utilise their samples. Furthermore, we are indebted to our laboratory colleagues for their invaluable assistance in the reception and processing of the samples.

Conflicts of Interest: The authors declare no conflicts of interest. The funders had no role in the design of this study; in the collection, analyses, or interpretation of data; in the writing of this manuscript; or in the decision to publish the results.

Abbreviations

CC: cervical cancer, CEICA: Ethics Committee of the Autonomous Community of Aragon, CT: *Chlamydia trachomatis*, EU: European Union, HPV: human papillomavirus, HR-HPV: high-risk human papillomavirus, IN: Indiana, TV: *Trichomonas vaginalis*, NG: *Neisseria gonorrhoeae*, MG: *Mycoplasma genitalium*, PCR: polymerase chain reaction, RT-PCR: real-time polymerase chain reaction, STIs: sexually transmitted infections, STIs-O: sexually transmitted infections other than HR-HPV, USA: United States of America, and WA: Washington.

References

1. Asociación Española Contra el Cáncer (AEECC). Dimensiones del Cáncer. 2024. Available online: https://observatorio.contraelcancer.es/explora/dimensiones-del-cancer (accessed on 19 December 2024).
2. Li, X.-Y.; Li, G.; Gong, T.-T.; Lv, J.-L.; Gao, C.; Liu, F.-H.; Zhao, Y.-H.; Wu, Q.-J. Non-Genetic Factors and Risk of Cervical Cancer: An Umbrella Review of Systematic Reviews and Meta-Analyses of Observational Studies. *Int. J. Public Health* **2023**, *68*, 1605198. [CrossRef]
3. Organisation for Economic Co-Operation and Development. *EU Country Cancer Profile: Spain 2023*; EU Country Cancer Profiles; OECD Publishing: Paris, France, 2023. [CrossRef]
4. Recomendaciones de la Sociedad Española de Enfermedades Infecciosas y Microbiología Clínica (SEIMC) para el Cribado de Cancer de Cuello de Útero. 2013. Available online: https://seimc.org/contenidos/inf_institucional/recomendacionesinstitucionales/seimc-rc-2013-1.pdf (accessed on 18 December 2024).
5. Mateos Lindemann, M.L.; Pérez-Castro, S.; Pérez-Gracia, M.T.; Rodríguez-Iglesias, M. *Diagnóstico Microbiológico de la Infección por el Virus del Papiloma Humano. 57*; Procedimientos en Microbiología Clínica, Cercenado Mansilla, E., Cantón Moreno, R., Eds.; Mateos Lindemann ML (coordinator); Sociedad Española de Enfermedades Infecciosas y Microbiología Clínica (SEIMC): Madrid, Spain, 2016; ISBN 978-84-608-7617-5.
6. Koster, S.; Gurumurthy, R.K.; Kumar, N.; Prakash, P.G.; Dhanraj, J.; Bayer, S.; Berger, H.; Kurian, S.M.; Drabkina, M.; Mollenkopf, H.-J.; et al. Modelling Chlamydia and HPV co-infection in patient-derived ectocervix organoids reveals distinct cellular reprogramming. *Nat. Commun.* **2022**, *13*, 1030. [CrossRef] [PubMed]
7. Yang, D.; Zhang, J.; Cui, X.; Ma, J.; Wang, C.; Piao, H. Status and epidemiological characteristics of high-risk human papillomavirus infection in multiple centers in Shenyang. *Front. Microbiol.* **2022**, *13*, 985561. [CrossRef] [PubMed]
8. Liu, Z.; Li, P.; Zeng, X.; Yao, X.; Sun, Y.; Lin, H.; Shen, P.; Sun, F.; Zhan, S. Impact of HPV vaccination on HPV infection and cervical related disease burden in real-world settings (HPV-RWS): Protocol of a prospective cohort. *BMC Public Health* **2022**, *22*, 2117. [CrossRef]
9. Gillet, E.; Meys, J.F.A.; Verstraelen, H.; Verhelst, R.; De Sutter, P.; Temmerman, M.; Broeck, D.V. Association between bacterial vaginosis and cervical intraepithelial neoplasia: Systematic review and meta-analysis. *PLoS ONE* **2012**, *7*, e45201. [CrossRef]
10. De Miranda Lima, L.; Hoelzle, C.; Toscano Simões, R.; de Miranda Lima, M.I.; Rodrigues Barbosa Fradico, J.; Cueva Mateo, E.C.; Comes Zauli, D.A.; Melo, V.H. Sexually Transmitted Infections Detected by Multiplex Real Time PCR in Asymptomatic Women and Association with Cervical Intraepithelial Neoplasia. *Rev. Bras. Ginecol. Obs.* **2018**, *40*, 540–546.
11. Brusselaers, N.; Shrestha, S.; van de Wijgert, J.; Verstraelen, H. Vaginal dysbiosis and the risk of human papillomavirus and cervical cancer: Systematic review and meta-analysis. *Am. J. Obstet. Gynecol.* **2019**, *221*, 9–18.e8. [CrossRef] [PubMed]
12. Mosmann, J.P.; Zayas, S.; Kiguen, A.X.; Venezuela, R.F.; Rosato, O.; Cuffini, C.G. Human papillomavirus and Chlamydia trachomatis in oral and genital mucosa of women with normal and abnormal cervical cytology. *BMC Infect Dis.* **2021**, *21*, 422. [CrossRef]
13. U.S. Centers for Diseases Control and Prevention. *Getting Tested for STIs*. Available online: https://www.cdc.gov/sti/testing/index.html (accessed on 17 December 2024).
14. Chesson, H.W.; Mayaud, P.; Aral, S.O. Sexually Transmitted Infections: Impact and Cost-Effectiveness of Prevention. In *Major Infectious Diseases*, 3rd ed.; Holmes, K.K., Bertozzi, S., Bloom, B.R., Jha, P., Eds.; The International Bank for Reconstruction and Development/The World Bank: Washington, DC, USA, 2017.
15. Mendoza, L.; Mongelos, P.; Paez, M.; Castro, A.; Rodriguez-Riveros, I.; Gimenez, G.; Araujo, P.; Echagüe, G.; Diaz, V.; Laspina, F.; et al. Human papillomavirus and other genital infections in indigenous women from Paraguay: A cross-sectional analytical study. *BMC Infect Dis.* **2013**, *13*, 531. [CrossRef] [PubMed]
16. Deng, D.; Shen, Y.; Li, W.; Zeng, N.; Huang, Y.; Nie, X. Challenges of hesitancy in human papillomavirus vaccination: Bibliometric and visual analysis. *Int. J. Health Plann. Manag.* **2023**, *38*, 1161–1183. [CrossRef] [PubMed]
17. De Cabezón, R.H.; Sala, C.V.; Gomis, S.S.; Lliso, A.R.; Bellvert, C.G. Evaluation of cervical dysplasia treatment by large loop excision of the transformation zone (LLETZ). Does completeness of excision determine outcome? *Eur. J. Obstet. Gynecol. Reprod. Biol.* **1998**, *78*, 83–89. [CrossRef]
18. Chen, M.M.; Mott, N.; Clark, S.J.; Harper, D.M.; Shuman, A.G.; Prince, M.E.P.; Dossett, L.A. HPV Vaccination Among Young Adults in the US. *JAMA* **2021**, *325*, 1673–1674. [CrossRef] [PubMed]
19. Robial, R.; Longatto-Filho, A.; Roteli-Martins, C.M.; Silveira, M.F.; Stauffert, D.; Ribeiro, G.G.; Linhares, I.M.; Tacla, M.; Zonta, M.A.; Baracat, E.C. Frequency of Chlamydia trachomatis infection in cervical intraepithelial lesions and the status of cytological p16/Ki-67 dual-staining. *Infect. Agents Cancer* **2017**, *12*, 3. [CrossRef]
20. Honey, E.; Augood, C.; Templeton, A.; Russell, I.; Paavonen, J.; Mårdh, P.-A.; Stary, A.; Stray-Pedersen, B. Cost effectiveness of screening for Chlamydia trachomatis: A review of published studies. *Sex Transm. Infect.* **2002**, *78*, 406–412. [CrossRef] [PubMed]

21. Lu, Z.; Zhao, P.; Lu, H.; Xiao, M. Analyses of human papillomavirus, *Chlamydia trachomatis*, *Ureaplasma urealyticum*, *Neisseria gonorrhoeae*, and co-infections in a gynecology outpatient clinic in Haikou area, China. *BMC Women's Health* **2023**, *23*, 117. [CrossRef] [PubMed]
22. ICO/IARC Information Centre on HPV and Cancer. Spain: Human Papillomavirus and Related Cancers, Fact Sheet. 2023. Available online: https://hpvcentre.net/statistics/reports/ESP_FS.pdf (accessed on 17 December 2024).
23. Puig, F.; Echavarren, V.; Yago, T.; Crespo, R.; Montañés, P.; Palacios, M.; Lanzón, R. Prevalencia del virus del papiloma humano en una muestra de población urbana en la ciudad de Zaragoza. *Prog. Obstet. Ginecol.* **2005**, *48*, 172–178. [CrossRef]
24. Rodriguez-Cerdeira, C.; Sanchez-Blanco, E.; Alba, A. Evaluation of Association between Vaginal Infections and High-Risk Human Papillomavirus Types in Female Sex Workers in Spain. *ISRN Obstet. Gynecol.* **2012**, *2012*, 240190. [CrossRef]
25. Castellsague, X.; Pawlita, M.; Roura, E.; Margall, N.; Waterboer, T.; Bosch, F.X.; De Sanjosé, S.; Gonzalez, C.A.; Dillner, J.; Gram, I.T.; et al. Prospective Seroepidemiologic Study on the Role of Human Papillomavirus and Other Infections in Cervical Carcinogenesis: Evidence from the EPIC Cohort. *Int. J. Cancer* **2014**, *135*, 440–452. [CrossRef]
26. Grupo de Trabajo Sobre Cribado de Cáncer de Cérvix. Documento de consenso sobre la modificación del Programa de Cribado de Cáncer de Cérvix. Ministerio de Sanidad. Dirección General de Salud Pública y Equidad en Salud. S.G. de Promoción de la Salud y Prevención. 2023. Available online: https://www.sanidad.gob.es/areas/promocionPrevencion/cribado/cribadoCancer/cancerCervix/docs/DocumentoconsensomodificacionCervix.pdf (accessed on 19 December 2024).
27. Bloch, S.C.M.; Jackson, L.J.; Frew, E.; Ross, J.D.C. Assessing the costs and outcomes of control programmes for sexually transmitted infections: A systematic review of economic evaluations. *Sex Transm. Infect.* **2021**, *97*, 334–344. [CrossRef] [PubMed]
28. Schnitzler, L.; Jackson, L.J.; Paulus, A.T.G.; Roberts, T.E.; Evers, S.M.A.A. Intersectoral costs of sexually transmitted infections (STIs) and HIV: A systematic review of cost-of-illness (COI) studies. *BMC Health Serv. Res.* **2021**, *21*, 1179. [CrossRef]
29. National Institute for Health and Care Excellence (NICE). *Effective and Cost-Effective Interventions to Increase Frequent STI Testing in Very High Risk Groups: Reducing Sexually Transmitted Infections (STIs): Evidence Review D*; NICE Evidence Reviews Collection: London, UK, 2022.
30. Daponte, N.; Valasoulis, G.; Michail, G.; Magaliou, I.; Daponte, A.-I.; Garas, A.; Grivea, I.; Bogdanos, D.P.; Daponte, A. HPV-Based Self-Sampling in Cervical Cancer Screening: An Updated Review of the Current Evidence in the Literature. *Cancers* **2023**, *15*, 1669. [CrossRef]
31. Maver, P.J.; Poljak, M. Primary HPV-based cervical cancer screening in Europe: Implementation status, challenges, and future plans. *Clin. Microbiol. Infect.* **2020**, *26*, 579–583. [CrossRef]
32. Banerjee, D.; Mittal, S.; Mandal, R.; Basu, P. Screening technologies for cervical cancer: Overview. *Cytojournal* **2022**, *19*, 23. [CrossRef] [PubMed]
33. Del Romero, J.; Guillén, S.M.; Rodríguez-Artalejo, F.; Ruiz-Galiana, J.; Cantón, R.; Ramos, P.D.L.; García-Botella, A.; García-Lledó, A.; Hernández-Sampelayo, T.; Gómez-Pavón, J.; et al. Sexually transmitted infections in Spain: Current status. *Rev. Española Quimioter.* **2023**, *36*, 444. [CrossRef] [PubMed]
34. Luvián-Morales, J.; Gutiérrez-Enríquez, S.O.; Granados-García, V.; Torres-Poveda, K. Risk factors for the development of cervical cancer: Analysis of the evidence. *Front. Oncol.* **2024**, *14*, 1378549. [CrossRef] [PubMed]
35. Fashedemi, O.; Ozoemena, O.C.; Peteni, S.; Haruna, A.B.; Shai, L.J.; Chen, A.; Rawson, F.; Cruickshank, M.E.; Grant, D.; Ola, O.; et al. Advances in human papillomavirus detection for cervical cancer screening and diagnosis: Challenges of conventional methods and opportunities for emergent tools. *Anal. Methods* **2024**. [CrossRef] [PubMed]
36. Gottlieb, S.L.; Spielman, E.; Abu-Raddad, L.; Aderoba, A.K.; Bachmann, L.H.; Blondeel, K.; Chen, X.-S.; Crucitti, T.; Camacho, G.G.; Godbole, S.; et al. WHO global research priorities for sexually transmitted infections. *Lancet Glob. Health* **2024**, *12*, e1544–e1551. [CrossRef] [PubMed]
37. Głowienka-Stodolak, M.; Bagińska-Drabiuk, K.; Szubert, S.; Hennig, E.E.; Horala, A.; Dąbrowska, M.; Micek, M.; Ciebiera, M.; Zeber-Lubecka, N. Human Papillomavirus Infections and the Role Played by Cervical and Cervico-Vaginal Microbiota-Evidence from Next-Generation Sequencing Studies. *Cancers* **2024**, *16*, 399. [CrossRef] [PubMed]
38. Nguyen, H.D.T.; Le, T.M.; Lee, E.; Lee, D.; Choi, Y.; Cho, J.; Park, N.J.-Y.; Chong, G.O.; Seo, I.; Han, H.S. Relationship between Human Papillomavirus Status and the Cervicovaginal Microbiome in Cervical Cancer. *Microorganisms* **2023**, *11*, 1417. [CrossRef] [PubMed]
39. Huang, R.; Liu, Z.; Sun, T.; Zhu, L. Cervicovaginal microbiome, high-risk HPV infection and cervical cancer: Mechanisms and therapeutic potential. *Microbiol. Res.* **2024**, *287*, 127857. [CrossRef] [PubMed]
40. Fong Amaris, W.M.; de Assumpção, P.P.; Valadares, L.J.; Moreira, F.C. Microbiota changes: The unseen players in cervical cancer progression. *Front. Microbiol.* **2024**, *15*, 1352778. [CrossRef] [PubMed]

Disclaimer/Publisher's Note: The statements, opinions and data contained in all publications are solely those of the individual author(s) and contributor(s) and not of MDPI and/or the editor(s). MDPI and/or the editor(s) disclaim responsibility for any injury to people or property resulting from any ideas, methods, instructions or products referred to in the content.

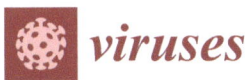

Article

Findings and Challenges in Replacing Traditional Uterine Cervical Cancer Diagnosis with Molecular Tools in Private Gynecological Practice in Mexico

José L. Castrillo-Diez [1], Carolina Rivera-Santiago [2,3], Silvia M. Ávila-Flores [1], Silvia A. Barrera-Barrera [4] and Hugo A. Barrera-Saldaña [3,4,5,*]

1. Leire Genomic Laboratories, León 37000, Mexico
2. Columbia Biotec, Columbia Laboratories, Tlalpan 14090, Mexico; crivera@gcolumbia.com
3. Columbia Laboratories, Basic Scientific Research Division, Mexico City 04000, Mexico
4. Innbiogem SC/Vitagenesis SA at National Laboratory for Services of Research, Development, and Innovation for the Pharma and Biotech Industries (LANSEIDI) of CONACyT Vitaxentrum Group, Monterrey 64630, Mexico; silviaabb92@gmail.com
5. Facultades de Medicina y Ciencias Biológicas, Universidad Autónoma de Nuevo León, San Nicolás de los Garza 66455, Mexico
* Correspondence: hbarrera@gcolumbia.com

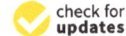

Citation: Castrillo-Diez, J.L.; Rivera-Santiago, C.; Ávila-Flores, S.M.; Barrera-Barrera, S.A.; Barrera-Saldaña, H.A. Findings and Challenges in Replacing Traditional Uterine Cervical Cancer Diagnosis with Molecular Tools in Private Gynecological Practice in Mexico. *Viruses* 2024, 16, 887. https://doi.org/10.3390/v16060887

Academic Editors: Hossein H. Ashrafi and Mustafa Ozdogan

Received: 11 April 2024
Revised: 29 May 2024
Accepted: 29 May 2024
Published: 31 May 2024

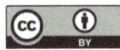

Copyright: © 2024 by the authors. Licensee MDPI, Basel, Switzerland. This article is an open access article distributed under the terms and conditions of the Creative Commons Attribution (CC BY) license (https://creativecommons.org/licenses/by/4.0/).

Abstract: We have been encouraging practicing gynecologists to adopt molecular diagnostics tests, PCR, and cancer biomarkers, as alternatives enabled by these platforms, to traditional Papanicolaou and colposcopy tests, respectively. An aliquot of liquid-based cytology was used for the molecular test [high-risk HPV types, (HR HPV)], another for the PAP test, and one more for p16/Ki67 dual-stain cytology. A total of 4499 laboratory samples were evaluated, and we found that 25.1% of low-grade samples and 47.9% of high-grade samples after PAP testing had a negative HR HPV-PCR result. In those cases, reported as Pap-negative, 22.1% had a positive HR HPV-PCR result. Dual staining with p16/Ki67 biomarkers in samples was positive for HR HPV, and 31.7% were also positive for these markers. Out of the PCR results that were positive for any of these HR HPV subtypes, n 68.3%, we did not find evidence for the presence of cancerous cells, highlighting the importance of performing dual staining with p16/Ki67 after PCR to avoid unnecessary colposcopies. The encountered challenges are a deep-rooted social reluctance in Mexico to abandon traditional Pap smears and the opinion of many specialists. Therefore, we still believe that colposcopy continues to be a preferred procedure over the dual-staining protocol.

Keywords: uterine cervical cancer screening; HPV genotyping; p16/Ki67 biomarkers; gynecology private practice

1. Introduction

The specific detection of the human papillomavirus (HPV) subtype has favored the reduction in the mortality and morbidity rate in women due to cervical cancer (CC) worldwide [1]. This reduction has been achieved due to the widespread use of liquid-based cytology preparations to obtain cervical samples and the implementation of new molecular technologies for HPV genotyping by polymerase chain reaction (PCR) [2–5].

Globally, CC is the fourth most common cancer in women, with 604,000 new cases in 2020 [5]. About 90% of the 342,000 deaths caused by CC occurred in low- and middle-income countries [6,7]. The highest rates of this tumor incidence and mortality are in sub-Saharan Africa (SSA), Central America, and South-East Asia. Regional differences in the CC burden are related to inequalities in access to vaccination, screening and treatment services, risk factors (including human immunodeficiency virus (HIV) prevalence and social and economic determinants such as sex), gender biases, and poverty. Women living with HIV are six times more likely to develop CC compared to the general population, with an estimated 5% of all cases attributable to this infection. The contribution of HIV to CC disproportionately affects younger women, and as a result, 20% of children who lose their mother to cancer do so due to this neoplasia [8].

In Mexico, this neoplasm represents the second cause of cancer in women, with 9440 new cases per year, and the second cause of death, with 4340 cases [9]. Among women with invasive CC, around 70% are diagnosed with locally advanced disease, which highlights deficiencies in timely diagnosis [9]. All these data reinforce the need to continue implementing early screening strategies for CC in Mexico and in other Latin American countries with similar incidences.

In recent years, the diagnosis of HPV infections by detection of viral DNA and PCR genotyping of high-risk (HR) variants in cervical samples has replaced the traditional Pap smear due to its higher sensitivity [1,10]. The improvement in the HR HPV detection capacity offered by PCR and its automation has led various countries, such as Australia, to abandon the Papanicolaou test as a CC screening tool [11]. On the other hand, in Latin America, the efforts to implement HPV genotyping by PCR continue to be limited, and greater awareness of this serious female health problem is necessary in public institutions and private hospitals [12].

HPV is a highly transmissible virus that leads to transient infections, with several factors increasing the risk of its persistence, including genetics, age, smoking, and the specific genomic sequence of the infecting virus [13]. To date, more than 150 subtypes of papillomavirus viruses have been described that, based on their association with CC, have been classified as very HR (HPV-16 and HPV-18), twelve HR subtypes (HR12), and other low-risk (LR) types that are associated with benign mucosal lesions [14]. The high- and very-HR HPV subtypes (16, 18, and HR12) are associated with malignant lesions and cause approximately 70% of CC cases worldwide [15,16].

The cytological course caused by transient HPV infection begins with low-grade squamous intraepithelial lesions, of which 90% revert to healthy epithelium. However, HR-HPV-specific infections aggravated by host risk factors are more difficult to reverse, and their persistence leads to high-grade squamous intraepithelial lesions (moderate or high dysplasia) that can progress to CC [15]. Cytological assessment by the expert cytotechnologist is highly relevant for predicting the course of HPV infection. However, it has its limitations, such as low sensitivity and the impossibility of distinguishing persistent infection from reinfection [17]. These are examples in which molecular tools such as PCR, given their greater sensitivity and ability to identify the subtype of HPV infection, outperform traditional diagnostics [4,5].

To date, seven PCR assays for the detection and genotyping of HPV from cervical cell samples have been validated. Three of them are tests aimed at amplifying a region of the L1 gene (Abbott Real-Time HR HPV Test, Anyplex II HPV HR Detection, and Cobas 4800 HPV Test). At the same time, another four are assays that amplify early-region genes (BD Onclarity HPV Assay, HPV-Risk Assay, PapilloCheck HPV-Screening Test, and Xpert HPV) [18].

In Mexico and the rest of Latin America, strategies have been developed to implement these molecular PCR tests for HPV detection in public and private institutions [12]. However, automated PCR methods, such as those used in our laboratories (Cobas 4800 HPV Test), stand out from other methods for their ability to process many simultaneous samples and their speed and diagnostic accuracy [19]. Using an internal control for co-amplification of a human gene makes it possible to practically eliminate the analysis of invalid samples and the presence of false negatives [19].

Although the specific detection of HPV genotyping by PCR is currently the "gold-standard" technique in the early diagnosis of CC, complementary technologies have been developed for diagnosing premalignant cervical lesions in liquid cytology samples [20]. The p16INK4a (p16) protein is a regulatory protein of the cell cycle under normal physiological conditions [21]. This biomarker is effective in histological samples and is widely used to improve the reproducibility of cervical biopsy assessment and accuracy in detecting premalignant lesions [20,22–24]. Likewise, the simultaneous detection of p16 and Ki67 (a proliferation biomarker) within the same cervical epithelial cell has been proposed as a marker of cellular transformation mediated by infections with the 12 HR HPV genotypes (HR12) [25]. This combination of biomarkers (p16/Ki67 dual-stain cytology, Cintec-Plus) has provided excellent results in cervical cytological samples where it has been used for the detection of premalignant and malignant lesions of CC [26–30].

Given the proven advantages of the herein-described molecular tests, we have been implementing them in our laboratories and boosting their adoption among private practicing gynecologists in Mexico.

2. Materials and Methods

2.1. Clinical Samples and Diagnostic Algorithms

A total of 4499 cervix samples received consecutively in our laboratories were analyzed using three strategies: (a) molecular PCR analyses (to screen for the presence of HPV infections); (b) liquid-based cytology to search for cellular alterations suggestive of HPV infections, and (c) finally, if the medical expert followed the triage, they requested the laboratory to perform dual-staining cytology (to assess if the cellular transformation process has already started). PCR was used to test all 4499 samples, 3806 were subjected to liquid-based cytology, and 567 samples were analyzed by p16/Ki67 dual-stain cytology.

2.2. Clinical Specimen Sampling

Cervical samples from the cervix were taken by gynecologists in private clinical practice using a cervix brush and deposited in a transport medium (ThinPrep or Roche Cell Collection Medium). The vials with the samples were sent at room temperature to the laboratory, where they were stored and refrigerated (4 degrees Celsius) until processing.

2.3. Liquid-Based Cytology (PAP Test)

Liquid-based cytology slides were prepared by a cytotechnologist and interpreted according to the Bethesda System for Reporting Cervical Cytology (third edition, 2017). In contrast, a pathologist reviewed 50% of negative samples and 100% of the positive ones for quality control and quality assurance.

2.4. HPV PCR Assay

The COBAS 4800 HPV Test (Roche) is an FDA-approved and validated qualitative test device for detecting HPV DNA in swabs from the cervical canal. This test amplifies target DNA isolated from cervical epithelium by real-time PCR to detect HPV 16 and HPV 18, along with a simultaneous pooled result for 12 other HR genotypes in a single test. The entire procedure is automated, and the manufacturer's instructions are followed. The COBAS 4800 HVPV Test Primers are used to amplify DNA from 14 HR-HPV types (16, 18, 31, 33, 35, 39, 45, 51, 52, 56, 58, 59, 66, and 68) in a single analysis, where probes with four different reporter dyes screen different targets in the multiplex reaction: dye 1 screens 12 pooled HR-HPVs (31, 33, 35, 39, 45, 51, 52, 56, 58, 59, 66, and 68), dyes 2 and 3 screen for HPV 16 and 18, respectively, while dye 4 targets the human β-globin gene to provide a control for uterine cervical cell adequacy for extraction and amplification.

2.5. p16/Ki67 Dual-Stain Cytology

One slide for each sample was prepared for PAP testing using a Cytospin chamber adapter and subjected to p16/Ki67 dual-stain cytology using the CINtec Plus Cytology Kit (Roche Laboratories, Indianapolis, USA), according to the manufacturer's instructions. Immunohistochemistry staining was performed using a BenchMark GX Stainer followed by evaluation by a trained cytotechnologist. An initial evaluation was performed to confirm the presence of the minimal criteria for squamous cellularity defined by the Bethesda terminology. Subsequently, the slide was checked for the presence of double-immunoreactive cervical epithelial cells, that is, cells with simultaneous brown cytoplasmic p16 immunostaining and Ki67 red nuclear immunostaining, which were interpreted as positive by double-stained cytological analysis regardless of the morphological interpretation. A pathologist reviewed all cases with positive cells for double-staining to confirm the result.

The PCR results were compared with the PAP findings using a contingency table and chi-square test. All data analyses were performed using Graph Pad Prism 10 (GraphPad Software, Inc. (Boston, MA, USA).

3. Results

Four thousand and four hundred ninety-nine liquid-based cervical samples were performed on samples from patients referred by private gynecologists mostly from central regions of Mexico. A molecular PCR study for genotyping of HPV was performed on all samples to detect the 14 most common HR genotypes of HPV to contribute to the early prevention of CC. In parallel, Pap tests were performed on 84.6% (n = 3806) of samples.

The global distribution of the results of the viral genotypes revealed by the PCR analysis is described in Figure 1. In 99.4% of cases, the samples received were considered adequate for this test, given that they rendered positive during the amplification of the internal control gene, i.e., the genomic β-globin gene. In cases where samples did not pass this control (0.6%), a second sample was requested from the gynecologist. This request was met on 53.8% of occasions (14/26). Thus, the final number of PCR results was 4487, or 99.7% of the samples received.

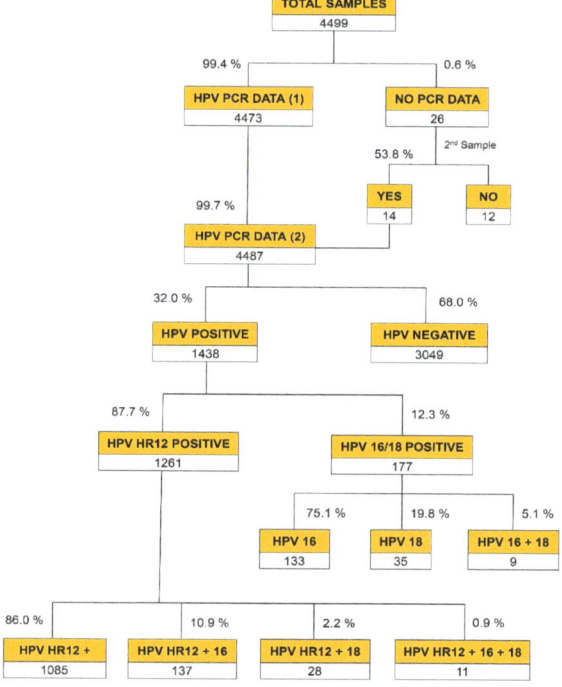

Figure 1. General distribution of HPV genotyping results by PCR. Findings are presented by type of virus: HPV-16 (16), HPV-18 (18), and a pool of other 12 HR-HPVs responsible for most cases of CC (HR12).

Out of the 4487 results obtained, 68% tested negative for any of the 14 HR HPV genotypes analyzed. Out of the 1438 samples that tested positive for HR HPV (32%), 1261 (87.7%) were positive for any of the 12 HR HPV subtypes present in the group. In 12.3%

of cases, the positive result corresponded to HPV16 and/or HPV18 subtypes, considered very HR for CC. It was observed that 86% of positive cases presented an isolated viral genotype without involving genotypes 16 or 18, while 14% showed co-infections with one of the two most oncogenic HR HPVs (viral genotype 16 or 18). Most of the positive samples yielded positive PCR results for the group of 12 HR subtypes (HR12). Overall, 24.5% of patients had PCR results involving very HR viruses (HPV16 and/or HPV18), alone or in combination with HR12 viral types. The results of PCR viral genotyping distributed by age range are shown in Table 1.

Table 1. Distribution of the different HPV subtypes by age groups.

Age (y)	Total PCR	Positivity by Viral Type				
		Total	HR-HPV12	HPV16	HPV18	Coinfections
<25	411	181	152	9	1	19
25–35	1724	614	450	57	16	91
>35	1691	409	296	44	12	57
Total	3826	1204	898	110	29	167

HPV: human papillomavirus; HR: high-risk; PCR: polymerase chain reaction; y: years.

The data shown in Table 1 correspond to 3826 samples for which data on the age of the patients were available. However, if the results are stratified by age ranges, the population under 25 years of age was the one that showed the highest percentage of overall positive HPV-PCR results: 44% (181/411) tested positive for one of the high or very HR subtypes.

If the results distributed by viral subtype are analyzed, the population between 25 and 35 years of age always shows a higher risk of infection with high or very HR genotypes. More than 50% of the results were positive in this age range for any viral genotype alone or in co-infection: 50.1% (450/898) for HR12, 51.8% (57/110) for HPV16, 55.2% (16/29) for HPV18, and 54.5% (91/167) for a viral co-infection.

If the different positive subtypes are analyzed by age range, the HR12 subgroup always shows the highest percentage: 84% (152/181) in patients younger than 25 years, 73.3% (450/614) for the age range of 25 to 35 years, and 72.4% (296/409) for those over 35 years. However, for the other subtypes, their behavior by age is vastly different. For HPV16, 5% (9/181) was obtained for those under 25 years of age, 9.3% (57/614) for the range of 25 to 35 years, and 10.8% (44/409) for others over 35 years of age. For HPV18, the data were 0.6% (1/181) for those under 25 years of age, 2.6% (16/614) for those 25 to 35 years of age, and 2.9% (12/409) for those over 35 years of age. The data for viral coinfections showed that 10.5% (19/181) correspond to those under 25 years of age, 14.8% (91/614) for the age range of 25 to 35 years, and 13.9% (57/409) for those over 35 years of age.

Analyzing the results globally, it stands out that: (a) The population under 25 years of age presented a higher percentage of positive results for HR12 viral types (84%), compared to 77.3% of the group between 25 and 35 years of age and a figure of 72.4% for those over 35 years of age. (b) The population between 25 and 35 years of age presented a higher percentage of results for co-infection, with 14.8%, compared to 13.9% in the group over 35 years of age and 10.5% in those under 25 years of age. (c) The population over 35 years of age presented a higher percentage of positive results for HPV16 with 10.8%, compared to 9.3% for the age range of 25 to 35 and 5% for those under 25. Likewise, the population over 35 years of age presented a higher percentage of positive results for HPV18 (2.9%), compared to 2.6% for the age range of 25 to 35 and 0.6% for those under 25 years of age.

The global distribution of the 3806 Pap test results, which represent 84.6% of the total of 4499 PCR tests, is shown in Figure 2. The positive results were sub-classified as low grade (69.1%) or high grade (30.9%). All negative and positive samples from the PAP test underwent PCR testing for the detection of high or very high-risk (HR) HPVs. Using a contingency table, we compared the results of the gold standard for HPV detection (PCR) with those of the PAP test. Within these findings, we noted that the percentage of false positives in cytology was 5.6% (*n* = 200) of the total samples assessed. Additionally, Figure 2 presents the results of HR HPV-PCR among the 3184 samples identified as negative in the PAP test. Notably, among these, 703 samples (22.1%) yielded positive results for viral genotypes of high or very HR for CC. Within this subset of false negatives from cytology for HPV detection, 85.9% (*n* = 604) corresponded to the 12 HR subtypes (HR12), while 14.1% (*n* = 99) were attributed to HPV16 or HPV-18, which are very HR genotypes.

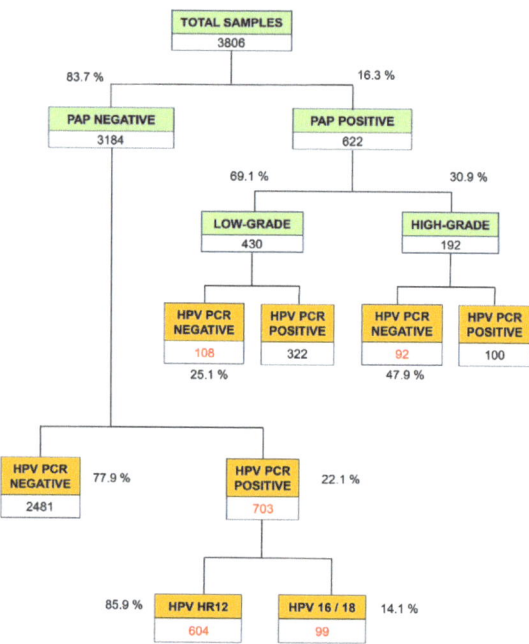

Figure 2. General distribution of PAP screening and HR HPV genotyping results by PCR.

Table 2 shows the distribution by age of the 622 samples with a positive result for PAP, and whether they are low- or high-grade. The most striking results correspond to patients over 35 years of age: 110 samples (45 low-risk and 65 HR) produced negative results in the PCR test, representing 45.6% of potential false positives (110/241). The percentages of the lack of correlation between PAP and HPV-PCR were lower in the other age ranges: 25.4% in the age range of 25 to 35 years [(53 + 21)/291] and 17.7% for those under 25 years [(10 + 6)/90].

Table 2. Distribution by age range of the positive PAP results (*n* = 622) with negative HPV PCR results (PCR NEG) versus positive (PCR POS).

	PAP LOW-GRADE		PAP HIGH-GRADE		
AGE (y)	PCR NEG	PCR POS	PCR NEG	PCR POS	Total
<25	10	64	6	10	90
25–35	53	170	21	47	291
>35	45	88	65	43	241
Total	108	322	92	100	622

PCR: polymerase chain reaction; y: years.

Table 3 shows the HR HPV-PCR genotyping results in the 422 double-positive samples in both the HPV-PCR and PAP tests (*n* = 322 low-grade and *n* = 100 high-grade). A total of

61.8% of the samples were positive for HR12, 16% were positive for HR12 plus HPV16, and 15.2% were positive for isolated HPV16. Overall, 79.6% of the analyses obtained an isolated infection [(261 + 64 + 11)/422], and 20.4% corresponded to double or triple co-infections [(4 + 67 + 1 + 41)/422].

Table 3. Distribution of the different HPV subtypes in coincident positive PAP and PCR results.

PAP + PCR Positivity	n = 422	%
HR12	261	61.8
HPV16	64	15.2
HPV18	11	2.6
HPV16 + HPV18	4	0.9
HR12 + HPV16	67	16.0
HR12 + HPV18	11	2.6
HR12 + HPV16 + HPV18	4	0.9

HPV: human papillomavirus; PCR: polymerase chain reaction; y: years.

Figure 3 shows the results of the confirmation tests for CC performed using p16/Ki67 dual-stain cytology (CINTEC PLUS). A total of 536 samples (37.3%) from the subgroup of 1438 positive results for 14 HR HPV types were tested. A total of 31.7% were positive for dual staining. These results also confirm that 68.3% of the positive results for any of the HR HPV subtypes do not present cellular transformation, which highlights the importance of performing p16/Ki67 dual-stain cytology after PCR to avoid unnecessary colposcopies in the screening of CC patients.

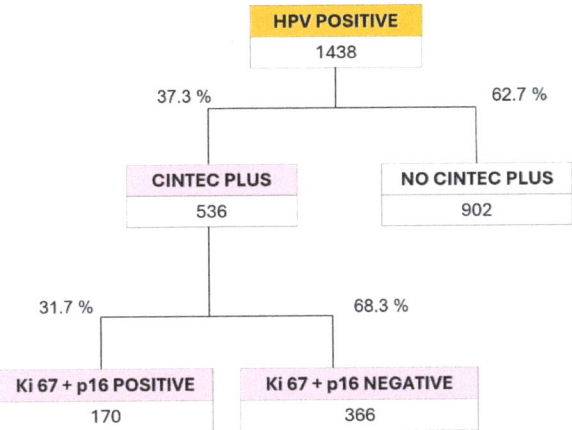

Figure 3. General distribution of CINTEC-PLUS results on samples with positive PCR results for the pool of 12 HPV subtypes at HR for CC (HR12).

These samples came from private practice gynecologists in private hospitals. In 100% of the cases, the gynecologists continued to perform the traditional Pap test in parallel with HPV genotyping analysis using PCR (Cobas). Although this double screening for the early diagnosis of CC represents an extra cost for their patients, gynecologists argue that the traditional Pap test allows them to identify other gynecological lesions (suspected infections by bacteria, fungi, or other viruses) that the PCR test alone does not allow. In Figure 4, we present a strategy to encourage the increased adoption of molecular methods, highlighting the benefits of employing these tools throughout the entire process, from sample collection to patient reporting. In our experience, gynecologists are aware of the good sensitivity and specificity of the molecular PCR test and the costs of the study for their patients are the only reason for not requesting the HPV genotyping test together with the traditional PAP test.

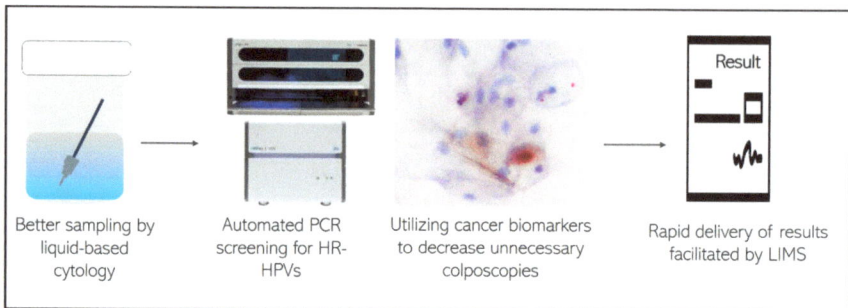

Figure 4. Ideal workflow for the adoption of molecular methods.

Regarding the possible reasons why the dual-stain test is not widely requested within the global detection program for CC in the private gynecology sector, we can include the following: (1) Extra costs for many of the patients, for whom the cost of the PCR study already represents a large increase over the expense of the traditional PAP; (2) Ignorance on the part of the patients of the objective and scope of the staining in CC screening, which implies a longer explanation time in private medical consultations; and (3) Reticence from a subgroup of gynecologists (colposcopists) since the positive/negative result of the dual-stain test determines (or relativizes) the need for surgical intervention (colposcopy) in their patients. This result seems to interfere with their area of expertise and business, which may be one of the causes of the low return rate in the confirmatory dual-stain test.

4. Discussion

The results presented here correspond to 4499 samples received in our laboratories during three years for CC screening. The distribution of HPV subpopulations in all samples is comparable to other results published internationally. However, this study shows for the first time the results in the Mexican population within the private medicine market [1,9].

It should be noted that if we analyze the results within each age range, the population under 25 years of age was the one that showed the highest percentage of overall positive HR HPV-PCR results: 44% tested positive for one of the risk subtypes, high or very high, compared to 35.6% of positive results in the population between 25 and 35 years of age and 24.2% of positive results in the population over 35 years of age.

Likewise, our results make it possible to highlight that the population between 25 and 35 years of age presented a higher percentage of results for viral co-infections with high or very HR for CC viral types at 14.8% compared to 13.9% in the group over 35 years of age and 10.5% in those under 25 years of age. On the other hand, the population over 35 years of age was the one that presented a higher percentage of positive results for HPV16 and HPV18.

Once we organized the PCR results into a contingency table alongside the PAP results, we identified 5.6% false positives and 18.5% false negatives for the PAP results. These findings strongly support the advantages of using PCR as the standard test for detecting the human papillomavirus and preventing CC. The most striking results correspond to patients older than 35 years, who show 45.6% potential false positives. The percentages of PAP vs. HR HPV-PCR non-correlation were lower in the other age ranges: 25.4% in the age range of 25 to 35 years and 17.7% for those younger than 25 years. These results may suggest the existence of an age bias when interpreting PAP results in the older population, who are theoretically more prone to presenting with CC.

Likewise, our data allowed us to detect a percentage of 68.3% negative results using confirmatory p16/Ki67 dual-stain cytology in the population of positive patients in the HR HPV group. These results made it possible to reassure the patients who had initially received a worrying result from the PCR test and to reduce the performance of unnecessary invasive tests (for example, colposcopy).

Although the PCR test for HPV screening is well known by gynecologists, p16/Ki67 dual-stain cytology is not a widely requested test for CC screening. Out of the total HR-HPV-positive samples, only 37.3% were claimed for re-analysis with confirmatory dual staining. PCR tests detect molecular changes within the cell that are not manifested in morphological changes. This premise supports the promotion of PCR and p16/Ki67 dual-stain cytology as primary screening methods for HPV detection and CC prevention, as they provide greater diagnostic sensitivity to the physician. It is worth noting that, although there are other sensitive methods for HPV detection, such as NGS (Next-Generation Sequencing), this option is costly and would take longer to obtain results (even weeks). In addition, this method is not validated for the clinical diagnosis of CC.

We acknowledge the limitations of our study in enhancing the robustness of our results. One limitation is the absence of clinical information or pathological tissue analysis of the patients, which is crucial for determining the sensitivity and specificity parameters, particularly within our study and the evaluated population sample. However, the most important challenges encountered after carrying out these works are: (1) Continue promoting, among gynecologists, that the papillomavirus PCR technique (HR HPV-PCR) is the best method for CC screening due to the lower presence of false negatives and false positives. (2) Stimulate the study of dual staining in HR12-positive patients to focus colposcopy procedures only on those patients who have cancer cells. (3) Promote the establishment of new protocols agreed between the Medical Societies of specialists (Gynecology and/or Colposcopy) for the better diagnosis and treatment of patients with CC [31,32]. (4) Recently, a new global WHO strategy to achieve the elimination of CC as a public health problem by 2030 has been launched. It is called "Strategy 90-70-90": 90% of girls (and boys in countries where resources allow) are to be fully vaccinated with the HPV vaccine by age 15, 70% of people are to be screened with a high-performance test, and 90% of persons identified with cervical disease will have received treatment [33]. However, there are large inequities still to be resolved. Significant disparities continue to increase between countries and within different regions of the same country. Large differences persist between sociodemographic groups, household income, and children's access to health insurance. The aspects in which we should improve to achieve these objectives are: (a) Accelerate the implementation of HPV screening programs, (b) Take advantage of diagnostic and therapeutic innovations, and (c) Focus on equity [33].

To address these challenges, we are considering and proposing to (1) Disseminate in gynecology congresses in our countries the benefits of molecular diagnosis of HR HPV by PCR, insisting on its greater speed, specificity, and sensitivity. (2) Carry out dissemination campaigns of these new technologies in social networks aimed at the neediest female population in the prevention of CC. (3) Inform and achieve scientific discussion in specialized societies on the clinical risks associated with the unnecessary performance of many colposcopy procedures, for example, infertility or miscarriages. (4) Implement two innovations in our countries: (a) Promote self-collection programs for HR HPV-PCR screening, and (b) Test and validate new detection procedures close to the patient, such as point-of-care (POC) testing. The self-collection programs have already been validated by many countries around the world [34]. The sensitivity and specificity of self-sample HPV tests are like provider-collected HPV tests, and some devices are excellently accepted by women from very different countries [34–36]. Regarding the accessibility of less expensive and convenient methodologies than automated laboratory machines, especially for developing countries, there is great interest in POC testing instruments that could be fast, low-cost, and with a minimal training requirement [33].

5. Conclusions

The HR HPV genotyping results by PCR show the low specificity and selectivity of the PAP test for CC screening. Up to 47.9% false positives have been observed in samples with a cytology diagnosed as high-grade positive. Likewise, 22.1% of false negatives have been observed in samples diagnosed as negative in the PAP test. The results of p16/Ki67 dual-stain cytology in positive PCR samples for any of the HR HPV subtypes show that 68.3% do not present with cancer cells, highlighting the importance of performing these tests to avoid unnecessary colposcopies after the screening of possible patients with CC.

The results of our interactions with practicing gynecologists can be summarized as follows. There is a deeply embedded societal reluctance to abandon traditional PAP tests given the long history of public relations campaigns to convince women and their doctors of their value as the preferred prevention tool for the diagnosis of CC. In the opinion of some specialists, colposcopy remains preferred to dual-staining protocols despite the invasive and frequently unnecessary practice.

Eradicating CC still is a challenge in Mexico due to poor prevention education and the inefficacy of current PAP technology. Our goal is to educate doctors and their patients about the benefits of the new molecular screening technologies for effective primary screening for HPV and the diagnosis of CC.

Author Contributions: Conceptualization, J.L.C.-D. and H.A.B.-S.; methodology, J.L.C.-D., C.R.-S., S.M.Á.-F., S.A.B.-B. and H.A.B.-S.; software, J.L.C.-D. and H.A.B.-S.; validation, J.L.C.-D., C.R.-S., S.M.Á.-F. and H.A.B.-S.; formal analysis, J.L.C.-D., C.R.-S., S.M.Á.-F. and H.A.B.-S.; investigation, J.L.C.-D., C.R.-S., S.M.Á.-F. and H.A.B.-S.; resources, J.L.C.-D. and H.A.B.-S.; data curation, J.L.C.-D. and H.A.B.-S.; writing—original draft preparation, J.L.C.-D. and H.A.B.-S.; writing—review and editing, J.L.C.-D. and H.A.B.-S.; visualization, J.L.C.-D., C.R.-S., S.M.Á.-F., S.A.B.-B. and H.A.B.-S.; supervision, J.L.C.-D. and H.A.B.-S.; project administration, J.L.C.-D. and H.A.B.-S.; funding acquisition, J.L.C.-D. and H.A.B.-S. All authors have read and agreed to the published version of the manuscript.

Funding: This research received no external funding.

Institutional Review Board Statement: Ethical review and approval were waived for this study due to the primary focus of the laboratories where all the authors are employed. Our main activities involve analyzing samples referred by gynecologists and gynecologists-oncologists, followed by reporting the results obtained. In this study, we conducted a retrospective analysis of our databases while ensuring the anonymization of patient information to protect their privacy. Such retrospective analyses, which do not involve direct patient interventions, typically do not require ethical committee approval.

Informed Consent Statement: Informed consent was obtained from all subjects involved in the study and their identification was protected by assigning a laboratory code. In the present study, we conducted a retrospective analysis of our databases, ensuring the anonymization of their content to safeguard the patients' personal information. This study had an exception for IRB approval.

Data Availability Statement: Data are contained within the article.

Acknowledgments: We wish to thank the staff of our laboratories for their valuable technical support, especially HD Cervantes Santiago, MA Mora-Jiménez, JI Andrade-Sashida, and Luis E Fernandez-Garza.

Conflicts of Interest: The authors declare no conflicts of interest.

References

1. Perkins, R.B.; Wentzensen, N.; Guido, R.S.; Schiffman, M. Cervical Cancer Screening: A Review. *JAMA* **2023**, *330*, 547–558. [CrossRef] [PubMed]
2. Weintraub, J.; Morabia, A. Efficacy of a liquid-based thin layer method for cervical cancer screening in a population with a low incidence of cervical cancer. *Diagn. Cytopathol.* **2000**, *22*, 52–59. [CrossRef]
3. Hoda, R.S.; Loukeris, K.; Abdul-Karim, F.W. Gynecologic cytology on conventional and liquid-based preparations: A comprehensive review of similarities and differences. *Diagn. Cytopathol.* **2013**, *41*, 257–278. [CrossRef] [PubMed]

4. Cuzick, J.; Arbyn, M.; Sankaranarayanan, R.; Tsu, V.; Ronco, G.; Mayrand, M.H.; Dillner, J.; Meijer, C.J. Overview of human papillomavirus-based and other novel options for cervical cancer screening in developed and developing countries. *Vaccine* **2008**, *26*, 29–41. [CrossRef] [PubMed]
5. Olivas, A.D.; Barroeta, J.E.; Lastra, R.R. Overview of Ancillary Techniques in Cervical Cytology. *Acta Cytol.* **2023**, *67*, 119–128. [CrossRef]
6. Arbyn, M.; Weiderpass, E.; Bruni, L.; de Sanjosé, S.; Saraiya, M.; Ferlay, J.; Bray, F. Estimates of incidence and mortality of cervical cancer in 2018: A worldwide analysis. *Lancet Glob. Health* **2020**, *8*, 191–203. [CrossRef] [PubMed]
7. Bruni, L.; Serrano, B.; Roura, E.; Alemany, L.; Cowan, M.; Herrero, R.; Poljak, M.; Murillo, R.; Broutet, N.; Riley, L.M.; et al. Cervical cancer screening programs and age-specific coverage estimates for 202 countries and territories worldwide: A review and synthetic analysis. *Lancet Glob. Health* **2022**, *10*, 1115–1127. [CrossRef] [PubMed]
8. World Health Organization. *Comprehensive Cervical Cancer Control. A Guide to Essential Practice*, 2nd ed.; WHO Library Cataloguing-in-Publication Data; World Health Organization: Geneva, Switzerland, 2014; pp. 1–364.
9. Arango-Bravo, E.A.; Cetina-Pérez, L.D.C.; Galicia-Carmona, T.; Castro-Equiluz, D.; Gallardo-Rincón, D.; Cruz-Bautista, I.; Duenas-Gonzalez, A. The health system and access to treatment in patients with cervical cancer in Mexico. *Front. Oncol.* **2022**, *12*, 1028291. [CrossRef] [PubMed]
10. Davies-Oliveira, J.C.; Smith, M.A.; Grover, S.; Canfell, K.; Crosbie, E.J. Eliminating Cervical Cancer: Progress and Challenges for High-income Countries. *Clin. Oncol.* **2021**, *33*, 550–559. [CrossRef]
11. Morris, B.J. The advent of human papillomavirus detection for cervical screening. *Curr. Opin. Obstet. Gynecol.* **2019**, *31*, 333–339. [CrossRef]
12. Rol, M.L.; Picconi, M.A.; Ferrera, A.; Sánchez, G.I.; Hernández, M.L.; Lineros, J.; Peraza, A.; Brizuela, M.; Mendoza, L.; Mongelós, P.; et al. Implementing HPV testing in 9 Latin American countries: The laboratory perspective as observed in the ESTAMPA study. *Front. Med.* **2022**, *9*, 1006038. [CrossRef]
13. Koliopoulos, G.; Arbyn, M.; Martin-Hirsch, P.; Kyrgiou, M.; Prendiville, W.; Paraskevaidis, E. Diagnostic accuracy of human papillomavirus testing in primary cervical screening: A systematic review and meta-analysis of non-randomized studies. *Gynecol. Oncol.* **2007**, *104*, 232–246. [CrossRef]
14. Tommasino, M. The human papillomavirus family and its role in carcinogenesis. *Semin. Cancer Biol.* **2014**, *26*, 13–21. [CrossRef]
15. Hareza, D.A.; Wilczyński, J.R.; Paradowska, E. Human Papillomaviruses as Infectious Agents in Gynecological Cancers. Oncogenic Properties of Viral Proteins. *Int. J. Mol. Sci.* **2022**, *23*, 1818. [CrossRef] [PubMed]
16. Muñoz-Bello, J.O.; Carrillo-García, A.; Lizano, M. Epidemiology and Molecular Biology of HPV Variants in Cervical Cancer: The State of the Art in Mexico. *Int. J. Mol. Sci.* **2022**, *23*, 8566. [CrossRef]
17. Scymonowicz, K.A.; Chen, J. Biological and clinical aspects of HPV-related cancers. *Cancer Biol. Med.* **2020**, *17*, 864–878. [CrossRef]
18. Arbyn, M.; Simon, M.; Peeters, E.; Xu, L.; Meijer, C.J.L.M.; Berkhof, J.; Cuschieri, K.; Bonde, J.; Ostrbenk Vanlencak, A.; Zhao, F.H.; et al. 2020 list of human papillomavirus assays suitable for primary cervical cancer screening. *Clin. Microbiol. Infect.* **2021**, *27*, 1083–1095. [CrossRef] [PubMed]
19. Arbyn, M.; Snijders, P.J.; Meijer, C.J.; Berkhof, J.; Cuschieri, K.; Kocjan, B.J.; Poljak, M. Which high-risk HPV assays fulfill criteria for use in primary cervical cancer screening? *Clin. Microbiol. Infect.* **2015**, *21*, 817–826. [CrossRef] [PubMed]
20. Galgano, M.T.; Castle, P.E.; Atkins, K.A.; Brix, W.K.; Nassau, S.R.; Stoler, M.H. Using biomarkers as objective standards in the diagnosis of cervical biopsies. *Am. J. Surg. Pathol.* **2010**, *34*, 1077–1087. [CrossRef]
21. Von Knebel Doeberitz, M.; Reuschenbach, M.; Schmidt, D.; Bergeron, C. Biomarkers for cervical cancer screening: The role of p16(INK4a) to highlight transforming HPV infections. *Expert Rev. Proteom.* **2012**, *9*, 149–163. [CrossRef]
22. Bergeron, C.; Ordi, J.; Schmidt, D.; Trunk, M.J.; Keller, T.; Ridder, R.; European CINtec Histology Study Group. Conjunctive p16INK4a testing significantly increases accuracy in diagnosing high-grade cervical intraepithelial neoplasia. *Am. J. Clin. Pathol.* **2010**, *133*, 395–406. [CrossRef] [PubMed]
23. Dijkstra, M.G.; Heideman, D.A.; de Roy, S.C.; Rozendaal, L.; Berkhof, J.; van Krimpen, K.; van Groningen, K.; Snijders, P.J.; Meijer, C.J.; van Kemenade, F.J. p16(INK4a) immunostaining as an alternative to histology review for reliable grading of cervical intraepithelial lesions. *J. Clin. Pathol.* **2010**, *63*, 972–977. [CrossRef] [PubMed]
24. Denton, K.J.; Bergeron, C.; Klement, P.; Trunk, M.J.; Keller, T.; Ridder, R.; European CINtec Cytology Study Group. The sensitivity and specificity of p16(INK4a) cytology vs HPV testing for detecting high-grade cervical disease in the triage of ASC-US and LSIL papa cytology results. *Am. J. Clin. Pathol.* **2010**, *134*, 12–21. [CrossRef] [PubMed]
25. Schmidt, D.; Bergeron, C.; Denton, K.J.; Ridder, R.; European CINtec Cytology Study Group. p16/ki-67 dual-stain cytology in the triage of ASCUS and LSIL Papanicolaou cytology: Results from the European equivocal or mildly abnormal Papanicolaou cytology study. *Cancer Cytopathol.* **2011**, *119*, 158–166. [CrossRef] [PubMed]
26. Petry, K.U.; Schmidt, D.; Scherbring, S.; Luyten, A.; Reinecke-Lüthge, A.; Bergeron, C.; Kommoss, F.; Löning, T.; Ordi, J.; Regauer, S.; et al. Triaging Pap cytology negative, HPV positive cervical cancer screening results with p16/Ki-67 Dual-stained cytology. *Gynecol. Oncol.* **2011**, *121*, 505–509. [CrossRef] [PubMed]
27. Wentzensen, N.; Schwartz, L.; Zuna, R.E.; Smith, K.; Mathews, C.; Gold, M.A.; Allen, R.A.; Zhang, R.; Dunn, S.T.; Walker, J.L.; et al. Performance of p16/Ki-67 immunostaining to detect cervical cancer precursors in a colposcopy referral population. *Clin. Cancer Res.* **2012**, *18*, 4154–4162. [CrossRef] [PubMed]

28. Edgerton, N.; Cohen, C.; Siddiqui, M.T. Evaluation of CINtec PLUS® testing as an adjunctive test in ASC-US diagnosed SurePath® preparations. *Diagn Cytopathol.* **2013**, *41*, 35–40. [CrossRef] [PubMed]
29. Tjalma, W.A.A. Diagnostic performance of dual-staining cytology for cervical cancer screening: A systematic literature review. *Eur. J. Obstet. Gynecol. Reprod Biol.* **2017**, *210*, 275–280. [CrossRef] [PubMed]
30. Ryu, A.; Honma, K.; Shingetsu, A.; Tanada, S.; Yamamoto, T.; Nagata, S.; Kamiura, S.; Yamasaki, T.; Ohue, M.; Matsuura, N. Utility of p16/Ki67 double immunocytochemistry for detection of cervical adenocarcinoma. *Cancer Cytopathol.* **2022**, *130*, 983–992. [CrossRef]
31. Kyrgiou, M.; Arbyn, M.; Bergeron, C.; Bosch, F.X.; Dillner, J.; Jit, M.; Kim, J.; Poljak, M.; Nieminem, P.; Sasieni, P.; et al. Cervical screening: ESGO-EFC position paper of the European Society of Gynaecologic Oncology (ESGO) and the European Federation of Colposcopy (EFC). *Br. J. Cancer* **2020**, *123*, 510–517. [CrossRef]
32. Sharma, J.; Yennapu, M.; Priyanka, Y. Screening Guidelines and Programs for Cervical Cancer Control in Countries of Different Economic Groups: A Narrative Review. *Cureus* **2023**, *15*, e41098. [CrossRef] [PubMed]
33. World Health Organization. *Global Strategy to Accelerate the Elimination of Cervical Cancer as A Public Health Problem and Its Associated Goals and Targets for the Period 2020-2030*; Seventy-third World Health Assembly. Agenda item 11.4. WHO Library Cataloguing-in-Publication Data; World Health Organization: Geneva, Switzerland, 2020; pp. 1–3.
34. Serrano, B.; Ibáñez, R.; Robles, C.; Peremiquel-Trillas, P.; de Sanjosé, S.; Bruni, L. Worldwide use of HPV self-sampling for cervical cancer screening. *Prev. Med.* **2022**, *154*, 106900. [CrossRef] [PubMed]
35. Arbyn, M.; Verdoodt, F.; Snijders, P.J.; Verhoef, V.M.; Suonio, E.; Dillner, L.; Minozzi, S.; Bellisario, C.; Banzi, R.; Zhao, F.H.; et al. Accuracy of human papillomavirus testing on self-collected versus clinician-collected samples: A meta-analysis. *Lancet Oncol.* **2014**, *15*, 172–183. [CrossRef] [PubMed]
36. Arbyn, M.; Latsuzbaia, A.; Castle, P.E.; Sahasrabuddhe, V.V.; Broeck, D.V. HPV testing of self-samples: Influence of collection and sample handling procedures on clinical accuracy to detect cervical precancer. *Lancet Reg. Health Eur.* **2022**, *14*, 100332. [CrossRef] [PubMed]

Disclaimer/Publisher's Note: The statements, opinions and data contained in all publications are solely those of the individual author(s) and contributor(s) and not of MDPI and/or the editor(s). MDPI and/or the editor(s) disclaim responsibility for any injury to people or property resulting from any ideas, methods, instructions or products referred to in the content.

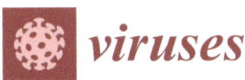

Article

Factors Associated with HPV Genital Warts: A Self-Reported Cross-Sectional Study among Students and Staff of a Northern University in Nigeria

Melvin Omone Ogbolu [1,*], Olanrewaju D. Eniade [2,3], Hussaini Majiya [4] and Miklós Kozlovszky [5,6]

1. BioTech Research Center, University Research and Innovation Center, Óbuda University, Bécsi Street 96/B, 1034 Budapest, Hungary
2. Department of Epidemiology and Medical Statistics, College of Medicine, University of Ibadan, CW22+H4W, Queen Elizabeth II Road, Agodi, Ibadan 200285, Nigeria; olanrewaju.eniade@ifain.org
3. International Foundation against Infectious Disease in Nigeria (IFAIN), 6A, Dutse Street, War College Estate, Gwarimpa, Abuja 900108, Nigeria
4. Department of Microbiology, Ibrahim Badamasi Babangida University, 3H89+XW3, Minna Road, Lapai 911101, Nigeria; hussainimajiya@ibbu.edu.ng
5. John von Neumann Faculty of Informatics, Óbuda University, Bécsi Street 96/B, 1034 Budapest, Hungary; kozlovszky.miklos@nik.uni-obuda.hu
6. Medical Device Research Group, LPDS, Institute for Computer Science and Control (SZTAKI), Hungarian Research Network (HUN-REN), 1111 Budapest, Hungary
* Correspondence: ogbolu.melvin@nik.uni-obuda.hu

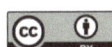

Citation: Ogbolu, M.O.; Eniade, O.D.; Majiya, H.; Kozlovszky, M. Factors Associated with HPV Genital Warts: A Self-Reported Cross-Sectional Study among Students and Staff of a Northern University in Nigeria. *Viruses* **2024**, *16*, 902. https://doi.org/10.3390/v16060902

Academic Editors: Hossein H. Ashrafi and Mustafa Ozdogan

Received: 29 April 2024
Revised: 30 May 2024
Accepted: 31 May 2024
Published: 2 June 2024

Copyright: © 2024 by the authors. Licensee MDPI, Basel, Switzerland. This article is an open access article distributed under the terms and conditions of the Creative Commons Attribution (CC BY) license (https://creativecommons.org/licenses/by/4.0/).

Abstract: The menace of human papillomavirus (HPV) infections among low- and middle-income countries with no access to a free HPV vaccine is a public health concern. HPV is one of the most common sexually transmitted infections (STIs) in Nigeria, while the most known types of HPV genotypes being transmitted are the high-risk HPV-16 and 18 genotypes. In this study, we explored the predictors of self-reported HPV infections and HPV genital warts infection among a population of students, non-academic staff, and academic staff of Ibrahim Badamasi Babangida (IBB) University located in Lapai, Nigeria. We also assessed their knowledge about HPV infections and genotypes, and sexual behaviors. An online cross-sectional study was conducted by setting up a structured questionnaire on Google Forms and it was distributed to the university community via Facebook and other social media platforms of the university. The form captured questions on HPV infection, and knowledge about HPV infection and genotypes, as well as the sexual health of the participants. All variables were described using frequencies and percentage distribution; chi-squared test statistics were used to explore the association between HPV infection (medical records of HPV infection) and the participants' profile, and a logistic regression analysis was performed to examine the factors associated with HPV genital warts infection among the population. This study reveals those participants between the ages of 26–40 years (81.3%) and those currently not in a sexually active relationship—single/divorced (26.4%)—who have self-reported having the HPV-16 and -18 genotypes. Moreover, participants between 26–40 years of age (OR: 0.45, 95%CI: 0.22–0.89) reported themselves to be carriers of HPV genital warts. Therefore, this study reveals the factors associated with HPV infection and genital warts peculiar to IBB university students and staff. Hence, we suggest the need for HPV awareness programs and free HPV vaccine availability at IBB university.

Keywords: HPV awareness programs; HPV infection; HPV genotypes; HPV genital warts; HPV knowledge; HPV vaccine

1. Introduction

Human papillomavirus (HPV) is one of the most common sexually transmitted infections (STIs) among adults, of which HPV 16, 18, 31, and 35 (high-risk types) [1] are the most prevalent HPV genotypes among sexually active adults in the northern part of Nigeria [2,3].

These high-risk HPV genotypes, especially HPV 16 and 18, have been clinically proven to be the leading cause of cervical cancer in women across low-income African countries [4,5]. However, the low-risk (11, 42, 61, 70, and 81) HPV genotypes are capable of causing HPV genital warts [6]. Numerous studies have revealed that HPV is also highly associated with the growth of HPV genital warts in both men and women [7,8]. In most cases, persons with a healthy immune system can be HPV-free over time even after being infected. An HPV vaccine-built immunity and other types of preventative vaccines (such as toxoids, messenger ribonucleic acid (mRNA), and subunit vaccines [9]), alongside with some other factors (such as healthy weight, healthy food, exercise, and staying away from excessive alcohol intake and smoking [10]) can effectively repel against persistent HPV infections within two years before it develops into a tumor [11] and other immunological diseases [12] in the presence of a healthy immune system. However, north-central Nigerian adults are faced with some challenges which have contributed to the spread of HPV infection such as the unavailability of some protective measures. Although this is associated with the lack of knowledge of HPV in general, the following are also factors: abject poverty (resulting in the inability to purchase HPV vaccines, eat healthy food, and attend paid HPV-related seminars), individuals' ethical imperatives, the unavailability of free medical services, and some national policies. In terms of national policies, this is a contributing factor such that the government does not put in place policies to make an HPV vaccine available at a low cost and enforce it as a part of the routine vaccination program in Nigeria [13]. Due to these challenges, there have been increases in the cases of HPV infection and the cervical cancer mortality rate among women in the north-central part of Nigeria yearly [14]. According to the statistical report gathered by the ICO/IARC Information Centre on HPV and Cancer (HPV Information Centre) in October 2021, among other kinds of cancers, the HPV-related (HPV 16 and 18) cancer occurrence in the female population of ages $\geq$ 15 years in Nigeria was 66.9% amidst 56.2 million total females who are at risk of cervical cancer [15].

Some epidemiological studies have also in the past revealed demographic variations among low-income settlements in Nigeria and its association with HPV infection [6]. For instance, a study conducted for 16 years in a rural area in Nigeria reveals that inaccessibility to childhood and adolescent routine immunization as a preventive measure for preventable diseases [16] is more prevalent in low- and middle-income areas in Nigeria and other sub-Saharan African (SSA) countries, causing severe infant mortality [17], thereby putting non-HPV vaccinated adults at risk of persistent HPV infections. Similarly, a study conducted among adolescent and young girls in Jos, Nigeria also shows that the lack of HPV vaccine and lack of knowledge about HPV enhanced the prevalence of HPV among the population [6]. Hence, it has been proven that the availability of free medical services to provide organized HPV programs, HPV vaccines, and HPV testing and cervical cancer screenings using cytology/visual inspection/colposcopic biopsy in low-income settlements would help to mitigate HPV infection cases and the cervical cancer mortality rate in Nigeria [2,5,18].

In this study, we explored the demographic predictors of self-reported [19] HPV infections and HPV genital warts infection among low-income students, and non-academic, and academic (lecturers) staff of Ibrahim Badamasi Babangida (IBB) University located in Lapai, Nigeria, considering their income rate as compared to the country's minimum wage and if they have reported to have had an HPV infection in the past. Furthermore, age as another demographic factor was also analyzed to observe if the population's age is likely to affect their monthly income rate. Abject poverty as one of the predictors of HPV infection was considered for analysis in this study, especially in low-income and lower-middle-income countries (LMICs) (as in Nigeria) [20], where the citizens cannot fend for their medical services in the presence of a Gross National Income (GNI) per capita at $2157 as recorded in 2019 by the World Bank collection of development indicators.

2. Motivation—Problem Definition

In the absence of knowledge about HPV and cervical cancer even in an academic/educational environment, there is a likelihood that there would be cases of HPV infection among a population. Sadly, the male population in the society are not aware of their HPV status, thereby causing females to harbor the risk of contracting HPV, which further develops into cervical cancer in the future [21]. Clinical research has revealed that HPV takes 10–15 years to develop into abnormal cells [22]. The purpose of this paper is to reveal the risk factors of HPV infection and genital warts in an academic environment and study those who have self-reported cases of HPV infection and genital warts using statistical methods. Our results can be adopted by the Niger State Ministry of Health for HPV awareness in an academic setting, healthcare sectors, and private organizations, and by individuals as a guide for safe sexual practices and knowledge about HPV.

3. Methods and Materials

3.1. Study Design and Setting

This was an online cross-sectional study among students, and non-academic and academic staff of Ibrahim Badamasi Babangida (IBB) University, Lapai, Niger State, Nigeria. IBB University comprises students and staff from various regions in Nigeria, which includes Igbo, Yoruba, and Hausa major ethnic groups. However, data to determine which regions the participants are from were not captured in our questionnaire. Taking into consideration the privacy of the participants, Nigerian citizens have right to their private data and the Nigerian constitution guarantees privacy protection to all citizens. Hence, the Nigeria Data Protection Regulation (NDPR) was enforced during data collection [23].

3.1.1. Sample Size

The sample size determination formula for a cross-sectional study was used in this study:

$$n = \frac{Z_\alpha^2 \times pq \times d_{eff}}{d^2} \quad (1)$$

where:

n = minimum sample size;

z = standard normal deviation of 95% confidence level—corresponds to a value of 1.96;

p = record of HPV genital warts from similar studies in southwestern Nigeria was (0.22) [24];

e = level of precision of 0.04;

$q = 1 - p$; $1 - 0.22 = 0.78$;

$d_{eff} = 1.98$—a design effect (d_{eff}) of 1.98 was factored because the study cut across clusters (i.e., cluster of students, and non-academic and academic staff);

$n = 1615$;

n_a (after adjusting for a 10% non-response rate) = 1860.

A total of 1860 eligible people who completed the online questionnaires were considered for/enrolled in this study (Figure 1).

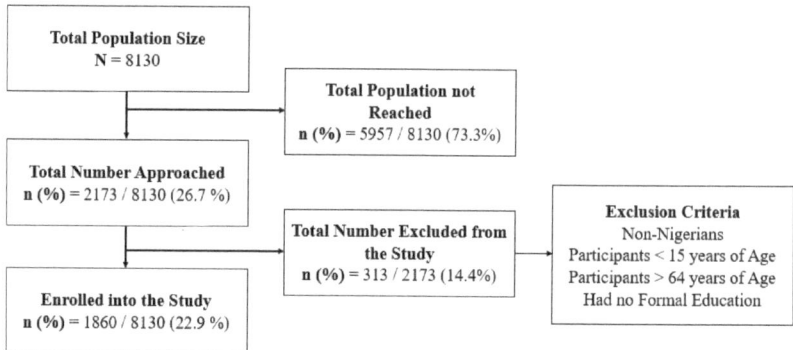

Figure 1. Study enrolment flowchart.

3.1.2. Sampling Method

Having established a high incidence of sexual behavior [25] which is a risk factor for HPV infection among university students and staff [26,27]. we, thus, carried out this study among the university community, at Ibrahim Badamasi Babangida University, Lapai in Niger State, Nigeria. IBB University is located in the north-central region of Nigeria and has a student capacity of about 7000, 820 non-academic staff, and 310 academic staff. The data were collected using an online data collection tool (Google survey form). The questionnaire was set up on the Google survey form and the function that restricts multiple responses from participants was enabled.

3.1.3. Study Instrument and Data Collection

A structured questionnaire was used, which captured the demographic characteristics, information about HPV and sexual health, and knowledge about early sex and HPV-16 and -18 genotype. In order to improve the response rate, we raised awareness (live event) about the study through the Facebook platform during the COVID-19 pandemic in 2019, but data collection lasted between 2019–2022. The lead investigator and a group of gynecologists in Nigeria and the United States of America facilitated the event. During the event, participants were asked to fill in an online questionnaire—the Human Papillomavirus (HPV) and Cervical Cancer Risk Assessment (HCRA) Tool (also known as the HPV Assessment Test (HAT) Tool [1]). The link to the online questionnaire (Google Forms) was distributed via Facebook and email address (it was sent to students who could not attend the online event). Google Forms is an electronic platform designed for creating surveys, quizzes, and knowledge evaluations. The Google Form can be created and administered on personal computers, and mobile devices, as well as tablets. Some of its important features are real-time data capturing, friendly user interface, the ability to limit responses to once per person, etc. The Google Form has proven to be effective for research data collection and other data-capturing activities [28].

3.1.4. Study Variables

The outcome variable for this study was self-reported medical record/history of HPV genital warts (Yes or No). The explanatory variables included the 1. Demographic variables: Gender [Male, Female]; Age group (15–25, 26–40, 41–64); Level of education [High school/equivalent, and BSc/MSc/Doctorate degree)]; Income in USD ($) [Below 100, 100–200, above 200], $100 ≡ #45,000 Nigerian currency; and Marital Status [Married—currently in a sexually active relationship, not in a sexually active relationship (single/divorced)]; 2. Sexual Health/Behavior: Sexual intercourse [Yes, No]; Age at first sex (15–20, 21–30, >30 years); Number of the sexual partner in a lifetime [1, 2–4, >4]; Kind of sex [vaginal only, others (anal, oral, and vaginal)]; Knowledge about early sex [Yes, No]; and Protected sex, defined as the use of condom for sexual intercourse [unprotected, protected]; and 3. Information on HPV factors:

Vaccinated against HPV [Yes, No]; HPV seminar attendance [Yes, No]; and Knowledge of HPV-16 and -18 genotypes [Yes, No].

3.2. Data Analysis

We summarized all the variables using frequencies and percentages (descriptive statistics). Moreover, a chi-square test of association was carried out to test the association between the participants' profiles and self-reported medical record/history of HPV genital warts. We examined the factors associated with HPV infection by fitting a binary logistic regression, and an adjusted odds ratio ($_{Adj}$OR) was reported.

Model Expression

The model expression implemented for statistical analysis is the logistic regression model [7]:

$$Log \frac{p_i}{1 - p_i} = \beta_0 + X_1\beta_1 + X_2\beta_2 + X_3\beta_3 + \varepsilon_i \qquad (2)$$

where:

$Log \frac{p_i}{1-p_i}$ is the probability of HPV genital warts up to ith participant;

X_1 denotes sexual health, X_2 represents the HPV factors (HPV vaccination, and HPV seminar), and X_3 denotes demographic variables;

β_0 is the model intercept, while β_1, β_2, and β_3 denote the coefficients for sexual health and demographic characteristics;

ε_i is the error term which was assumed to follow the binomial distribution.

Stata MP version 15 was used for statistical analysis, and p-values < 0.05 were considered significant at a 95% confidence interval (CI).

3.3. Ethical Considerations

The ethical approval for this study was obtained from the Niger State Ministry of Health Review Committee (protocol number: ERC PIN/2022/08/17 and approval number: ERC PAN/2022/08/17) in Minna, Niger State, Nigeria. Participants provided consent by clicking the "accept to participate" button after reading the informed consent statement on the first page. In order to assure the privacy and confidentiality of the participants, all participants voluntarily participated in this study and no identifying information was captured. Since data were collected online, the study has no/minimal risk to the health of the participants, their environment, and their relatives.

4. Results

4.1. Demographic Characteristics of the Study

The results in Table 1 below reveal the demographic characteristics of the students, non-academic staff, and academic staff who participated in this study ($n = 1860$). The participants' age ranged between 15–64 years with Mean 32.1 ± 7.13 SD. The study contained more female than male participants, whereby 1750 (94.1%) of them were females and 110 (5.9%) were males. Most of the participants were millennials; thus, 1512 (81.3%) were aged 26–40 years, while 151 (8.1%) and 197 (10.6%) were aged 15–25 years and >40 years, respectively. Only 136 (7.3%) had a high school education and 1724 (92.7%) had a BSc or MSc or Doctoral Degree. Most of the participants recorded having an average livelihood, where 739 (39.7%) earned below 100 USD monthly, 27.4% earned between 100–200 USD, and 32.9% earned above 200 USD monthly. The majority of the population of 1369 (73.6%) were in a marital, sexually active relationship, and 26.4% were not in a marital, sexually active relationship.

Table 1. Demographic characteristics of the participants.

Variables	Frequency (n = 1860)	Percent (%)
Gender		
Male	110	5.9
Female	1750	94.1
Age		
15–25	151	8.1
26–40	1512	81.3
41–64	197	10.6
Education		
High School/Equivalent	136	7.3
BSc, MSc, Doctorate Degree	1724	92.7
Income (USD)		
Below 100	739	39.7
100–200	509	27.4
Above 200	612	32.9
Marital status		
Currently married	1369	73.6
Not in a sexually active relationship (Single/Divorced)	491	26.4

4.2. Information about HPV and Sexual Health of Participants

The results in Table 2 below present the information about the participants' self-reported HPV infection and sexual health. Mostly, 1843 (99.1%) were sexually exposed, where about a half (49.4%) had an early sexual debut from the ages of 15–20 years, 875 (47.5%) experienced a sexual debut between the ages of 21–30 years, and 57 (3.1%) had a sexual debut at age ≥31 years. It was observed that 569 (30.9%) participants have had only one sexual partner in a lifetime, 636 (34.5%) have had 2–4 sexual partners, and 638 (34.6%) have had ≥4 sexual partners. Among those who had more than one sexual partner, 934 (73.3%) practiced unprotected sex and 340 (26.7%) practiced protected sex, 1790 (97.1%) practiced vaginal sexual intercourse, and 53 (2.9%) practiced other (anal, oral, and vaginal) sexual intercourse. Furthermore, only 528 (28.4%) have attended an HPV seminar. Moreover, the rate of HPV vaccination was low, where just 107 (5.8%) among the participants have been vaccinated against HPV infection. Finally, 74 (4.0%) of the participants reported that they have had medical records of HPV genital warts, while 55 (3.0%) have had medical records of HPV-16 and -18 genotype infections.

Table 2. Sexual health and HPV information.

Variables	Frequency (n = 1860)	Percent (%)
Have you ever had sex?		
Yes	1843	99.1
No	17	0.9
Age at first sexual intercourse (n = 1843)		
15–20	911	49.4
21–30	875	47.5
31 and above	57	3.1
Number of sexual partners in lifetime (n = 1843)		
1 sexual partner in a lifetime	569	30.9
2–4 sexual partners in a lifetime	636	34.5
>4 sexual partners in a lifetime	638	34.6
Protected sex (n = 1274)		
Unprotected sex	934	73.3
Protected sex	340	26.7

Table 2. Cont.

Variables	Frequency (n = 1860)	Percent (%)
Kind of sex practiced (n = 1843)		
Vaginal sex	1790	97.1
Others (anal, oral, vaginal)	53	2.9
HPV seminar		
No	1332	71.6
Yes	528	28.4
Ever received HPV vaccine?		
No	1753	94.2
Yes	107	5.8
Medical record of HPV-16 and -18 genotypes		
No	1805	97.0
Yes	55	3.0
Medical record of HPV genital warts infection		
No	1786	96.0
Yes	74	4.0

4.3. The Participants' Knowledge about the Association between Early Sex and HPV-16 and -18 Genotypes

Figure 2 below shows the population's level of knowledge about the association between early sex and the HPV-16 and -18 genotypes. Quite a number of the participants agreed that early sex is associated with HPV infection, which means that 822 (44.2%) have knowledge about early sex, but knowledge about the HPV-16 and -18 genotypes was low as the statistical analysis revealed that only 149 (8.0%) among the participants agreed that they have any knowledge about the HPV-16 and -18 genotypes.

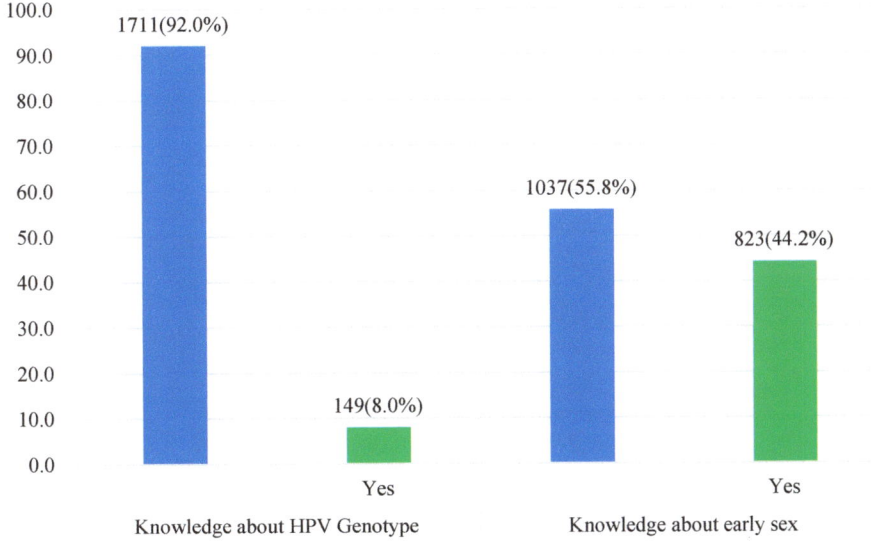

Figure 2. Knowledge about early sex and HPV-16 and -18 genotypes.

4.4. Association between HPV Infection and Participants' Profile

At the time of the survey distribution, the results in Table 3 below show the association between participants who recorded self-reported HPV infection and the participants' profile using chi-square test. The rate of HPV infection was 13 (8.6%) among those aged 15–25 years compared to the 56 (3.7%) and 5 (2.5%) rate among participants aged between 26–40 years and 41–64 years, respectively; $p = 0.007$. There was a preponderance of 27 (5.5%) of HPV infection among those who were not in a marital, sexually active relationship compared to married participants; $p = 0.045$. Similarly, more 48 (5.1%) of those who practiced unprotected sexual intercourse had HPV infection compared to those who practiced protected sexual intercourse; $p = 0.096$. Moreover, HPV infection was more common—5 (9.4%)—among those who practiced other (anal, oral, and vaginal) kinds of sex compared to those who practiced vaginal sex only; $p = 0.083$. HPV infection was 14 (9.4%) among those who have knowledge about the HPV-16 and -18 genotype compared to those—60 (3.5%)—who do not; $p < 0.001$. The proportion of HPV infection was slightly higher—42 (5.1%)—among participants who had knowledge about early sex compared to those who did not have knowledge about early sex; $p = 0.027$.

Table 3. Association between HPV infection (medical records of HPV infection) and the participants' profile.

Variables	Self-Reported HPV Infection		Test Statistics (Chi-Square/ Fisher's Exact)	p-Value
	No	Yes		
Gender			0.67	0.414
Male	104 (94.5)	6 (5.5)		
Female	1682 (96.1)	68 (3.9)		
Age			9.85	0.007 **
15–25	138 (91.4)	13 (8.6)		
26–40	1456 (96.3)	56 (3.7)		
41–64	192 (97.5)	5 (2.5)		
Education			0.04	0.852
Elementary School and High School	131 (96.3)	5 (3.7)		
BSc, MSc, Doctorate Degree	1655 (96.0)	69 (4.0)		
Income			1.41	0.495
Below 100	706 (95.5)	33 (4.5)		
100–200	493 (96.9)	16 (3.1)		
Above 200	587 (95.9)	25 (4.1)		
Marital status			4.07	0.045
Married	1322 (96.6)	47 (3.4)		
Not in a sexually active relationship (single/divorced)	464 (94.5)	27 (5.5)		
Have you ever had sexual intercourse?			0.71	0.645
No	17 (100.0)	0 (0.0)		
Yes	1769 (96.0)	74 (4.0)		
Age at first sexual intercourse			1.07	0.585
15–20	876 (96.2)	35 (3.8)		
21–30	837 (95.7)	38 (4.3)		
$\geq$31	56 (98.2)	1 (1.8)		
Number of sexual partners in lifetime			3.4	0.182
1 sexual partner in a lifetime	553 (97.2)	16 (2.8)		
2–4 sexual partners in a lifetime	609 (95.8)	27 (4.2)		
$\geq$4 sexual partners in a lifetime	607 (95.1)	31 (4.9)		

Table 3. Cont.

	Self-Reported HPV Infection			
Variables	No	Yes	Test Statistics (Chi-Square/ Fisher's Exact)	p-Value
Protected sex			2.77	0.096 *
Unprotected sex	886(94.9)	48(5.1)		
Protected sex	330(97.1)	10(2.9)		
Kind of sex practiced			4.97	0.083 *
Vaginal sex only	1721(96.1)	69(3.9)		
Others (anal, oral, vaginal)	48(90.6)	5(9.4)		
HPV seminar			0.28	0.600
No	1281(96.2)	51(3.8)		
Yes	505(95.6)	23(4.4)		
Knowledge about HPV-16 and -18 genotype			12.44	0.000 **
No	1651(96.5)	60(3.5)		
Yes	135(90.6)	14(9.4)		
HPV vaccine?			1.95	0.162
No	1686(96.2)	67(3.8)		
Yes	100(93.5)	7(6.5)		
Knowledge about early sex			4.89	0.027 **
No	1005(96.9)	32(3.1)		
Yes	781(94.9)	42(5.1)		

* p-value is significant at 10% level of significance. ** p-value is significant at 5% level of significance.

4.5. Factors Associated with HPV Genital Warts Infection among Students, Non-Academic Staff, and Academic Staff in North-Central Nigeria

The results in Table 4 represent the factors associated with HPV infection among the study participants using the logistic regression model. Only two variables had a significant association with HPV infection. The likelihood of HPV infection was lower among those aged between 26–40 years ($_{Adj}$OR = 0.45, CI: 0.22–0.89, p = 0.024) and 41–64 years ($_{Adj}$OR = 0.31, CI: 0.10–0.95, p = 0.041) compared to those aged 15–25 years.

Table 4. Factors associated with HPV genital warts infection among students, non-academic staff, and academic staff in north-central Nigeria.

Self-Reported HPV Genital Warts	Odds Ratio	95% CI		p-Value
		Lower	Upper	
Gender				
Male	ref			
Female	0.80	0.32	1.99	0.630
Age				
15–25	ref			
26–40	0.45	0.22	0.89	0.024
41–64	0.31	0.10	0.95	0.041
Marital status				
Married	ref			
Not in a sexually active relationship (Single/Divorced)	1.39	0.81	2.40	0.233
Kind of sex practiced				
Vaginal sex	ref			
Others (anal, oral, vaginal)	2.13	0.77	5.84	0.143
Protected sex				
Unprotected sex	ref			
Protected sex	0.59	0.32	1.09	0.095

5. Discussion

This study examined 1860 students, non-academic staff, and academic staff in north-central Nigeria on their demographic characteristics, their awareness/knowledge about HPV infections and HPV genotypes, and their sexual health and practices. The findings observed are a concern to public health.

Considering the demographic characteristics, we observed that the study sample was representative as it includes both high school/equivalent (low-levelled) and BSc, MSc, and Doctorate Degree (high-levelled) elite participants between the ages of 15–64 years, whereas most were between the age of 26–40 years. However, the gender distribution was not even as there were fewer males than females in the study. However, the survey also included some questions about cervical cancer, and this might be why male participants were not interested in taking the survey. The distribution of the participants based on their monthly income was fairly even. The distribution of the participants' based on their marital status was skewed, where most of the participants indicated that they were in a sexually active relationship (married or separated), which is because the rate of divorce among ever married couples is low in the north-central region of Nigeria as compared to other regions [29]. This skewedness is expected because the north-central part of Nigeria is mostly populated by Muslims who believe that their religion detests divorce, according to Sunan Abu-Dawud, Book 6:2173 [30]. Moreover, a study conducted to examine cancer of the cervix in Zaria [31] and Lagos [32] revealed that most of the study participants were married which validates our result for having more participants who are currently in a marriage.

The result of the participants' sexual behavior shows that a large majority of the participants reported having had sexual intercourse in their lifetime, and having their first experience between the age of 15–20 years, and more having had >4 partners in a lifetime. These results corroborate with other studies' results that have explored the predictors of HPV among the male and female population, where early sex ($\leq$20 years) is common among early and late adolescents in Nigeria [33], having 1 or more sexual partners before the age of 20 years [15], and having >4 sexual partners in a lifetime [34]. Furthermore, a vast number of the participants were also not concerned about practicing safe sex before they entered into a sexually active relationship. We excluded those who indicated having had only one sexual partner and analyzed those who have had >1 sexual partners (1274 participants) in a lifetime; the result revealed that most of the participants (73.3%) who fall under these group do not practice safe sex (with the use of condoms). This aligns with results from other studies that have reported that condoms are not widely used among non-married people in Nigeria [35]. A survey distributed by NOIpolls, in alliance with the National Agency for the Control of AIDS (NACA) and AIDS HealthCare Foundation (AHF) in 2020 to mitigate the spread of HIV/AIDS, reveals that only 34% of Nigerians indicated that they use condoms during sexual intercourse [36]. This study also reveals that the combination of anal, oral, and vaginal sex was low among the population, as 97.1% participants mostly practiced vaginal sex only. This is because the population under study might be affected by religious beliefs and detest the act of oral and anal sex. Another study also revealed that vaginal sex (95.2%) was mostly practiced among adolescents in Nigeria who were examined for self-reported HIV transmission [37].

The proportion of the participants with awareness of HPV-related seminars and the HPV vaccine was low (28.4% and 5.8%, respectively), similar to the corresponding percentage from a study that revealed that only 9.0% have had knowledge about HPV and cervical cancer programs/seminars [38], while another study examined secondary school female teachers in Lagos who have had an HPV vaccine (2.2%) given to their teenage children [32].

The chi-square test was used to measure the association between self-reported HPV infection and the participants' profile. A statistical analysis shows that there was a significant association between HPV infection and the participants aged between 26–40 years (Fisher's exact, $p = 0.007$), not in a marital sexually active relationship (Fisher's exact, $p = 0.045$), who had no knowledge about HPV-16 and -18 genotypes (Fisher's exact, $p < 0.001$), and who had no knowledge about early sex (Fisher's exact, $p = 0.027$). The result about the participants who have self-reported having HPV infection correlated with the results from other studies where there exists an association between the population under study aged ≤ 30 years (Fisher's exact, $p = 0.006$) [39], those with an unstable marital status or are single with multiple sexual partners (Fisher's exact, $p = 0.022$ and $p = 0.001$, respectively) [40], and lack of knowledge about HPV (Fisher's exact, $p < 0.0001$) [41] as predictors of HPV infection.

A regression analysis also reveals the factors predicting HPV genital warts among the population under study. The result shows that participants between the ages of 26–64 years have reported that they were likely carriers of HPV genital warts: 26–40 years with $_{Adj}OR = 0.45$, CI: 0.22–0.89; and 41–64 years with $_{Adj}OR = 0.31$, CI: 0.10–0.95). Thus, the participants between the ages of 26–40 years have higher odds as compared to those between the ages of 41–64 years (p-value, $p = 0.024$ and $p = 0.041$, respectively). This result aligns with previous studies where ages lower than or equal to 30 years are more likely to be infected than those whose ages are over 45 years [15,39,42,43]. Conversely, the variables of gender, marital status, kind of sex practiced, protected sex, and knowledge about early sex were not significantly associated with HPV infection in this study.

5.1. Study Strength and Limitations

The availability of a large sample size is one of the strengths of this study and it is also the first study to be conducted in Lapai, Niger State. It was also an achievement to include the male population in this study. However, one of the limitations faced by the study is that we had an extremely low sample size of the male population as compared to the female population. Therefore, we acknowledge that the male population in this study was not well-represented. An additional significant limitation of this study is that we have conducted the study based on self-reported data only. Hence, some responses provided by the participants to sensitive questions may have been biased. Furthermore, during data collection, we did not provide categorization for students, non-academic staff, and academic staff; thus, the *Human Papillomavirus (HPV) and Cervical Cancer Risk Assessment (HCRA) Tool (questionnaire)* has been modified and currently used for the last phase of the research field work for data collection.

5.2. Conclusions

HPV infection was high among participants (who have self-reported having a medical/history of the HPV-16 and -18 genotype) between the ages of 26–40 years, currently not in a sexually active relationship, and who had no knowledge about the HPV-16/-18 genotypes and the consequences of an early sexual debut. Moreover, participants > 26 years of age are likely to be carriers of HPV genital warts. These factors have been revealed as the most important predictors peculiar to IBB university students, non-academic staff, and academic staff in this study. Hence, the need for awareness about HPV is required/a must for the safety and well-being of the IBB university community. As a concern and solution, this situation, therefore, suggests the need for free routine HPV vaccination and programs in universities in Nigeria, as well as stresses the importance of sex education among adults through awareness programs in the academic environment populated with low- and middle-income earners in Nigeria.

Author Contributions: Conceptualization of research: M.O.O. and M.K.; methodology: M.O.O., O.D.E. and M.K.; software: M.O.O. and O.D.E.; formal analysis: M.O.O. and O.D.E.; investigation: M.O.O.; resources: M.O.O. and M.K.; data curation: M.O.O.; writing—original draft preparation: M.O.O., O.D.E. and H.M.; writing—review and editing: M.O.O., O.D.E., H.M. and M.K.; visualization: M.O.O., O.D.E., H.M. and M.K.; supervision: M.K.; project administration: M.O.O. and M.K.; funding acquisition: M.K. All authors have read and agreed to the published version of the manuscript.

Funding: This research was funded by the Eötvös Loránd Research Network Secretariat (Development of cyber-medical systems based on AI and hybrid cloud methods), the GINOP-2.2.1-15-2017-00073 "Telemedicina alapú ellátási formák fenntartható megvalósítását támogató keretrendszer kiala-kítása és tesztelése" project, and the 2019-1.3.1-KK-2019-00007 "Innovációs szolgáltató bázis létrehozása diagnosztikai, terápiás és kutatási célú kiberorvosi rend-szerek fejlesztésére" projects.

Institutional Review Board Statement: The ethical approval for this study was obtained from the Niger State Ministry of Health Ethical Review Committee (NSMOH ERC) (protocol number: ERC PIN/2022/08/17 and approval number: ERC PAN/2022/08/17) in Minna, Niger State, Nigeria. Participants provided consent by clicking the "accept to participate" button after reading the informed consent statement on the first page of the online survey. In order to assure the privacy and confidentiality of the participants, all participants voluntarily participated in this study and no identifying information was captured. Since the data were collected online, the study has no/minimal risk to the health of the participants, their environment, and their relatives.

Informed Consent Statement: Informed consent was obtained from all subjects involved in the study.

Data Availability Statement: The HPV and CC data collected during this project and processed for this research publication as part of this study were submitted to the Niger State Ministry of Health Ethical Review Committee (NSMOH ERC) and are available upon request. Data is contained within the article.

Acknowledgments: We acknowledge the Niger State Ministry of Health Ethical Review Committee (NSMOH ERC) in Minna, Niger State, Nigeria for their support in granting us permission for data collection in Niger State and their support during the dissemination of the first part of this project.

Conflicts of Interest: The authors declare no conflicts of interest.

References

1. Omone, O.M.; Kozlovszky, M. HPV and Cervical Cancer Screening Awareness: A Case-control Study in Nigeria. In Proceedings of the 2020 IEEE 24th International Conference on Intelligent Engineering Systems (INES), Reykjavík, Iceland, 8–10 July 2020; pp. 145–152. [CrossRef]
2. Emeribe, A.U.; Abdullahi, I.N.; Etukudo, M.H.; Isong, I.K.; Emeribe, A.O.; Nwofe, J.O.; Umeozuru, C.M.; Shuaib, B.I.; Ajagbe, O.R.O.; Dangana, A.; et al. The pattern of human papillomavirus infection and genotypes among Nigerian women from 1999 to 2019: A systematic review. *Ann. Med.* **2021**, *53*, 944–959. [CrossRef] [PubMed]
3. Manga, M.M.; Fowotade, A.; Abdullahi, Y.M.; El-nafaty, A.U.; Adamu, D.B.; Pindiga, H.U.; Bakare, R.A.; Osoba, A.O. Epidemiological patterns of cervical human papillomavirus infection among women presenting for cervical cancer screening in North-Eastern Nigeria. *Infect. Agents Cancer* **2015**, *10*, 39. [CrossRef] [PubMed]
4. Ramogola-Masire, D.; Luckett, R.; Dreyer, G. Progress and challenges in human papillomavirus and cervical cancer in southern Africa. *Curr. Opin. Infect. Dis.* **2022**, *35*, 49–54. [CrossRef] [PubMed]
5. Louie, K.S.; de Sanjose, S.; Mayaud, P. Epidemiology and prevention of human papillomavirus and cervical cancer in sub-Saharan Africa: A comprehensive review. *Trop. Med. Int. Health* **2009**, *14*, 1287–1302. [CrossRef] [PubMed]
6. Cosmas, N.T.; Nimzing, L.; Egah, D.; Famooto, A.; Adebamowo, S.N.; Adebamowo, C.A. Prevalence of vaginal HPV infection among adolescent and early adult girls in Jos, North-Central Nigeria. *BMC Infect. Dis.* **2022**, *22*, 340. [CrossRef] [PubMed]
7. Omone, O.M.; Gbenimachor, A.U.; Kovács, L.; Kozlovszky, M. Knowledge Estimation with HPV and Cervical Cancer Risk Factors Using Logistic Regression. In Proceedings of the 2021 IEEE 15th International Symposium on Applied Computational Intelligence and Informatics (SACI), Timisoara, Romania, 19–21 May 2021; pp. 000381–000386. [CrossRef]
8. McBride, K.R.; Singh, S. Predictors of Adults' Knowledge and Awareness of HPV, HPV-Associated Cancers, and the HPV Vaccine: Implications for Health Education. *Health Educ. Behav.* **2018**, *45*, 68–76. [CrossRef] [PubMed]
9. What Are the Different Types of Vaccines? *News-Medical.net*, 28 July 2020. Available online: https://www.news-medical.net/health/What-are-the-Different-Types-of-Vaccines.aspx (accessed on 2 November 2022).
10. CDC. *Enhanced Immunity*; Centers for Disease Control and Prevention: Atlanta, GA, USA, 21 January 2022. Available online: https://www.cdc.gov/healthy-weight-growth/about/enhancing-immunity.html?CDC_AAref_Val=https://www.cdc.gov/nccdphp/dnpao/features/enhance-immunity/index.html (accessed on 2 November 2022).
11. Song, D.; Li, H.; Li, H.; Dai, J. Effect of human papillomavirus infection on the immune system and its role in the course of cervical cancer. *Oncol. Lett.* **2015**, *10*, 600–606. [CrossRef] [PubMed]
12. Childs, C.E.; Calder, P.C.; Miles, E.A. Diet and Immune Function. *Nutrients* **2019**, *11*, 1933. [CrossRef] [PubMed]
13. Brown, B.; Folayan, M. Barriers to uptake of human papilloma virus vaccine in Nigeria: A population in need. *Niger. Med. J.* **2015**, *56*, 301. [CrossRef]
14. Musa, J.; Nankat, J.; Achenbach, C.J.; Shambe, I.H.; Taiwo, B.O.; Mandong, B.; Daru, P.H.; Murphy, R.L.; Sagay, A.S. Cervical cancer survival in a resource-limited setting-North Central Nigeria. *Infect. Agents Cancer* **2016**, *11*, 15. [CrossRef]

15. Bruni, L.; Albero, G.; Serrano, B.; Mena, M.; Collado, J.J.; Gómez, D.; Muñoz, J.; Bosch, F.X.; de Sanjosé, S. ICO/IARC Information Centre on HPV and Cancer (HPV Information Centre). Human Papillomavirus and Related Diseases in Nigeria. Summary Report 22 October 2021.pdf. Available online: https://hpvcentre.net/statistics/reports/NGA.pdf (accessed on 11 November 2022).
16. CDC. *Immunization Schedules for 18 & Younger*; Centers for Disease Control and Prevention: Atlanta, GA, USA, 17 February 2022. Available online: https://www.cdc.gov/vaccines/schedules/hcp/imz/child-adolescent.html (accessed on 4 November 2022).
17. Ahonkhai, A.A.; Odusanya, O.O.; Meurice, F.P.; Pierce, L.J.; Durojaiye, T.O.; Alufohai, E.F.; Clemens, R.; Ahonkhai, V.I. Lessons for strengthening childhood immunization in low- and middle-income countries from a successful public-private partnership in rural Nigeria. *Int. Health* **2022**, *14*, 632–638. [CrossRef] [PubMed]
18. National Cancer Institute (NCI). Epidemiologic and Molecular Features of Cervical Cancer in Nigeria-Project Itoju (Care). Available online: https://clinicaltrials.gov/ct2/show/NCT00804466 (accessed on 9 November 2022).
19. Beszédes, B.; Széll, K.; Györök, G. A Highly Reliable, Modular, Redundant and Self-Monitoring PSU Architecture. *Acta Polytech. Hung.* **2020**, *17*, 233–249. [CrossRef]
20. Brisson, M.; Kim, J.J.; Canfell, K.; Drolet, M.; Gingras, G.; Burger, E.A.; Martin, D.; Simms, K.T.; Bénard, É.; Boily, M.-C.; et al. Impact of HPV vaccination and cervical screening on cervical cancer elimination: A comparative modelling analysis in 78 low-income and lower-middle-income countries. *Lancet* **2020**, *395*, 575–590. [CrossRef] [PubMed]
21. Australia, C. What Are the Risk Factors for Cervical Cancer? 18 December 2019. Available online: https://www.canceraustralia.gov.au/cancer-types/cervical-cancer/awareness (accessed on 10 March 2022).
22. Cervical Cancer. Available online: https://www.who.int/news-room/fact-sheets/detail/cervical-cancer (accessed on 14 March 2022).
23. Law in Nigeria—DLA Piper Global Data Protection Laws of the World. Available online: https://www.dlapiperdataprotection.com/index.html?t=law&c=NG (accessed on 8 August 2022).
24. Schnatz, P.F.; Markelova, N.V.; Holmes, D.; Mandavilli, S.R.; O'Sullivan, D.M. The prevalence of cervical HPV and cytological abnormalities in association with reproductive factors of rural Nigerian women. *J. Womens Health* **2008**, *17*, 279–285. [CrossRef] [PubMed]
25. Garai-Fodor, M. The Impact of the Coronavirus on Competence, from a Generation-Specific Perspective. *Acta Polytech. Hung.* **2022**, *19*, 111–125. [CrossRef]
26. Uthman, O.A. Does it really matter where you live? A multilevel analysis of social disorganization and risky sexual behaviours in sub-Saharan Africa. In *DHS Working Papers*; ICF Macro: Calverton, MD, USA, 2010; pp. 1–29.
27. Menon, J.A.; Mwaba, S.O.C.; Thankian, K.; Lwatula, C. Risky sexual behaviour among university students. *Int. STD Res. Rev.* **2016**, *4*, 1–7. [CrossRef]
28. Jain, M.N.; Karnad, V. Online Forms for Data Collection and its Viability in Fashion and Consumer Buying Behavior Survey—A Case Study. ESSENCE—International Journal for Environmental Rehabilitation and Conservation 2017, Volume 8: Special No. 1, 66–71. ISSN 0975-6272. Available online: https://www.academia.edu/32807943/Online_Forms_for_Data_Collection_and_its_Viability_in_Fashion_and_Consumer_Buying_Behavior_Survey_A_Case_Study (accessed on 20 August 2017).
29. Ntoimo, L.F.C.; Akokuwebe, M.E. Prevalence and Patterns of Marital Dissolution in Nigeria. *NJSA* **2014**, *12*. [CrossRef]
30. SUNAN ABU-DAWUD, Book 6: Divorce (Kitab Al-Talaq). Available online: https://www.iium.edu.my/deed/hadith/abudawood/006_sat.html (accessed on 18 November 2022).
31. Oguntayo, O.; Zayyan, M.; Kolawole, A.; Adewuyi, S.; Ismail, H.; Koledade, K. Cancer of the cervix in Zaria, Northern Nigeria. *Ecancermedicalscience* **2011**, *5*, 219. [CrossRef] [PubMed]
32. Toye, M.A.; Okunade, K.S.; Roberts, A.A.; Salako, O.; Oridota, E.S.; Onajole, A.T. Knowledge, perceptions and practice of cervical cancer prevention among female public secondary school teachers in Mushin local government area of Lagos State, Nigeria. *Pan Afr. Med. J.* **2017**, *28*, 221. [CrossRef]
33. Makwe, C.C.; Anorlu, R.I.; Odeyemi, K.A. Human papillomavirus (HPV) infection and vaccines: Knowledge, attitude and perception among female students at the University of Lagos, Lagos, Nigeria. *JEGH* **2012**, *2*, 199. [CrossRef]
34. Adebamowo, S.N.; Olawande, O.; Famooto, A.; Dareng, E.O.; Offiong, R.; Adebamowo, C.A. Persistent Low-Risk and High-Risk Human Papillomavirus Infections of the Uterine Cervix in HIV-Negative and HIV-Positive Women. *Front. Public Health* **2017**, *5*, 178. [CrossRef] [PubMed]
35. Bolarinwa, O.A.; Ajayi, K.V.; Sah, R.K. Association between knowledge of Human Immunodeficiency Virus transmission and consistent condom use among sexually active men in Nigeria: An analysis of 2018 Nigeria Demographic Health Survey. *PLoS Glob. Public Health* **2022**, *2*, e0000223. [CrossRef] [PubMed]
36. Nike Adebowale-Tambe Only 34% of Nigerians Use Condoms–Survey: Premiumtimesng. 2020. Available online: https://www.premiumtimesng.com/health/health-news/377202-only-34-of-nigerians-use-condoms-survey.html (accessed on 18 November 2022).
37. Folayan, M.O.; Odetoyinbo, M.; Brown, B.; Harrison, A. Differences in sexual behaviour and sexual practices of adolescents in Nigeria based on sex and self-reported HIV status. *Reprod. Health* **2014**, *11*, 83. [CrossRef] [PubMed]
38. Enebe, J.T.; Enebe, N.O.; Agunwa, C.C.; Nduagubam, O.C.; Okafor, I.I.; Aniwada, E.C.; Aguwa, E.N. Awareness, acceptability and uptake of cervical cancer vaccination services among female secondary school teachers in Enugu, Nigeria: A cross-sectional study. *Pan Afr. Med. J.* **2021**, *39*, 62. [CrossRef] [PubMed]

39. Akarolo-Anthony, S.N.; Famooto, A.O.; Dareng, E.O.; Olaniyan, O.B.; Offiong, R.; Wheeler, C.M.; Adebamowo, C.A. Age-specific prevalence of human papilloma virus infection among Nigerian women. *BMC Public Health* **2014**, *14*, 656. [CrossRef] [PubMed]
40. Kero, K.M.; Rautava, J.; Syrjänen, K.; Kortekangas-Savolainen, O.; Grenman, S.; Syrjänen, S. Stable marital relationship protects men from oral and genital HPV infections. *Eur. J. Clin. Microbiol. Infect. Dis.* **2014**, *33*, 1211–1221. [CrossRef]
41. Iliyasu, Z.; Galadanci, H.S.; Muhammad, A.; Iliyasu, B.Z.; Umar, A.A.; Aliyu, M.H. Correlates of human papillomavirus vaccine knowledge and acceptability among medical and allied health students in Northern Nigeria. *J. Obstet. Gynaecol.* **2022**, *42*, 452–460. [CrossRef] [PubMed]
42. Vahle, K.; Gargano, J.W.; Lewis, R.M.; Querec, T.D.; Unger, E.R.; Bednarczyk, R.A.; Markowitz, L.E. Prevalence of Human Papillomavirus Among Women Older than Recommended Age for Vaccination by Birth Cohort, United States 2003–2016. *J. Infect. Dis.* **2022**, *225*, 94–104. [CrossRef]
43. Okunade, K.S.; Nwogu, C.M.; Oluwole, A.A.; Anorlu, R.I. Prevalence and risk factors for genital high-risk human papillomavirus infection among women attending the out-patient clinics of a university teaching hospital in Lagos, Nigeria. *Pan Afr. Med. J.* **2017**, *28*, 227. [CrossRef]

Disclaimer/Publisher's Note: The statements, opinions and data contained in all publications are solely those of the individual author(s) and contributor(s) and not of MDPI and/or the editor(s). MDPI and/or the editor(s) disclaim responsibility for any injury to people or property resulting from any ideas, methods, instructions or products referred to in the content.

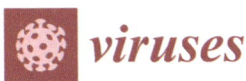

Communication

Short Communication: Understanding the Barriers to Cervical Cancer Prevention and HPV Vaccination in Saudi Arabia

Jobran M. Moshi [1], Aarman Sohaili [2], Hassan N. Moafa [3], Ahlam Mohammed S. Hakami [4], Mohsen M. Mashi [5] and Pierre P. M. Thomas [2,*]

1 Department of Medical Laboratory Technology, Faculty of Applied Medical Sciences, Jazan University, P.O. Box 114, Jazan 45142, Saudi Arabia; jmoshi@jazanu.edu.sa
2 Institute of Public Health Genomics, Genetics and Cell Biology Cluster, GROW Research School for Oncology and Development Biology, Maastricht University, 6229 ER Maastricht, The Netherlands; aarman.sohaili@outlook.com
3 Department of Epidemiology, College of Public Health and Tropical Medicine, Jazan University, P.O. Box 114, Jazan 45142, Saudi Arabia; moafa@jazanu.edu.sa
4 Department Obstetrics and Gynecology, Jazan University, P.O. Box 114, Jazan 45142, Saudi Arabia; ahlamhakami@jazanu.edu.sa
5 Department of Microbiology, Jazan Armed Forces Hospital, Jazan 1568422, Saudi Arabia; mohsen-mashi@hotmail.com
* Correspondence: p.thomas@maastrichtuniversity.nl

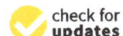

Citation: Moshi, J.M.; Sohaili, A.; Moafa, H.N.; Hakami, A.M.S.; Mashi, M.M.; Thomas, P.P.M. Short Communication: Understanding the Barriers to Cervical Cancer Prevention and HPV Vaccination in Saudi Arabia. *Viruses* **2024**, *16*, 974. https://doi.org/10.3390/v16060974

Academic Editors: Hossein H. Ashrafi and Mustafa Ozdogan

Received: 19 April 2024
Revised: 11 June 2024
Accepted: 13 June 2024
Published: 18 June 2024

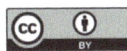

Copyright: © 2024 by the authors. Licensee MDPI, Basel, Switzerland. This article is an open access article distributed under the terms and conditions of the Creative Commons Attribution (CC BY) license (https:// creativecommons.org/licenses/by/ 4.0/).

Abstract: Cervical cancer, along with other sexual and reproductive health and rights (SRHR) conditions, poses a significant burden in the Kingdom of Saudi Arabia (KSA). Despite the availability of effective preventive methods such as vaccinations, particularly against the Human Papillomavirus (HPV), awareness about such preventive methods and HPV vaccination remains alarmingly low in the KSA, even with governmental effort and support. While many women are aware of the risks, the uptake of the HPV vaccine remains below 10% (7.6%) at the country level. This highlights the urgent need for Knowledge, Attitude, and Practice (KAP) at the community level to raise awareness, dispel misconceptions, and empower women to embrace vaccinations. Additionally, there is a need to revitalize the cancer registry system to better track and monitor cervical cancer cases. This short communication aims to map these barriers while identifying opportunities for impactful research. Drawing from the scientific literature, government reports, and expert insights, we highlight the challenges surrounding the tackling of HPV. By exploring diverse sources of knowledge, this paper not only highlights current obstacles but also proposes actionable solutions for future interventions.

Keywords: HPV; cervical cancer; HPV vaccine; prevention; Saudi Arabia

1. Introduction

Cancers and neoplasia stand out as major contributors to the global burden of mortality and morbidity. Cervical cancer is the fourth most common cancer in women worldwide, with an estimated 660,000 new cases and 350,000 attributable deaths annually as of 2022 [1]. Furthermore, cervical cancer disproportionately impacts the Global South, necessitating urgent public health action [2].

A significant portion of the burden of cervical cancer is preventable, given that one of the major contributing factors is the presence of carcinogenic strains of the Human Papilloma Virus [HPV]. Particular HPV strains, especially subtypes 16 and 18, have, in fact, been documented to be involved in the development of precancerous cervical lesions and neoplasia. The implementation of preventive measures, notably HPV vaccination, could potentially avert up to 70% of these cases [3].

Countries located in the Middle East are explicitly affected by the burden of cancers, which holds true for Saudi Arabia. The KSA is home to 37 million inhabitants [4]. Alongside other nations in the Middle Eastern and Northern African Region (MENA), the KSA is experiencing a shift in the mortality and morbidity patterns [5]. The Saudi healthcare system is facing increased strain due to the rising prominence of cancer and other non-communicable diseases.

While the burden of mortality and morbidity from cervical cancer is low in the KSA when compared with other regions in the world, it is swiftly evolving into a matter of significant public health concern [6]. Numerous barriers impede prevention, screening and treatment of cervical cancer, leading to a complex challenge for the healthcare system [7]. There exists multiple knowledge and research gaps, particularly in the realm of preventive efforts such as HPV vaccination [8].

Recognizing the preventable morbidities and mortalities associated with cervical cancer, as well as the global efforts and resources dedicated to combatting HPV, it is crucial to address the current barriers to cervical cancer and HPV vaccination efforts in the KSA. The aim of this paper is to map the current barriers to cervical cancer and HPV vaccination efforts in KSA, and to outline opportunities for impactful research. This paper aims to bring findings from the scientific literature, government reports, and the experience of experts on the ground to the forefront in order to shed light on the challenges and outline solutions for the future. Additionally, this study aims to provide a comprehensive overview of the existing knowledge gaps and methodological limitations surrounding HPV and cervical cancer, thereby directing future research efforts towards generating the data needed to inform more effective public health strategies.

By enriching the literature with comprehensive data on these aspects, this study seeks to provide valuable insights that can inform the development of a detailed national strategy to eliminate cervical cancer in the KSA.

2. Materials and Methods

The study utilized a dual approach to examine the burden of cervical cancer and vaccination efforts in the KSA. The first part involved a mapping review that integrated both qualitative and quantitative data to chart the KSA's progress in tackling cervical cancer and in their vaccination efforts.

To guide and contextualize the research, a mapping review framework established by Paré and Kitsiou [9] was used to identify extensive literature across multiple electronic databases. To ensure broad coverage and minimize potential gaps, the following combination of databases was used: ("Human Papillomavirus" [MeSH] OR HPV [Title/Abstract]) AND ("Cervical Neoplasms" [MeSH] OR "Cervical Cancer" [Title/Abstract]) AND ("Papillomavirus Vaccines" [MeSH] OR "HPV Vaccine" [Title/Abstract]) AND "Saudi Arabia" [MeSH]. The search was aimed at identifying relevant articles, with an emphasis on randomized controlled trials, systematic reviews, and reputable grey literature from sources like the WHO and the Saudi Ministry of Health.

Following the literature search, a meticulous screening process was employed to manage the references efficiently, eliminate duplicates, and select studies that aligned with the research question. Articles selected for a full-text review were individually assessed by the authors to determine their alignment with the inclusion criteria. This was supplemented by 'reverse snowballing' to capture any additional relevant studies.

The inclusion criteria for this review were defined as follows:

- (1) The types of articles considered included empirical research studies conducted in Saudi Arabia.
- (2) The review was limited to articles published from 2015 onward to ensure the relevance of the data in reflecting current trends and developments in HPV trends.
- (3) The focus of the review was on studies that analyzed specific variables related to HPV in the KSA.
- (4) Only articles originally written in English and Arabic were included, to accommodate the linguistic scope of the study.

The selected studies were then systematically charted and recorded, detailing the citation, location, method of evaluation, and key HPV indicators assessed.

As a complement to the analysis, expert opinions were gathered from notable Saudi Arabian experts across different fields. These experts were chosen for their extensive experience in addressing HPV from the perspective of various disciplines (epidemiology, microbiology, and public health). Their broad expertise provided unique and valuable perspectives on the challenges and strategies related to cervical cancer and HPV vaccination. Written informed consent was secured from the experts before the beginning of the study.

3. Results

3.1. Awareness

Sexual and Reproductive Health and Rights [SRHR] awareness is consistently low in the MENA region, including the KSA, with a particular deficiency in understanding cervical cancer among women, as noted in [10]. The overall awareness levels remain largely undocumented at the population level [10]. Notably, prior to 2022, SRHR topics, including cervical cancer, were absent from the school curricula in Saudi Arabia. Subsequent updates introduced a modest inclusion of these subjects in high school, primarily within the health fields at universities [11].

Despite these efforts, some awareness gaps persist, extending to medical professionals. Recent data highlight a significant lack of information and referrals for cervical cancer screening among women. Although the Ministry of Health aims for implementation, there remain challenges in realizing these intentions.

Questions arise about the integration of cervical cancer prevention, such as HPV vaccination, into the healthcare system. A recent nationwide study in the KSA focused on sexually active Saudi women aged 21 to 65, revealing concerning trends in cervical cancer screening and HPV vaccine uptake [8]. The findings showed that only 22.1% of participants had undergone cervical cancer screening, with merely 7.6% receiving the HPV vaccine. Despite some positive attitudes towards screening and vaccination, a significant 84.1% of participants lacked the essential knowledge about cervical cancer screening.

These observed gaps in the uptake of preventive measures are associated with suboptimal communication between primary care physicians and the target population, insufficient educational campaigns, and a lack of health promotion programs. This trend continues to persist, with 40% of those declining the HPV vaccine citing reasons like limited awareness and concerns about injection-related adverse events [10].

Insufficient awareness, even among healthcare professionals, leaves women without the essential knowledge about cervical cancer and screening. Addressing these challenges is vital for enhancing awareness of SRHR and promoting preventive measures in the region. Furthermore, there is a public inquiry regarding the incorporation of HPV vaccination into the Saudi healthcare system, ensuring its availability for young women at general practices without charge.

3.2. Vaccine Hesitancy

The prevention of cervical cancer faces additional challenges beyond awareness, with vaccine hesitancy standing out as a significant hurdle [10]. In 2020, a study uncovered that only 2% of Saudi females had received the HPV vaccine [12]. Surprisingly, even among populations with a solid comprehension of cervical cancer risks, the vaccine uptake remains low, with less than 10% of females having received any form of HPV vaccination [13]. Surprisingly, this hesitancy extends to healthcare students, including those in medical, nursing, and dentistry fields. Cultural and religious factors also appear to play a role in shaping attitudes, with the factor of traditional medicine holding importance within communities [14].

Informal networks, such as family and friends, seem to play a vital role in disseminating information and encouraging vaccination [15]. Leveraging these networks could contribute to overcoming the hesitancy surrounding vaccines, especially in communities where cultural and religious factors heavily influence decision-making.

It is worth noting that the KSA approved the commercial vaccines Gardasil and Cervarix in 2010, with widespread implementation occurring in 2017. The Ministry of Health then began integration of the vaccines into the national immunization schedule, making them available to girls aged 9–13 [16]. However, the implementation seems to currently be in the pilot phase, limited to selected regions of the KSA, and lacks a comprehensive overview.

3.3. Treatment

Cancer is increasingly recognized as a major public health concern and economic burden in the KSA. The Saudi government has prioritized the healthcare system, investing in infrastructure, and providing education and training opportunities for health professionals. Currently, there are 15 specialized oncology care settings situated in major cities, catering to around 80% of the Saudi population, with ongoing efforts to extend such services to less populated areas [17,18].

Cancer care in the KSA is accessible to all Saudi citizens free of charge, and non-citizens can avail themselves of these services through health insurance and non-profit organizations. The current cancer care model in the country follows a "find it and fix it" approach, lacking comprehensive risk factor surveillance programs and proactive interventions [19]. Patients usually access cancer care settings through various routes, including primary or secondary healthcare referrals, screening centers diagnosis, or emergency room presentations [20].

Aligned with the Saudi Vision 2030, a new care model is being developed, focusing on the prevention of non-communicable diseases [NCDs] and involving the private sector more actively in cancer care [19]. Despite this, several challenges to cervical cancer exist in the KSA. Improving the quality of cancer care is a continuous process. One area of improvement would be the strengthening of current cancer registries. The Saudi health authority would, in fact, benefit from more capability to track and monitor current cancer trends, care outcomes, and survival rates [21]. This is especially true for the cases where Saudi citizens seek healthcare outside of the country. A rigorous registry would, in fact, help tailor current outreach efforts and understand current needs.

4. Way Ahead and Conclusions

In light of the current barriers to cervical cancer prevention and HPV vaccination in the KSA, a multidimensional approach ought to be outlined. A pervasive challenge is the lack of awareness, with certain segments of the Saudi population vaguely acknowledging the risk of cervical cancer, while overall community-level awareness remains low. Additionally, awareness of HPV vaccination options is consistently limited, emphasizing the need for innovative strategies to educate adolescents and the individuals of reproductive age.

To enhance awareness, health authorities should delve into current knowledge gaps, identify contentious ideas, and understand the influence of traditional and religious beliefs. Recent data indicate suboptimal awareness among healthcare professionals, highlighting the importance of targeted efforts to inform medical practitioners, nurses, and healthcare providers. This, in turn, can create a ripple effect, empowering patients to make informed decisions about their sexual and reproductive health.

A holistic approach to raising awareness, coupled with an understanding of community-level health-seeking behavior, presents a significant intervention opportunity. Furthermore, existing shortcomings in cervical cancer screening in the KSA, exacerbated by underutilized screening opportunities and insufficient referrals from primary care practitioners, require attention. A thorough examination of the current care pathway is essential to structuring strategies for optimal outcomes.

Augmenting screening efforts could involve incorporating HPV testing, potentially as part of pre-marital screenings for sexually transmitted infections. This approach aligns with a broader strategy to improve reproductive health outcomes. The healthcare sector's deficiencies extend to the cancer registration infrastructure, where gaps in gathering accurate and up-to-date cancer epidemiology data at the national level persist. Establishing a well-functioning database for cervical cancer cases in the KSA is crucial for tracking trends, identifying high-risk groups, and developing evidence-based prevention strategies. A robust information system would contribute significantly to improving the overall effectiveness of cervical cancer prevention initiatives in the KSA.

Author Contributions: Conceptualization, J.M.M. and P.P.M.T.; methodology J.M.M., P.P.M.T. and A.S.; writing—original draft preparation, P.P.M.T. and A.S.; writing—review and editing, P.P.M.T., J.M.M., A.S., H.N.M., A.M.S.H. and M.M.M.; supervision, J.M.M. and P.P.M.T.; project administration, J.M.M., A.S. and P.P.M.T. All authors have read and agreed to the published version of the manuscript.

Funding: This research received no external funding.

Institutional Review Board Statement: Not applicable.

Informed Consent Statement: Not applicable.

Data Availability Statement: No new data were created for this paper; the literature and documents used can be made available upon reasonable request.

Acknowledgments: The authors gratefully acknowledge the funding of the Deanship of Graduate Studies and Scientific Research, Jazan University, Saudi Arabia, through Project Number: GSSRD-24.

Conflicts of Interest: The authors declare no conflicts of interest.

References

1. World Health Organization: WHO. Cervical Cancer. Who.int. 2024. Available online: https://www.who.int/news-room/fact-sheets/detail/cervical-cancer#:~:text=Key%20facts,-%20and%20middle-income%20countries (accessed on 5 March 2024).
2. Lin, S.; Gao, K.; Gu, S.; You, L.; Qian, S.; Tang, M.; Wang, J.; Chen, K.; Jin, M. Worldwide Trends in Cervical Cancer Incidence and Mortality, with Predictions for the next 15 Years. *Cancer* **2021**, *127*, 4030–4039. [CrossRef] [PubMed]
3. Viveros-Carreño, D.; Fernandes, A.; Pareja, R. Updates on Cervical Cancer Prevention. *Int. J. Gynecol. Cancer* **2023**, *33*, 394–402. [CrossRef] [PubMed]
4. Worldometer. Saudi Arabia Population (2024)—Worldometer. worldometers.info. 2024. Available online: https://www.worldometers.info/world-population/saudi-arabia-population (accessed on 5 March 2024).
5. Mansour, R.; Al-Ani, A.; Al-Hussaini, M.; Abdel-Razeq, H.; Al-Ibraheem, A.; Mansour, A.H. Modifiable Risk Factors for Cancer in the Middle East and North Africa: A Scoping Review. *BMC Public Health* **2024**, *24*, 223. [CrossRef] [PubMed]
6. Momenimovahed, Z.; Mazidimoradi, A.; Maroofi, P.; Allahqoli, L.; Salehiniya, H.; Alkatout, I. Global, Regional and National Burden, Incidence, and Mortality of Cervical Cancer. *Cancer Rep.* **2023**, *6*, e1756. [CrossRef] [PubMed]
7. Alkhalawi, E.; Allemani, C.; Al-Zahrani, A.S.; Coleman, M.P. Cervical Cancer in Saudi Arabia: Trends in Survival by Stage at Diagnosis and Geographic Region. *Ann. Cancer Epidemiol.* **2022**, *6*, 7. [CrossRef]
8. Alkhamis, F.H.; Alabbas, Z.A.S.; Al Mulhim, J.E.; Alabdulmohsin, F.F.; Alshaqaqiq, M.H.; Alali, E.A. Prevalence and Predictive Factors of Cervical Cancer Screening in Saudi Arabia: A Nationwide Study. *Cureus* **2023**, *15*, e49331. [CrossRef] [PubMed]
9. Paré, G.; Kitsiou, S. Methods for Literature Reviews. In *Handbook of eHealth Evaluation: An Evidence-Based Approach*; Lau, F., Kuziemsky, C., Eds.; University of Victoria: Victoria, BC, Canada, 2017.
10. Gari, A.; Ghazzawi, M.A.; Ghazzawi, S.A.; Alharthi, S.M.; Yanksar, E.A.; Almontashri, R.M.; Batarfi, R.; Kinkar, L.I.; Baradwan, S. Knowledge about Cervical Cancer Risk Factors and Human Papilloma Virus Vaccine among Saudi Women of Childbearing Age: A Community-Based Cross-Sectional Study from Saudi Arabia. *Vaccine X* **2023**, *15*, 100361. [CrossRef] [PubMed]
11. Zahid, H.M.; Qarah, A.B.; Alharbi, A.M.; Alomar, A.E.; Almubarak, S.A. Awareness and Practices Related to Cervical Cancer among Females in Saudi Arabia. *Int. J. Environ. Res. Public Health* **2022**, *19*, 1455. [CrossRef] [PubMed]
12. Akkour, K.; Alghuson, L.; Benabdelkamel, H.; Alhalal, H.; Alayed, N.; AlQarni, A.; Arafah, M. Cervical Cancer and Human Papillomavirus Awareness among Women in Saudi Arabia. *Medicina* **2021**, *57*, 1373. [CrossRef] [PubMed]
13. Sahoo, S.K.; Awinashe, V.; Bhati, M.; Chougule, P.G.; Mathar, M.I.; Thomas, T.; Garg, R. Assessment of Various Post Systems' Fracture Resistance after Endodontic Treatment. *J. Pharm. Bioallied. Sci.* **2024**, *16*, S699–S701. [CrossRef] [PubMed]
14. Alrasheed, A.A.; Irfan, U.M. Knowledge, Attitude and Practices Regarding Cervical Cancer and Screening among Saudi Women in Ar Rass, Qassim. *J. Biosci. Med.* **2023**, *11*, 456–479. [CrossRef]
15. Alsanafi, M.; Salim, N.A.; Sallam, M. Willingness to Get HPV Vaccination among Female University Students in Kuwait and Its Relation to Vaccine Conspiracy Beliefs. *Hum. Vaccin. Immunother.* **2023**, *19*, 2194772. [CrossRef] [PubMed]
16. Aldawood, E.; Dabbagh, D.; Alharbi, S.; Alzamil, L.; Faqih, L.; Alshurafa, H.; Dabbagh, R. HPV Vaccine Knowledge and Hesitancy Among Health Colleges' Students at a Saudi University. *J. Multidiscip. Healthc.* **2023**, *16*, 3465–3476. [CrossRef] [PubMed]

17. Al-Mandeel, H.M.; Sagr, E.; Sait, K.; Latifah, H.M.; Al-Obaid, A.; Al-Badawi, I.A.; Alkushi, A.O.; Salem, H.; Massoudi, N.S.; Schunemann, H.; et al. Clinical Practice Guidelines on the Screening and Treatment of Precancerous Lesions for Cervical Cancer Prevention in Saudi Arabia. *Ann. Saudi. Med.* **2016**, *36*, 313–320. [CrossRef] [PubMed]
18. Alsalmi, S.F.; Othman, S.S. Cervical Cancer Screening Uptake and Predictors Among Women in Jeddah, Saudi Arabia. *Cureus* **2022**, *14*, e24065. [CrossRef] [PubMed]
19. Alessy, S.A.; AlWaheidi, S. Moving Cancer Prevention and Care Forward in Saudi Arabia. *J. Cancer Policy* **2020**, *26*, 100250. [CrossRef]
20. Khoja, T.; Rawaf, S.; Qidwai, W.; Rawaf, D.; Nanji, K.; Hamad, A. Health Care in Gulf Cooperation Council Countries: A Review of Challenges and Opportunities. *Cureus* **2017**, *9*, e1586. [CrossRef] [PubMed]
21. Ministry of Education KSA. Features-of-the-Development-of-the-Saudi-Curriculum. moe.gov.sa. 2022. Available online: https://moe.gov.sa/ar/education/generaleducation/StudyPlans/Documents/Features-of-the-development-of-the-Saudi-curriculum.pdf (accessed on 5 March 2024).

Disclaimer/Publisher's Note: The statements, opinions and data contained in all publications are solely those of the individual author(s) and contributor(s) and not of MDPI and/or the editor(s). MDPI and/or the editor(s) disclaim responsibility for any injury to people or property resulting from any ideas, methods, instructions or products referred to in the content.

MDPI AG
Grosspeteranlage 5
4052 Basel
Switzerland
Tel.: +41 61 683 77 34

Viruses Editorial Office
E-mail: viruses@mdpi.com
www.mdpi.com/journal/viruses

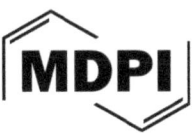

Disclaimer/Publisher's Note: The title and front matter of this reprint are at the discretion of the Guest Editors. The publisher is not responsible for their content or any associated concerns. The statements, opinions and data contained in all individual articles are solely those of the individual Editors and contributors and not of MDPI. MDPI disclaims responsibility for any injury to people or property resulting from any ideas, methods, instructions or products referred to in the content.

www.ingramcontent.com/pod-product-compliance
Lightning Source LLC
LaVergne TN
LVHW072356090526
838202LV00019B/2562